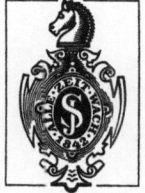

W. Hacke   M. Hennerici
H. J. Gelmers   G. Krämer

Cerebral Ischemia

With 107 Figures and 34 Tables

Springer-Verlag
Berlin Heidelberg New York
London Paris Tokyo
Hong Kong Barcelona

Werner Hacke, MD
Professor and Chairman
Department of Neurology
University of Heidelberg
Im Neuenheimer Feld 400
6900 Heidelberg
Federal Republic of Germany

Michael Hennerici, MD
Professor and Chairman
Department of Neurology
Klinikum Mannheim
University of Heidelberg
Theodor-Kutzer-Ufer
6800 Mannheim
Federal Republic of Germany

Herman J. Gelmers, MD
Department of Neurology
Streekziekenhuis
7606 PP Almelo
The Netherlands

Günter Krämer, MD
Department of Neurology
University of Mainz
Langenbeckstraße 1
6500 Mainz 1
Federal Republic of Germany

This translation is a revised and extended version of the original German edition:
Zerebrale Ischämien.© Springer-Verlag Berlin Heidelberg 1989.ISBN-13:978-3-642-75550-7

ISBN-13: 978-3-642-75550-7   e-ISBN-13: 978-3-642-75548-4
DOI: 10.1007/978-3-642-75548-4

Library of Congress Cataloging-in-Publication Data
Zerebrale Ischämien. English. Cerebral Ischemia / W. Hacke ... [et al.]. Translation of:
Zerebrale Ischämien. Includes bibliographical references. Includes index.
ISBN-13:978-3-642-75550-7 (alk. paper): DM 128.00. ISBN-13:978-3-642-75550-7 (alk. paper)
1. Cerebral ischemia. I. Hacke, W. (Werner), 1948- . II. Title. [DNLM: 1. Cerebral Ischemia.
WL 355 Z585] RC388.5.Z4413 1990 616.8'1--dc20

2125/3130/543210 – Printed on acid-free paper

Preface

Despite a worldwide reduction in its incidence, stroke remains one of the most common diseases generally and the most important cause of premature and persistent disability in the industrialized countries.

The most frequent cause of stroke is a localized disturbance of cerebral circulation, i.e., cerebral ischemia. Less common are spontaneous intracerebral and subarachnoid hemorrhages and sinus venous thromboses. The introduction of new diagnostic procedures such as cranial computed tomography, magnetic resonance imaging, digital subtraction radiologic techniques, and various ultrasound techniques has led to impressive advances in the diagnosis of stroke. Through the planned application of these techniques, it is even possible to identify the pathogenetic mechanisms underlying focal cerebral ischemia in humans. However, these diagnostic advances have made the gap between diagnostic accuracy and therapeutic implications even greater than before. This fact can be easily explained. In the past, therapeutic studies had to be based on the symptoms and temporal aspects of stroke; it was impossible for early investigations to consider the various pathogeneses of cerebral ischemia. Inevitably, stroke patients were treated as suffering from a uniform disease.

Hence, it is not surprising – and no fault of the neurologists – that a reliable therapeutic approach has still not been found to manage an acute ischemic episode, and that only a few treatment strategies can be considered effective in prophylaxis. On the contrary, in view of the great diversity of ischemic episodes, it is really quite surprising that a common prophylactic concept has been achieved at all.

We have proceeded from the assumption that even the data from quite recent studies lose their validity if the studies were not performed according to today's diagnostic standards. To be able to use comparative data on the spontaneous course of the various types of cerebral ischemia, it is necessary to devise an epidemiologic basis that also considers the pathogenesis.

Our goal in this book is to present the current concepts of the development, pathogenesis, course, and therapeutic approaches in cerebral ischemia. Starting from the functional anatomy of the cerebral arteries and a classification of cerebral ischemia based on morphology and pathogenesis, we describe the pathophysiologic mechanisms responsible. After discussing the epidemiologic data, the various approaches for classifying cerebral ischemias, and the clinical syndromes, including their pathogenesis and differential diagnosis, we describe the use of clinical findings and data from diagnostic equipment in making diagnoses. This includes a description of the new investigative techniques and a review of their clinical relevance. Treatment and prophylaxis are dealt with in the final chapter; consideration is given to the differential therapeutic concepts for particular types of cerebral ischemia, based on pathogenetic considerations.

Although the four authors are from different centers, this text has been prepared according to a common concept. While the individual chapters have each been written primarily by one or two of us, we have discussed, elaborated, and organized them in common. Thus despite some apparent differences in personal style and content, we agree on the essential concepts of the new pathogenetic and morphologic interpretation of cerebral ischemia. We therefore decided not to attribute authorship for individual chapters. We have limited the references to current review articles and important original publications.

We felt it very important to provide a thorough description and examples of the diagnostic imaging techniques, and in this we received the energetic support of our colleagues in neuroradiology. We express our thanks to Prof. Hermann Zeumer of Hamburg, MD, Prof. Armin Thron, MD, of Aachen, Albrecht Aulich, MD, of Düsseldorf, Wolfgang Rautenberg, MD, of Mannheim, Klaus Sartor, MD, of Heidelberg, and Rüdiger von Kummer, MD, of Heidelberg for supplying a large number of the figures. We are also grateful to Dr. V. Hömberg of Düsseldorf for contributing the section on rehabilitation in cerebrovascular disorders.

For their work on the many drafts for this text, which covered nearly 2½ years, we are grateful to our secretaries, Mrs. Böhler and Mrs. Seidel of Aachen, Mrs. Kosemetzky of Düsseldorf, Mrs. Ehlert of Mainz, and Mrs. Wilczek of Heidelberg. We acknowledge the support provided by Bayer Leverkusen, specifically by Dr. Ingedoh and Dr. Hartmann. We are indebted to Springer-Verlag, particularly Victor P. Oehm, for·support and motivation, especially in the final phases of the preparation of this book.

Heidelberg, October 1990

Werner Hacke
Michael Hennerici
Herman J. Gelmers
Günter Krämer

Contents

1 Applied Anatomy of the Cerebral Arteries

Four arteries supply the brain with blood: the two carotid and the two vertebral arteries. Although these four vessels are ultimately interlinked via a basal arterial network, the circle of Willis, and anastomoses at the brain surface, Heubner's anastomoses, it is useful to distinguish anterior (carotid anterior and middle cerebral) and posterior (vertebrobasilar posterior cerebral) vascular territories (Gillian 1957, 1968; Lazorthes 1961; Kaplan and Ford 1966; Gänshirt 1972; Seeger 1978; Dorndorf 1983; Duus 1983).

The structure of the walls of the extracranial arteries supplying the brain does not differ from that of the other arteries of the body, but the structure of the arterial walls changes after these large vessels penetrate the skull base. The walls become markedly thinner, partly by a reduction in the diameter of the tunica media (muscularis) but mainly by means of a substantial reduction in the tunica externa (adventitia).

In the large intracranial arteries (long and short circumferential arteries) in the subarachnoid space, the media is only about half as thick as in extracranial arteries of comparable lumen. This is primarily the result of a loss of elastic elements and a consequent relative increase in muscular components. The adventitia is reduced to one-fifth that of extracranial arteries. This loss of supportive tissue is compensated by the fact that the arteries pass specifically within the only slightly compressible CSF space and through the rigid cranial capsule. In the perforating arteries the thickness of the muscular layer is still further reduced (Lehrer 1968).

The vessels supplying the brain possess no vasa vasorum and are nourished via gaps in the internal elastic membrane, through which the muscle cells of the muscularis obtain their nutrients. The muscle fibers of the middle layer of the vessel wall are arranged transversely to the direction of the vessel. This arrangement is disturbed at the sites of junction of the basal vessels and at the origins of the directly penetrating paramedian arteries, as the central vessels such as the lenticulostriate arteries arise almost at right angles from the main vessels. This gives rise to an irregularity in muscle development, with the development of sites of muscle weakness and actual gaps which are the preferential sites for the formation of aneurysms. The origins of the central vessels are also particularly liable to hemorrhages.

1.1 Extracranial Anatomy

The right common carotid artery arises from the division of the brachiocephalic trunk into the subclavian and common carotid arteries, while the left common carotid arises directly from the aortic arch. The vertebral arteries arise from the subclavian arteries (Fig. 1.1). Variant origins of the large cerebral vessels from the aortic arch are not uncommon: the left carotid may arise from the (right) brachiocephalic trunk; the vertebral arteries may arise directly from the aortic arch on one or both sides, or they may be hypoplastic or even quite undeveloped on one side. The descriptive anatomy of the cerebral arteries is only briefly summarized here; one can refer to the relevant anatomic and neuroradiologic textbooks for a detailed description.

The common carotid artery divides at about the level of the thyroid cartilage into the internal and external carotids, a site frequently affected by arteriosclerotic plaques and stenoses. Whereas the external carotid very soon divides into its main branches, the internal carotid usually continues to the carotid canal in the skull base without further branching. This portion is designated as the extracranial or cervical segment. Subsequently the carotid first extends through its bony canal in the petrous part of the temporal bone and then arrives at the cavernous sinus in the vicinity of the clivus

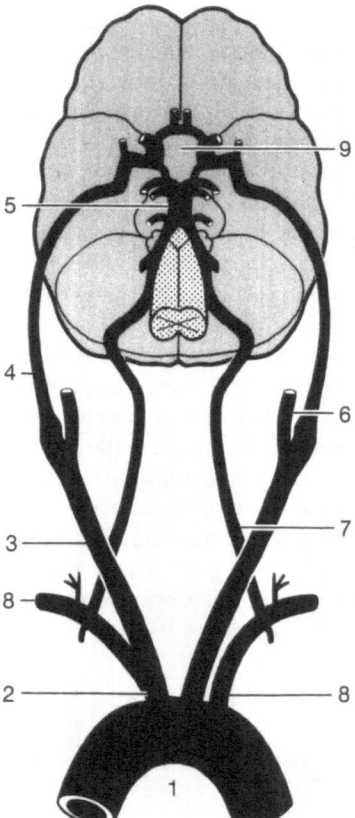

Fig. 1.1. Diagram of aortic arch and main cerebral arterial trunks. *1*, Aorta; *2*, brachiocephalic trunk; *3*, common carotid artery; *4*, internal carotid artery; *5*, basilar artery; *6*, external carotid artery; *7*, vertebral artery; *8*, subclavian artery; *9*, circle of Willis. (From Dorndorf 1983)

(intracavernous sinus). In the cavernous sinus the carotid forms a loop, known as the carotid siphon, from which arteries to the hypophysis and the mammillary bodies arise. At about the level of the anterior clinoid process the carotid penetrates the dura mater and subsequently runs through the subarachnoid space.

The two vertebral arteries arise from the subclavian arteries. After they pass through the transverse foramina of the upper six cervical vertebrae, around the lateral part of the atlas (atlantal loop), they enter the posterior cranial fossa through the foramen magnum (Takahashi 1974). Often one vertebral artery (usually the left) is increased in caliber; sometimes one is hypoplastic or absent. Variations may also occur in the intracranial segment. Thus, one vertebral artery may end in the posterior inferior cerebellar artery without any junction with the other vertebral artery. This variant, in which one vertebral completely supplies the basilar, does not give rise to symptoms.

1.2 Intracranial Anatomy

The four principal arteries are interconnected at the skull base by means of the circle of Willis. Basically, the cerebral arteries may be divided into long circumferential, short circumferential, and paramedian perforating arteries (Duvernoy 1978). The long circumferential arteries arise from the circle of Willis and run on the cerebral surface, mostly in the cortical sulci, over the lateral and anterior convexity towards the vertex, giving off small branches to the adjacent cortical regions as they do so. They span very long distances and enter an extensive meningeal anastomotic plexus (Heubner's meningeal anastomoses; Fig. 1.2). From the long circumferential arteries the short circumferential arteries arise, and after a markedly shorter course these give off their intracerebral terminal branches in the lateral or laterobasal cortical regions. They likewise enter, albeit to a lesser degree, leptomeningeal anastomoses, partly also with the long circumferential arteries.

From the proximal intracranial vessels, the circle of Willis, and the basal portions of the long circumferential arteries the third group of cerebral arteries arise: the paramedian perforating vessels, also known as the central arteries. These very thin vessels, arising almost at right angles to the main trunks, immediately take an intracerebral course, one which is very long in relation to their lumen (Fig. 1.3). They have no anastomoses and are functional end-arteries. In the hemispheres the penetrating arteries supply the subcortical nuclear zones and large portions of the medullary layer, whereas short medullary arteries originating from the surface branches in the anterior circulation supply mainly the cerebral cortex and a thin layer of adjacent white matter. The allocation of the different vascular territories to particular types of arteries is seen particularly well in the brainstem (Fig. 1.4).

With regard to the vascular supply of the posterior circulation, the description of the course of the intracranial arteries to the brainstem and cerebellum distinguishes between the median penetrating arteries (medial group), the short circumferential arteries (anterolateral group), and the long circumferential arteries (posterior group). The penetrating arteries arise directly from the basilar, the vertebral, or the proximal segment of a cerebellar artery and enter the brainstem ventrally after only a few millimeters. They are virtually noncollateralized and constitute functional end-arteries which have a relatively long intracerebral course in terms of the size of the

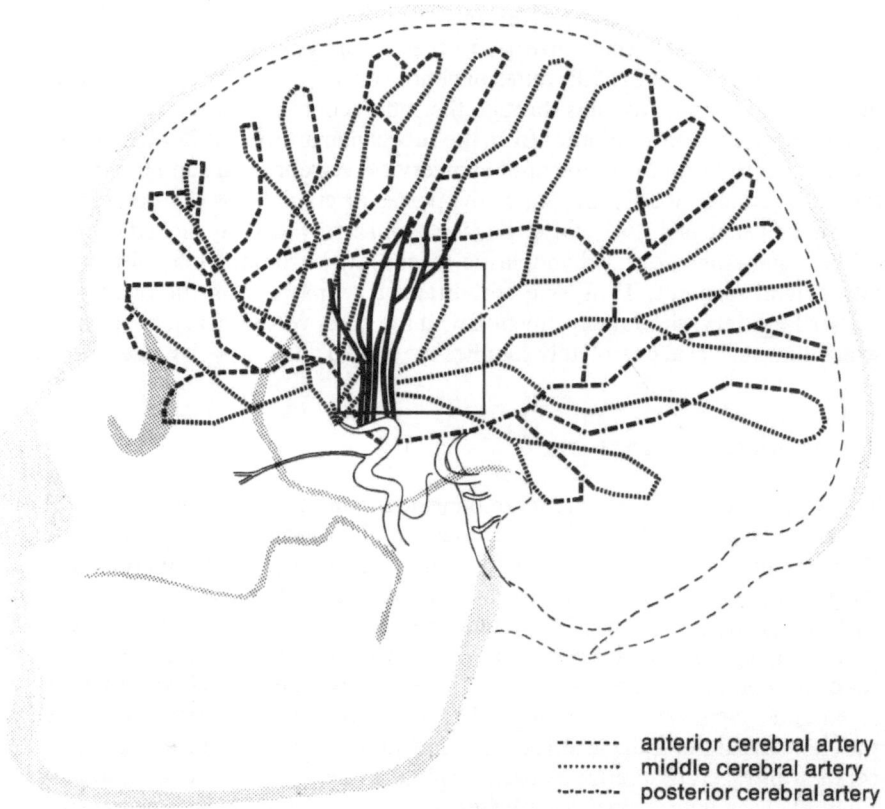

- - - - - - anterior cerebral artery
·············· middle cerebral artery
·-·-·-·-· posterior cerebral artery

Fig. 1.2. Diagram of the leptomeningeal anastomoses of the anterior, middle, and posterior cerebral arteries. In the *central insert* the lenticulostriate arteries are shown diagrammatically as examples of noncollateralized end-arteries. (From Toole 1984)

brainstem. The thalamoperforating arteries (from the posterior communicating artery) and the posterior choroidal arteries also constitute medial penetrating arteries. The large main cerebellar branches and the collicular arteries are circumferential vessels. They give off the short circumferential branch to the lateral brainstem, whereas the long circumferential branch gives dorsolateral branches only to the brainstem. The circumferential branches enter profuse collaterals (see above).

1.2.1 Carotid, Middle, and Anterior Cerebral Territory

The intra-arachnoidal (or cisternal) portion of the carotid extends to the carotid bifurcation (carotid T junction), the division of the vessel into the middle and anterior cerebral arteries. Neuroradiologically, the cisternal and cavernous portions of the carotid are subdivided from distal to proximal into segments labeled C1–C5 (Fig. 1.5; Huber 1979; Salomon and Huang 1976). Up to the division at the carotid T important

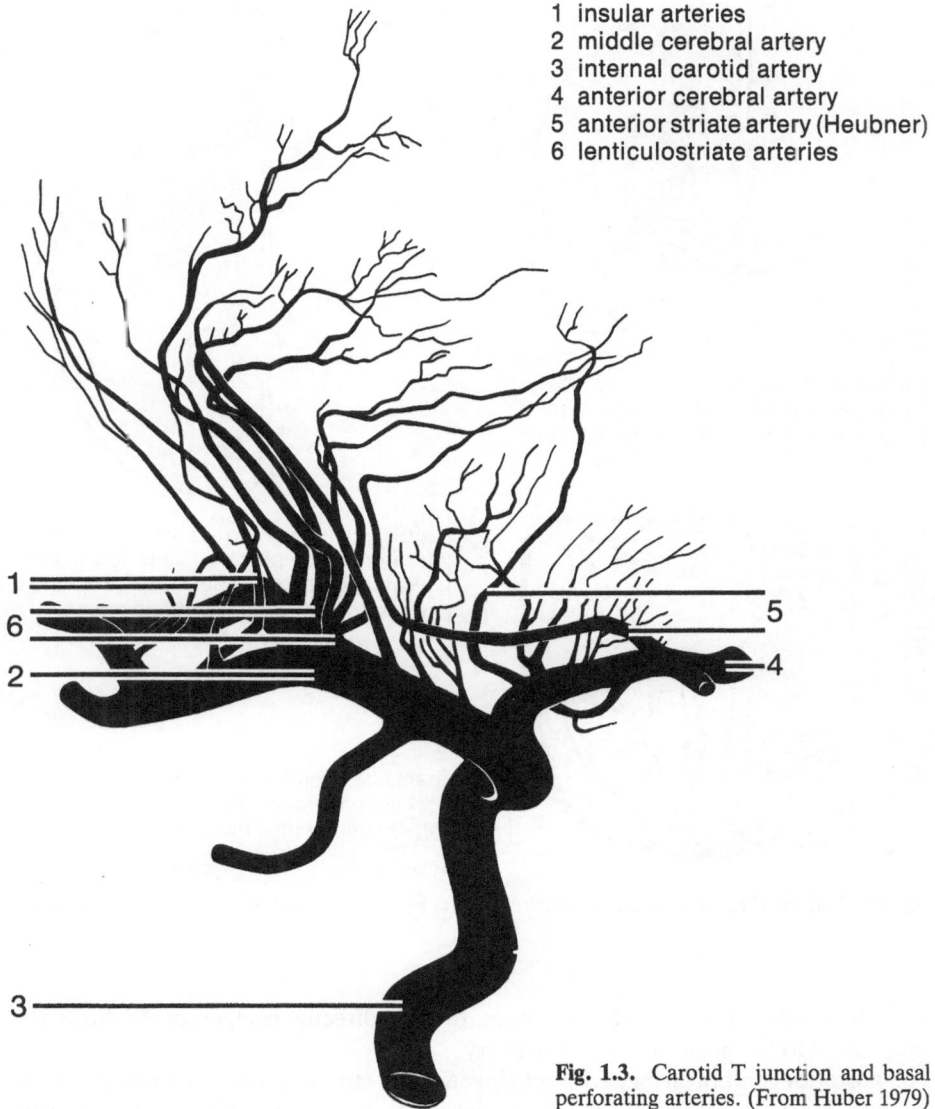

1 insular arteries
2 middle cerebral artery
3 internal carotid artery
4 anterior cerebral artery
5 anterior striate artery (Heubner)
6 lenticulostriate arteries

Fig. 1.3. Carotid T junction and basal perforating arteries. (From Huber 1979)

vessels arise from the intracranial course of the internal carotid: the ophthalmic artery, the posterior communicating artery, and the anterior choroidal artery.

After the carotid has crossed the oculomotor and optic nerves in its cisternal portion, the ophthalmic artery arises at the junction of the C2 und C3 segments. This provides important anastomoses to the branches of the external carotid. Its end-branch is the central retinal artery, a cerebral artery that can be examined directly by ophthalmoscopy. From a lateral view the internal carotid then describes a curve with backward convexity (C1 segment), with the posterior communicating artery branching off the

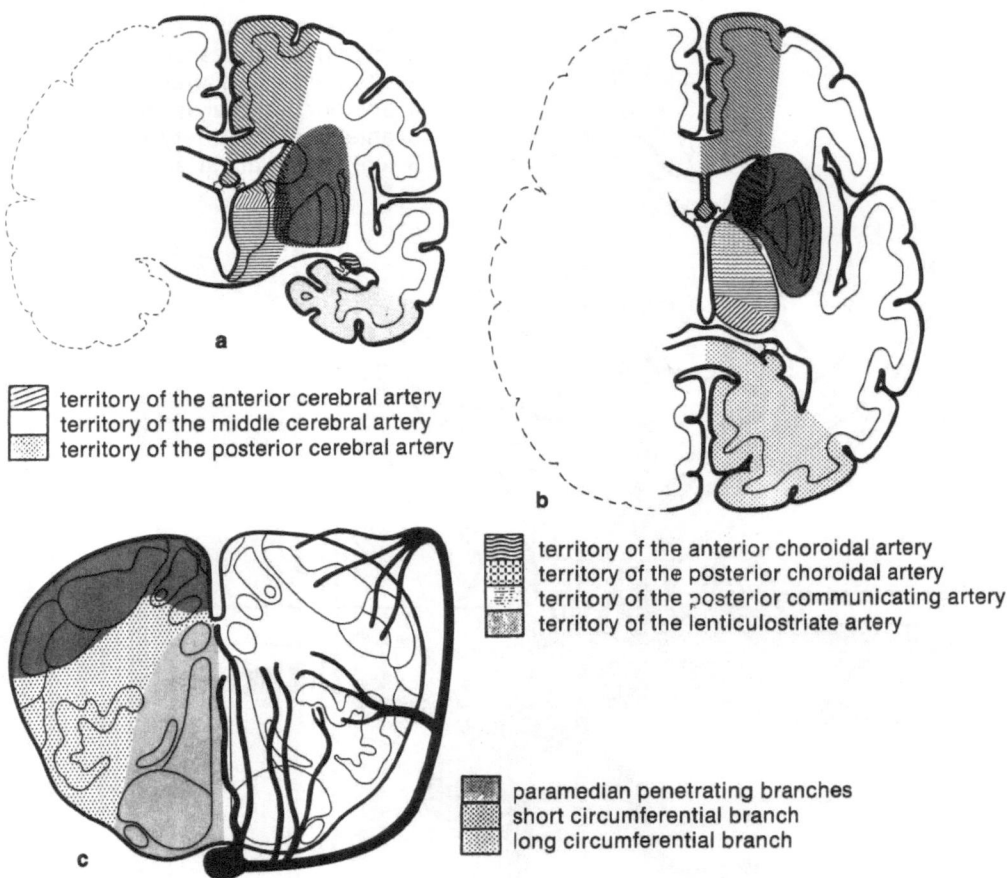

territory of the anterior cerebral artery
territory of the middle cerebral artery
territory of the posterior cerebral artery

territory of the anterior choroidal artery
territory of the posterior choroidal artery
territory of the posterior communicating artery
territory of the lenticulostriate artery

paramedian penetrating branches
short circumferential branch
long circumferential branch

Fig. 1.4. Pattern of vascularization of the cerebrum (**a, b**) and brainstem (**c**). (From Duvernoy 1978)

ascending limb. This vessel runs more or less directly backwards to form the connection to the posterior cerebral artery.

The posterior cerebral artery arises phylogenetically from the carotid territory, but in primates it usually belongs to the vertebrobasilar territory. The caliber and expression of the posterior communicating artery vary greatly. Sometimes it is absent on one side; in other, rare cases both posterior vessels arise directly from the internal carotid and have no connection with the basilar. From the posterior communicating artery and the proximal part of the posterior cerebral a series of perforating branches arise, which supply inter alia the thalamus and hypothalamus and also participate by individual branches in the blood supply of the posterior internal capsule (among others, the posterior thalamoperforators; see also the vertebrobasilar system). A few millimeters further distally, but still in the C1 segment, there are branches off the anterior choroidal artery which in rare cases may arise directly from the middle cerebral artery. This is a further instance of a perforating artery supplying important

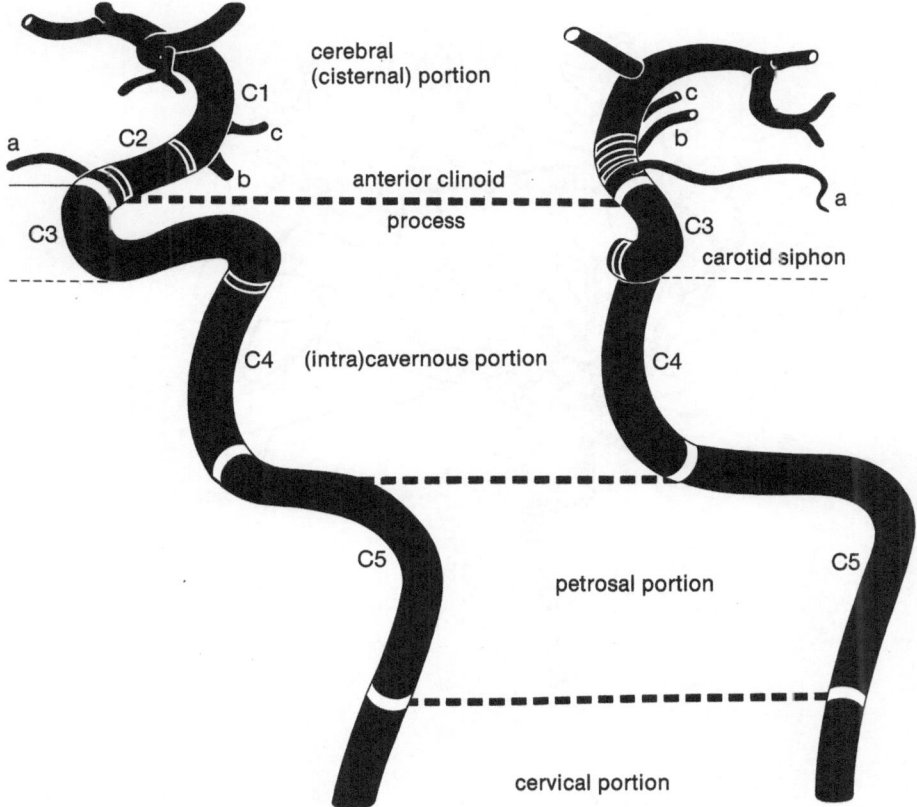

Fig. 1.5. The portions of the internal carotid artery in lateral and anteroposterior view. *a,* Ophthalmic artery; *b,* posterior communicating artery; *c,* anterior choroidal artery. (From Huber 1979)

parts of the central optic tract, the limbic system, the basal ganglia, and the posterior limb of the internal capsule. However, in contrast to most other perforating arteries, it enters a close connection via its branches with its twin artery derived from the posterior circulation, the posterior choroidal artery. This anastomosis explains why obstructions in the distribution of the anterior choroidal artery rarely lead to clinically relevant symptoms.

At the carotid T junction the internal carotid divides into its two terminal branches, the middle and anterior cerebral arteries. In terms of caliber, the middle cerebral constitutes the true continuation of the internal carotid. It runs laterally in the direction of the lateral (sylvian) fissure, which it then follows. In its proximal, horizontally directed portion the middle cerebral gives off a series of parenchymal branches, which are sometimes so densely packed as they enter the brain that this region is designated anatomically as the anterior perforated substance. Although the individual vascular clusters can be exactly identified anatomically, they are generally grouped together for clinical purposes as the lenticulostriate arteries. As direct penetrating arteries they are virtually noncollateralized. Large portions of the basal

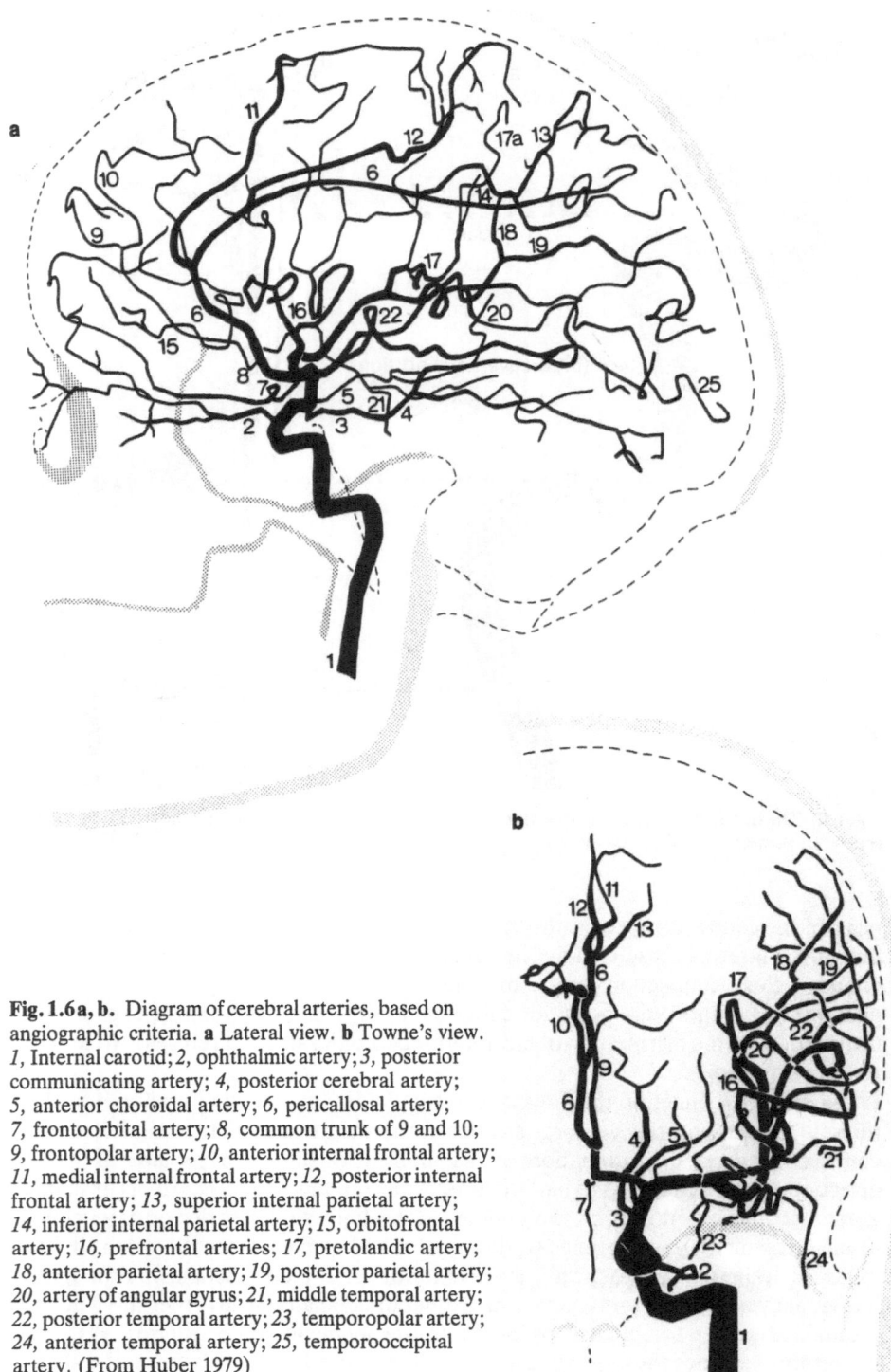

Fig. 1.6a, b. Diagram of cerebral arteries, based on angiographic criteria. **a** Lateral view. **b** Towne's view. *1,* Internal carotid; *2,* ophthalmic artery; *3,* posterior communicating artery; *4,* posterior cerebral artery; *5,* anterior choroidal artery; *6,* pericallosal artery; *7,* frontoorbital artery; *8,* common trunk of 9 and 10; *9,* frontopolar artery; *10,* anterior internal frontal artery; *11,* medial internal frontal artery; *12,* posterior internal frontal artery; *13,* superior internal parietal artery; *14,* inferior internal parietal artery; *15,* orbitofrontal artery; *16,* prefrontal arteries; *17,* pretolandic artery; *18,* anterior parietal artery; *19,* posterior parietal artery; *20,* artery of angular gyrus; *21,* middle temporal artery; *22,* posterior temporal artery; *23,* temporopolar artery; *24,* anterior temporal artery; *25,* temporooccipital artery. (From Huber 1979)

ganglia, internal capsula, and paraventricular medullary layer are supplied by these arteries, whereas the thalamus and hypothalamus obtain their blood from comparable branches of the posterior communicating artery. Also, there arise from the anterior cerebral artery some more rostrally positioned vessels, among them Heubner's artery which has a particularly long intracerebral course (see Fig. 1.3). The middle cerebral artery is also divided neuroradiologically into several segments: the M1 segment corresponding to the horizontal portion, M2 the insular portion, and M3–M5 the further branching of the middle cerebral.

In the lateral cerebral fissure the middle cerebral divides into its various terminal branches at about the level of the insular cortex (M2 segment). These branches run frontally, parietally, and temporally as long circumferential arteries. It is fairly typical that the first bifurcation or trifurcation is at this site, from which the terminal branches arise. The names, course, and territories of the individual vessels are shown in Fig. 1.6. Thus, the anterior temporal artery supplies the anterior temporal pole. It is the first constant branch of the middle cerebral, arising already from its horizontal portion. The frontal (orbitofrontal) artery supplies the anterior convexity and runs over the frontal lobes, entering extensive anastomoses with branches of the anterior cerebral. This results in an elongated borderzone, which is discussed in detail below. Other branches travel in the direction of the central region, to the parietal lobes, and finally to the posterior and lateral parts of the temporal lobe. Here there are also anastomoses with the circumferential arteries from the anterior and posterior distribution territories. About 70% of the two cerebral hemispheres are supplied by the two middle cerebral arteries.

The two anterior cerebral arteries are connected by the anterior communicating artery. In their horizontal course (A1) they branch off the direct paramedian branches already mentioned, such as those supplying the head of the caudate nucleus, the putamen, and the anterior commissure. The individual terminal branches of the anterior cerebral artery are again long circumferential arteries. It is particularly from the examples of the callosomarginal and pericallosal arteries that the European term "circumferential arteries" has derived.

Marked individual variations are not uncommonly found in the anatomy of the anterior cerebral artery, produced particularly by deviations of the anterior communicating artery from the norm. Sometimes both pericallosal arteries arise from an anterior segment, while the other horizontal anterior portion is hypoplastic or absent. There are sometimes three pericallosal arteries and sometimes multiple communicating arteries.

1.2.2 Vertebrobasilar and Posterior Cerebral Territory

Before the fusion of the two vertebral arteries to form the basilar at the base of the pons, but already intradurally, they give off branches to form the anterior spinal artery and the posterior inferior cerebellar arteries (PICA; Fig. 1.7). These arteries arising from the intracranial segment of the vertebral artery supply the lateral and dorsal cerebellar hemispheres as far as the vermis, the cerebellar nuclei, and the choroid plexus of the fourth ventricle. Some quite proximal efferent branches supply the brainstem ventrally (paramedian branches), while a circumferential branch

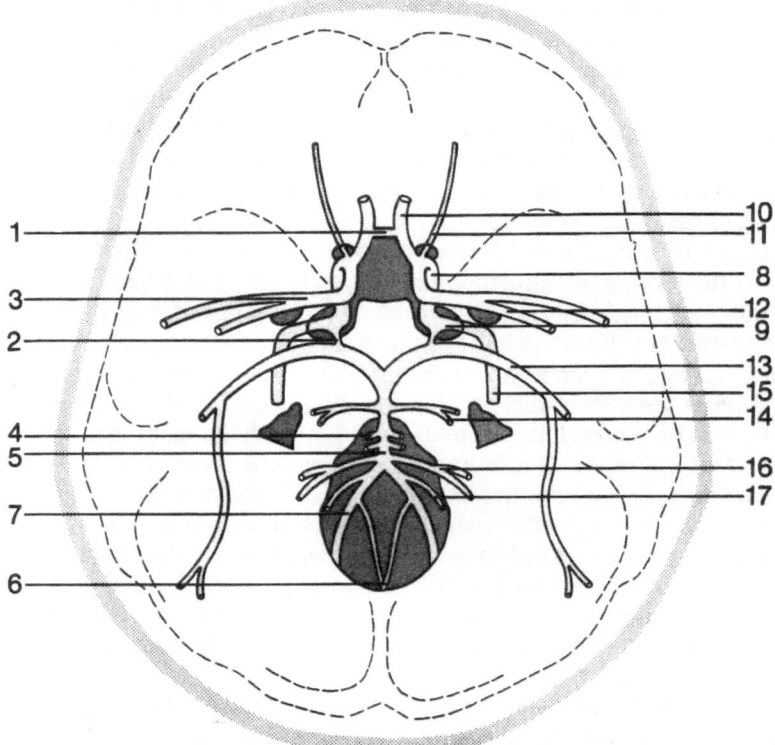

Fig. 1.7. Diagram of cerebral arteries at the skull base with the arterial circle of Willis. *1*, Anterior communicating artery; *2*, posterior communicating artery; *3*, middle cerebral artery; *4*, pontine branches; *5*, basilar artery; *6*, anterior spinal artery; *7*, vertebral artery; *8*, carotid T junction; *9*, carotid siphon; *10*, anterior cerebral artery; *11*, ophthalmic artery; *12*, median banches; *13*, posterior cerebral artery; *14*, superior cerebellar artery; *15*, internal carotid artery; *16*, anterior inferior cerebellar artery; *17*, posterior inferior cerebellar artery

(Wallenberg's artery) reaches the dorsolateral portion of the medulla oblongata. At a variable level, sometimes even differing between left and right, the basilar artery gives off the anterior inferior cerebellar arteries (AICA) which supply the ventral part of the cerebellar cortex, part of the cerebellar medullary layer, and the cerebellar nuclei. This branch also gives off small proximal branches to the medulla and pons. It also usually gives off the internal auditory artery, although this may arise directly from the basilar, the intracranial portion of the vertebral, or from the PICA. The basilar subsequently gives off a series of direct branches to the brainstem (Duvernoy 1978). The next largest branches are the collicular arteries and the upper cerebellar arteries (superior cerebellar), which arise from the basilar immediately before its termination. These supply the dorsorostral portions of the cerebellum, the superior cerebellar peduncle, and the ventral portions of the midbrain and the pons. The basilar divides finally into the two posterior cerebral arteries. In this region the posterior choroidal, posterior communicating, posterior thalamoperforating, and posterior geniculate arteries also arise. The posterior communicating arteries constitute the connection with the carotid territory. Here, too, marked intraindividual variations are common. Sometimes the posterior vessels arise directly via a large-caliber communicating artery from the carotid siphon (carotid type of posterior cerebral origin; see p. 4), and this may also be the case only unilaterally.

1.3 Collaterals and Anastomoses

(see Fields et al. 1965; van der Eecken 1959; Zülch 1985)

The collateral supply is an essential factor in understanding the etiology of strokes; physiologic anastomoses with extracranial vessels constitute an additional safeguard to the cerebral blood supply. The most important collaterals are formed between the external carotid and the carotid siphon, via the facial, angular, and ophthalmic arteries. Likewise, there is very often a collateral between the external carotid, the external occipital artery, and muscular branches to the vertebral artery. Direct connections to the vertebral artery may be formed via the thyrocervical trunk. In individual cases, collaterals also exist via the ascending pharyngeal artery or via meningeal branches (Fig. 1.8).

Whether and to what extent these anastomoses are really helpful when a supplying vessel is obstructed presumably depends on a range of factors whose individual significance cannot be conclusively defined. The possible effectiveness of an anastomosis depends on the lumen of the vascular connection and presumably on the pressure gradient. It may also be important whether a vascular occlusion has developed gradually, whether therefore a collateral can "grow into" its function, or whether the occlusion is acute, e. g., embolic. It must also be considered that up to a luminal constriction of more than 70% no decisive fall in pressure develops behind the stenosis, so that "training" of the collateral probably occurs only with high-grade stenoses. It is also surprising that functionally developed anastomoses can quickly increase their lumen according to the needs for blood supply.

The circle of Willis connects the vessels of the carotid and vertebral systems on both sides (Fig. 1.7). This is subject to considerable variations. Sometimes individual components of this circle are absent. With an intact basal plexus, the obstruction of one and sometimes even two efferent extracranial vessels can be tolerated for a long time. The meningeal connections function as a second essential anastomotic system between the anterior and middle cerebral arteries (parasagittal borderzone), between the middle, posterior, and anterior territories (parieto-occipital borderzone), and over the cerebellar hemispheres. In addition to these collaterals that commonly exist between intracranial vessels, others are sometimes also found, such as when the anterior spinal artery or dural connecting branches contribute to maintenance of function. A weak point in this system consists of the direct penetrating arteries (central branches) which, as functional end-arteries, are poorly collateralized, so that occlusion of these vessels virtually always leads to infarction.

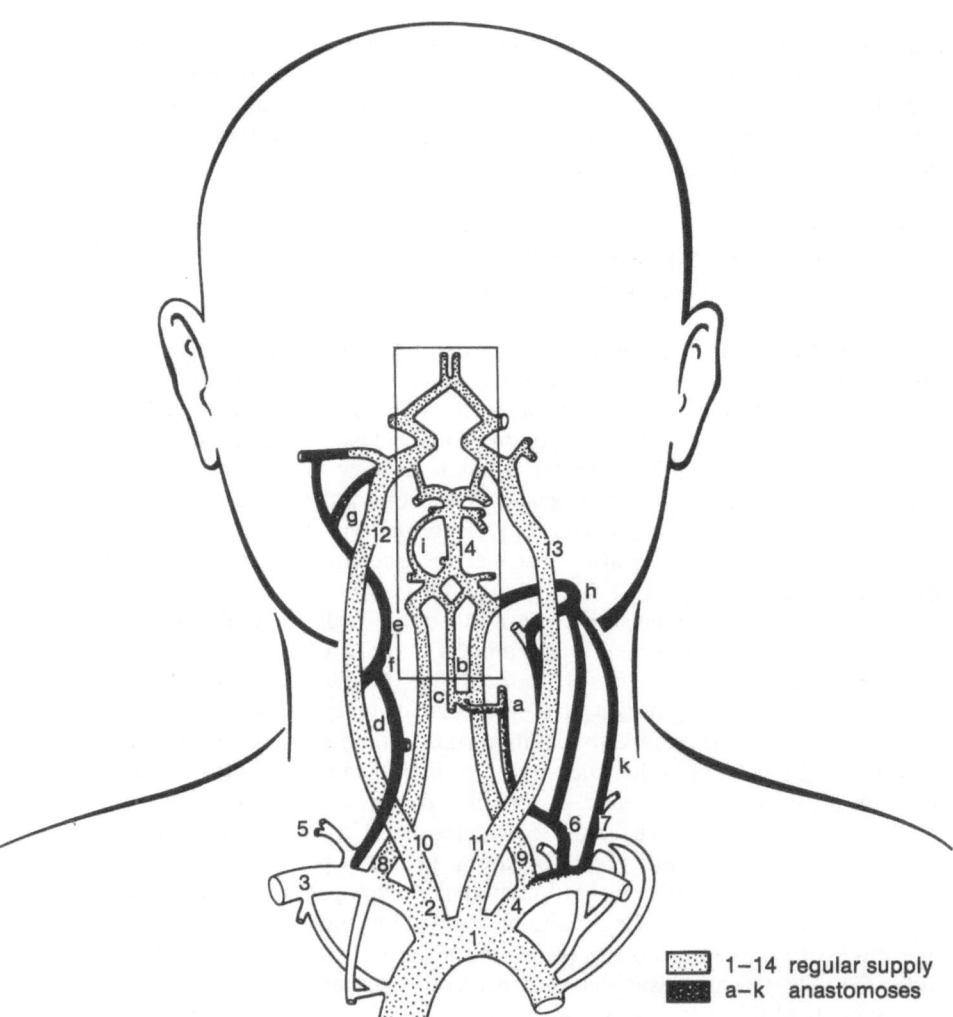

Fig. 1.8. Collaterals ascending from the aortic arch (*a–k*). *1,* Aortic arch; *2,* brachiocephalic trunk; *3, 4,* subclavian artery; *5, 6,* thyrocervical trunk; *7,* costocervical trunk; *8, 9,* vertebral artery; *10, 11,* common carotid artery; *12, 13,* internal carotid artery; *14,* basilar artery; *a,* ascending cervical artery; *b,* radicular and spinal arteries; *c,* anterior spinal artery; *d,* occipital artery, descending branch; *e,* superior thyroid artery; *f,* external carotid; *g,* ophthalmic artery; *h,* caroticotympanic artery; *i,* inferior and superior cerebellar arteries; *k,* deep cervical artery. (Modified from Gänshirt 1972)

1.4 Arterial Anatomy and Infarct Types

Pathologic, angiologic, and CT morphologic findings often provide evidence as to the mechanism of development of an ischemic infarct. The various types of infarcts can be distinguished particularly on the basis of the morphologic description of an infarcted area obtained intravitally from CT and MRI information. The degree and extent of

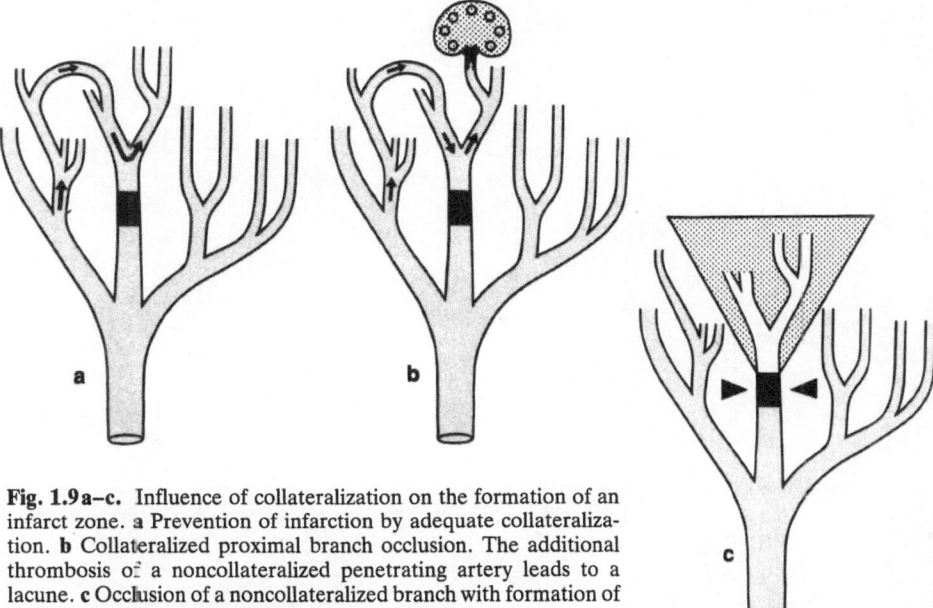

Fig. 1.9 a–c. Influence of collateralization on the formation of an infarct zone. **a** Prevention of infarction by adequate collateralization. **b** Collateralized proximal branch occlusion. The additional thrombosis of a noncollateralized penetrating artery leads to a lacune. **c** Occlusion of a noncollateralized branch with formation of a territorial infarct. (Modified from Zülch 1985)

individual infarct zones are defined not only by the site of the lesion or the degree of construction of the afferent vessels but also by the nature and quality of the anastomoses (Fig. 1.9). The section on CT findings deals with the various infarct patterns in detail (shown here diagrammatically in Fig. 1.10). It is essential to determine whether the lesions are related predominantly to disease or obstruction of noncollateralized, penetrating, small intracerebral arteries (microangiopathies) or to that of the large cerebral arteries (macroangiopathies), or both. Many infarcts may lie in the supply territory of a short or long circumferential artery (territorial infarction) or occur in the borderzone between two interanastomosing vascular zones (extraterritorial infarction; Ringelstein et al. 1985; Zeumer and Hacke 1988; Zülch 1985).

Macroangiopathies may arise hemodynamically (loss of pressure gradients) through thromboembolism or local thrombosis. Among the hemodynamically produced infarcts it is possible to distinguish low-flow infarcts (in the distal distribution zone of the noncollateralized middle cerebral arteries; in German, *letzte Wiese*) and the borderzone infarcts in the border area of supply zones between two or three large vessels (see pp. 66, 139).

Territorial infarcts develop through embolic or local thrombotic occlusion of large superficial cerebral arteries. They are often wedge shaped and limited to the territory of the affected arteries. With partial collateralization of the marginal zone of such a territorial infarct, central infarcts develop. In our view, occlusion of the lenticulostriate arteries constitutes a special form of these territorial infarcts.

Microangiopathies develop when there is isolated or multiple thrombosis of the small arteries penetrating deep into the brain substance. They correspond to the infarct pattern of lacunes and are the expression of a "systemic disease" of the small cerebral

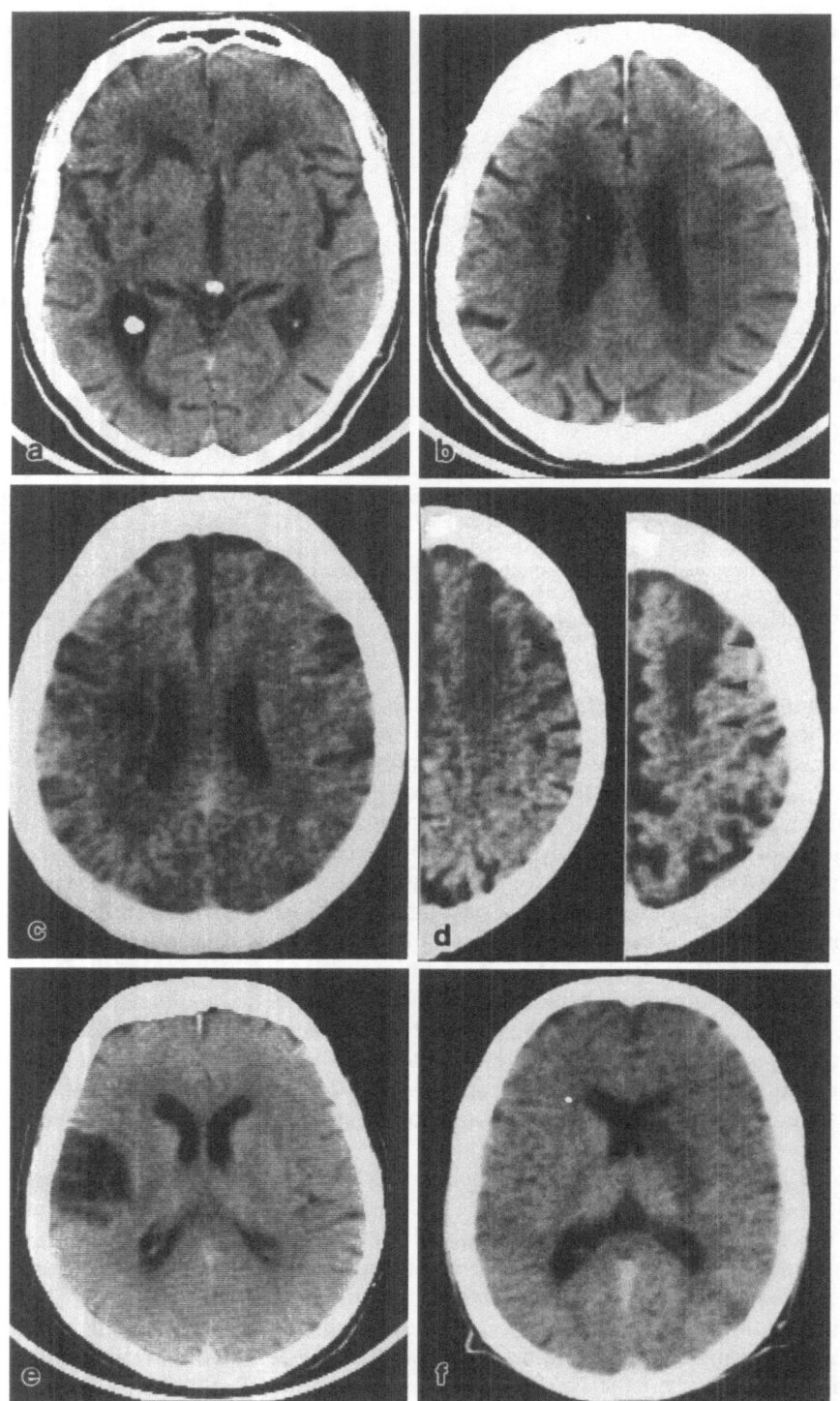

Fig. 1.10

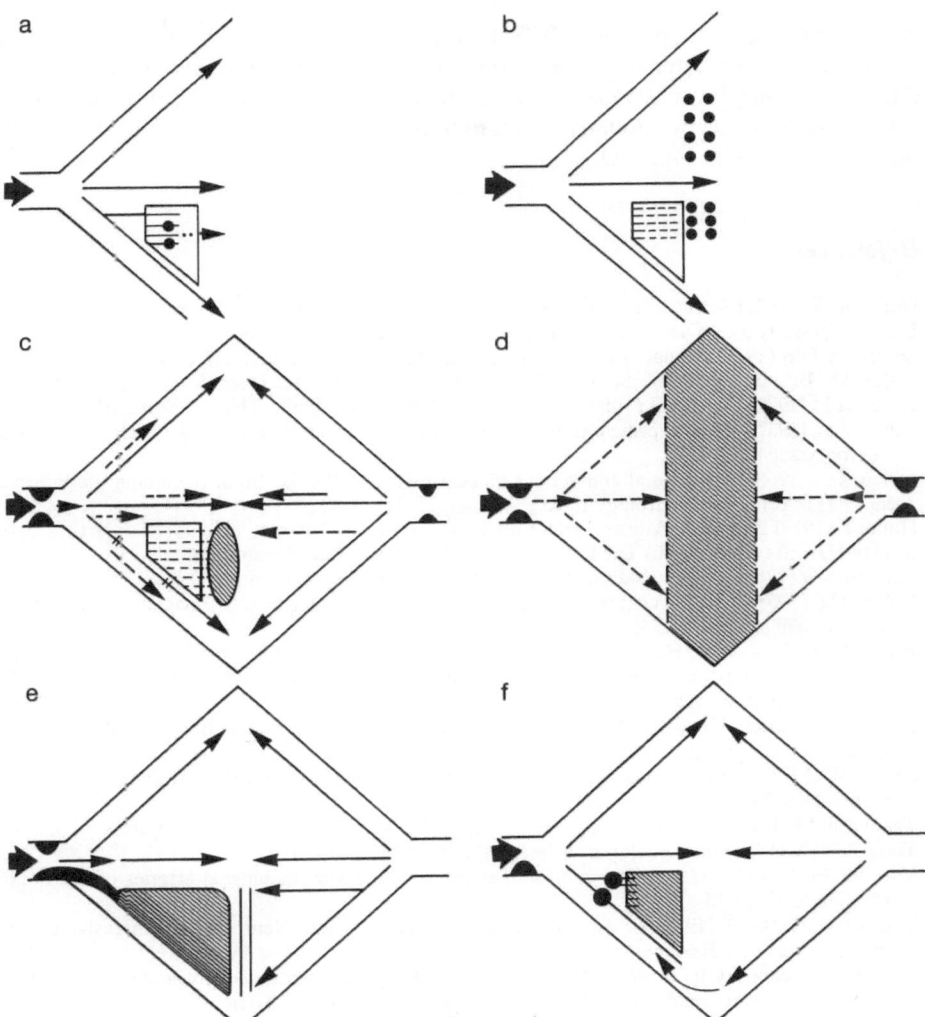

Fig. 1.11a–f. Schematic illustration of the pathogenetic concepts underlying the infarcts shown in Fig. 1.10

Fig. 1.10a–f. Characteristic examples of the various types of micro- and macroangiopathic lesions. **a** Status lacunaris in cerebral microangiopathy with bilateral lacunes in the basal ganglia. **b** Diffuse reduction in thickness of the medullary layer with individually formed paraventricular lacunes (subcortical arteriosclerotic encephalopathy, Binswanger's disease). **c** Subcortical paraventricular lesion (low-flow infarct). **d** Extraterritorially situated subcortical lesion in borderzone between anterior and middle cerebral territories (borderzone infarct). **e** Territorial infarct of central middle cerebral group of branches. **f** Typical infarct in territory of lenticulostriate arteries. Each of the lesions produces a similar clinical picture, i.e., a central hemiparesis with mainly right brachiofacial expression. At the same time, the existing infarct extension may be associated with any type of course: transient, completely or partly reversible, irreversible, or completed strokes. Accurate conclusions as to the underlying angiopathy are obtained only by combining the clinical picture and the temporal evolution of the stroke

vessels (risk factor: hypertension). Subcortical arteriosclerotic encephalopathy is a special type of this systemic disease of the small vessels, in which lacunar lesions and a diffuse medullary layer hypodensity are both found on CT (Zeumer et al. 1980, 1981). The etiologic concepts underlying infarctions, as shown in Fig. 1.10, are shown diagrammatically in Fig. 1.11.

References

Dorndorf W (1983) Schlaganfälle, Klinik und Therapie, 2nd edn. Thieme, Stuttgart

Duus P (1983) Topical Diagnosis in Neurology, 3rd edn. Thieme, Stuttgart

Duvernoy HM (1978) Human brainstem vessels. Springer, Berlin Heidelberg New York

Fields WS, Bruetman ME, Weibel J (1965) Collateral circulation of the brain. Monogr Surg Sci 2:183

Gänshirt H (1972) Der Hirnkreislauf. Physiologie, Pathologie, Klinik. Thieme, Stuttgart

Gillian LA (1957) General principles of the arterial blood vessels pattern to the brain. Trans Am Neurol Assoc 82:65

Gillian LA (1968) The arterial and venous blood supplies to the forebrain (including the internal capsule) of primates. Neurology 18:653

Huber P (1979) Zerebrale Angiographie für Klinik und Praxis, 3rd edn. Thieme, Stuttgart

Kaplan HA, Ford DH (1966) The brain vascular system. Elsevier, Amsterdam

Lazorthes G (1961) Vascularisation et circulation cerebrale. Masson, Paris

Lehrer HZ (1968) Relative calibre of the cervical internal carotid artery; normal variation with the circle of Willis. Brain 91:339

Ringelstein EB, Zeumer H, Schneider R (1985) Der Beitrag der zerebralen Computertomographie zur Differentialtypologie und Differentialtherapie des ischämischen Großhirninfarktes. Fortschr Neurol Psychiatr 53:315

Salomon G, Huang YP (1976) Radiologic anatomy of the brain. Springer, Berlin Heidelberg New York

Seeger W (1978) Atlas of topographical anatomy of the brain and surrounding structures. Springer, Vienna New York

Takahashi M (1974) Atlas of vertebral angiography. University Park Press, Baltimore

Toole JF (1984) Cerebrovascular disorders, 3rd edn. Raven, New York

Van der Eecken HM (1959) The anastomoses between the leptomeningeal arteries of the brain. Thomas, Springfield

Zeumer H, Hacke W (1988) Ischämische Insulte. In: Hacke W (ed) Neurologische Intensivmedizin, 2nd edn. Perimed, Erlangen, p 89

Zeumer H, Schonsky B, Sturm KW (1980) Predominant white matter involvement in subcortical arteriosclerotic encephalopathy (Binswanger's disease). J Comput Tomogr 4:14

Zeumer H, Hacke W, Hündgen R (1981) Subkortikale arteriosklerotische Enzephalopathie: klinische, CT-morphologische und elektrophysiologische Befunde. Fortschr Neurol Psychiatr 49:223

Zülch KJ (1985) The cerebral infarct. Pathology, pathogenesis, and computed tomography. Springer, Berlin Heidelberg New York

2 Pathophysiology of Cerebral Ischemia

2.1 Introduction

The weight of the brain amounts to only 2% of total body weight, but it receives 15% of the cardiac output and uses 20% of the oxygen consumed by the body. The energy supply is provided almost exclusively by glucose metabolism. The substrate for this is stored in the brain in the form of glucose or glycogen and is sufficient to cover the energy requirements for only about 1 min. Consequently, there is a delicate equilibrium between oxygen and nutrient supply from the blood and the energy requirements of the brain. Disturbances in neurologic function appear after a few seconds of ischemia, although they are not necessarily persistent at first.

2.2 General Aspects of Brain Cell Metabolism

Like every other living cell, the brain cell is characterized by its energy turnover. Three different types of turnover can be distinguished. Maintenance turnover corresponds to the minimal energy conversion which is absolutely necessary for the preservation of cell structures. If this is not sustained, irreversible cell damage occurs, and the cell dies. "Stand-by" turnover corresponds to that needed by a cell for maintaining its immediate, unlimited preparedness for function. This includes, for instance, the maintenance of specific concentration gradients for sodium and calcium ions (ion channels, ion pumps). Activity turnover corresponds to the energy turnover of a biologically and functionally active cell (Fig. 2.1).

In the resting state the human brain consumes about 3.35 ml oxygen per minute for each 100 g brain tissue. The chief source of energy is glucose; under physiologic conditions about 90% of the glucose is subject to complete oxidative metabolism while the residual 10% is converted anaerobically to pyruvate. Only in negligibly small amounts and practically only under pathologic conditions can other substrates such as amino acids or ketone bodies be transformed in cerebral metabolism. Limitation of the substances potentially available rests on the blood-brain barrier.

It is because of the physicochemical properties of the blood-brain barrier that most of the hydrophilic substances circulating in the plasma are excluded from transfer into the brain. In addition to diffusion according to the concentration gradients for some molecules, there is carrier-mediated transport (glucose, amino acids; Lund-Anderson 1979). Ions can be transported by special energy-consuming transporting agents (ion pumps) against the concentration gradients.

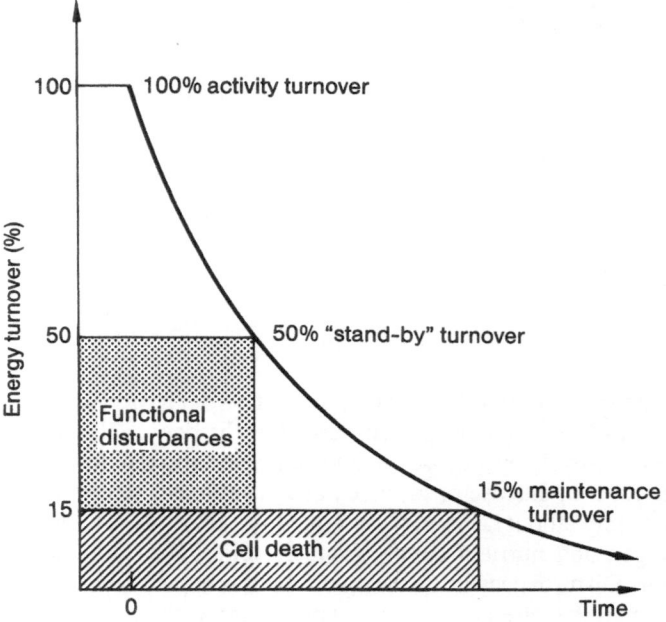

Fig. 2.1. Diagram illustrating the concepts of maintenance turnover, "stand-by" turnover, and activity turnover

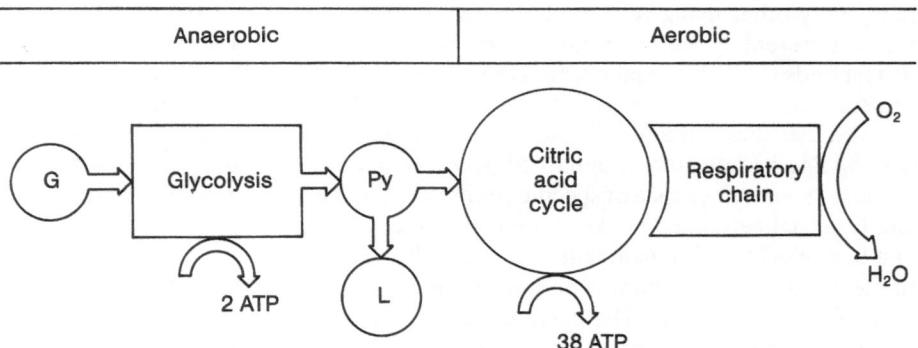

Fig. 2.2. Anaerobic oxygen utilization in glycolysis and oxidative conversion of glucose in the respiratory chain. *ATP*, adenosine triphosphate; *G*, glucose; *L*, lactate; *Py*, pyruvate

Energy is liberated by glycolysis and the citric acid cycle (Fig. 2.2), which balance aerobically 38 mol ATP as energy-rich phosphate per mole glucose. The glucose is converted by complete oxidation, i.e., under aerobic conditions, into CO_2 and H_2O. In normal brain functioning only about 10% of the glucose is converted to pyruvate and lactate and therefore does not participate in the further conversion in the citric acid cycle. Thus some 33 mol ATP is formed per mole glucose. From the citric acid cycle there not only results the overwhelming part of the energy output in the form of energy-rich phosphate, but a spectrum of syntheses such as for amino acids and transmitter substances also have their origin here. Under anaerobic conditions the respiratory chain and citric acid cycle fail, and the residual anaerobic glycolysis gives rise to only 2 mol ATP per mole glucose. Part of the free energy is consumed by the numerous synthetic processes which keep the cell structurally and functionally intact. These include the preservation of the cell membrane and the regulation of the intracellular milieu, which is very labile because of the development of a series of intermediate metabolic products. Principal among these are the free fatty acids formed by the breakdown of phospholipids and from which, depending on the situation of the intracellular milieu, prostaglandins and leukotrienes, potent precursors of free radicals, can be formed. A special function of the neurone is the (re)synthesis of transmitter substances responsible for the transmission of bioelectric processes from cell to cell and hence for the function of the central nervous system. Finally, energy is required for the maintenance of ionic disequilibrium (rest potential), the essential prerequisite for bioelectric irritability of the neurone. The intracellular concentration of potassium is 20–100 times higher than the extracellular concentration, and the intracellular sodium concentrations 5–15 times lower than the extracellular. Finally, the intracellular chloride concentration is lower than the extracellular by a factor of 20–100 (Katzman and Pappius 1973).

2.2.1 Significance of Calcium

Ca^{2+} ions also occupy a central position in the regulation of cell function, with a precisely regulated disequilibrium.

Acting synergistically with cyclic adenosine monophosphate, Ca^{2+} ions exert a further regulatory effect. An increase in the intracellular Ca^{2+} concentration acts directly to promote the formation of energy-rich phosphate via an increased activation of various intracellular enzymes, raises the concentration of substrate for the respiratory chain, and leads to a higher ATP concentration. This mechanism may be regarded as one of feedback since the energy-dependent exclusion of Ca^{2+} from the cell is supported by the increased ATP production. The concentration gradient that must be preserved amounts to about 10^{-7} mol/l within the cell as against 10^{-3} mol/l extracellularly for Ca^{2+} (Carafoli and Crompton 1978).

Ca^{2+} transmits electrical and chemical signals arriving at the cell surface to the biochemical systems within the cell. Via phospholipase A, calcium activates the breakdown of the phospholipids of the cell membrane. The metabolic path to arachidonic acid is particularly important, as with a rise in concentration of arachidonic acid increased prostaglandins and leukotrienes are formed. The course of this catabolism leads to the formation of unstable peroxides, from which so-called free radicals are formed (hydroxyl radicals, OH^-). Free radicals are also formed in the respiratory chain as peroxide radicals (O_2^-). Because of their high reactivity, the hydroxyl radicals may lead to damage of cell structure and membrane defects. The cell disposes of various radical-capture systems such as enzymes (dysmutases, catalases, peroxidases), antioxidants (tocopherol or ascorbic acid), and thio-containing amino acids and peptides (e. g., glutathione; Demopoulos et al. 1980). Therefore no danger to the cell arises from free radical formation under physiologic conditions. So that the processes in the cell may be effectively regulated, the calcium concentration is regulated in the physiologic state by several systems (pumps, exchangers, and channels). This also involves intracellular organelles and the cell membrane. The intracellular organelles have a double function. On the one hand, they remove the Ca^{2+} ions after sequestration in the mitochondria; on the other, they can regulate activation of the cell by short-term expulsion of Ca^{2+} ions. An exchange system is interposed in the membranes for the exclusion of Ca^{2+} ions which eliminates the ions from the cell by exploitation of the Na^+ concentration gradient without energy consumption. In the resting state the low intracellular Ca^{2+} level is regulated by the calcium-transport ATPases contained in the plasma membrane. To replace the Ca^{2+} ions eliminated, $2H^+$ ions are admitted to the cell so that this pump is electroneutrally operated. Hence it is functionally independent of the actual membrane potential (Schweitzer and Blaustein 1980). In depolarization there is a short-term massive entry of calcium ions into the cell. This calcium influx takes place via specific transfer structures in the membrane, the calcium channels. On the basis of in vitro studies, two calcium channels of differing capacity for stimulation have been identified, designated

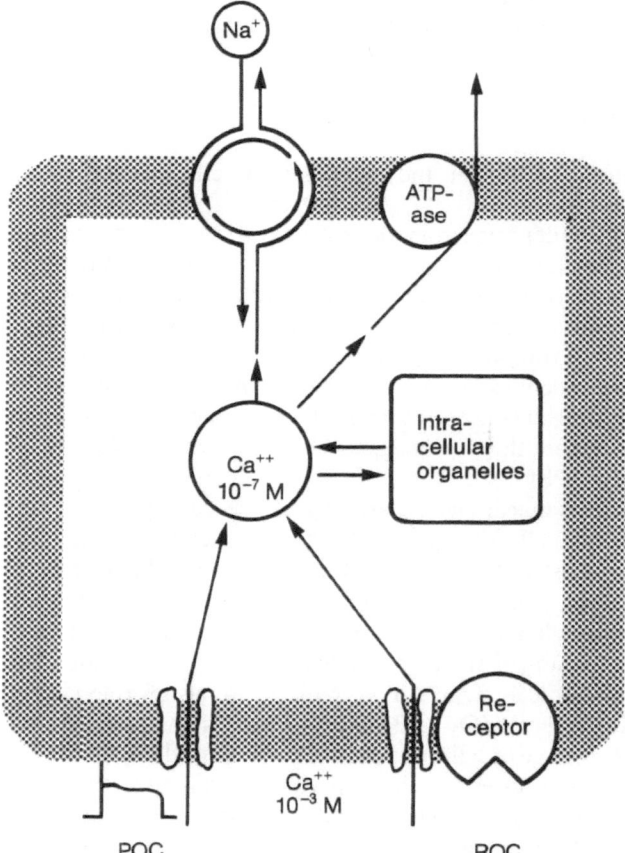

Fig. 2.3. Regulation of intracellular Ca^{2+} concentration. Calcium can enter the cell interior via potential-operated channels (*POC*) or receptor-operated channels (*ROC*). Calcium is transported into the extracellular space by the sodium-potassium antiport system and by the calcium-transport ATPase contained in the plasma membrane. In addition, the cellular calcium concentration is influenced by sequestration in the mitochondria and sarcoplasmic reticulum

as potential-operated and receptor-operated channels (Nayler and Horowitz 1983). It has not yet been finally determined whether there are in fact two different channels, or whether there is only a single channel of differential reactivity. In principle, only the potential-operated channel should be opened by a change in membrane potential, whereas in the case of the receptor-dependent channel an additional activation of a receptor adjacent to the channel is promoted (Fig. 2.3).

2.3 Regulation of Cerebral Circulation

2.3.1 Cerebral Perfusion Pressure and Vascular Resistance

The driving force for the circulation is the blood pressure, and as in every vascular bed the cerebral circulation is determined by the hydraulic analog of Ohm's law ($Q = P/R$). Q corresponds here to the blood volume per unit of time (also termed the cerebral blood flow, CBF), P to the perfusion pressure, and R to the vascular resistance. The difference between the mean arterial pressure in the arteries supplying the brain, on the one hand, and the intracranial and venous pressure, on the other, determines the cerebral perfusion pressure. As the venous pressure is normally small (only 2 mmHg higher than the pressure in the right atrium), this can usually be neglected. However, the situation changes in upper influx obstruction, thrombosis of the cerebral veins and sinuses, or even in positive end-expiratory pressure (PEEP) ventilation. Although the intracranial pressure is low under physiologic conditions (0–10 mmHg), it can increase markedly in pathologic conditions such as space-occupying lesions or cerebral edema (see Sect. 2.5).

Under normal conditions the cerebral perfusion pressure can be equated approximately with the mean arterial blood pressure. The vascular resistance (R) is determined by three factors: the length of the vessel (l), the viscosity of the blood (η), and the vascular caliber (r). By the Hagen-Poiseuille law this relationship is expressed as: $R = l \cdot \eta \cdot 8/r^4$. The vascular resistance is greatest in the small arteries and arterioles. About 30% of the vascular resistance comes from arteries with a caliber of over 100 μm and 40% from arterioles with a diameter of 40–100 μm.

The blood viscosity is determined, among other factors, by the protein concentration of the blood and its erythrocyte content. The viscosity is not constant but depends on the flow velocity of the blood and the caliber of the vessels. In large and medium-sized vessels, in which the blood flows rapidly, the viscosity is comparatively low; it increases in the small vessels because of increasing erythrocyte aggregation, and falls again in the very small vessels (Fahraeus-Lindquist effect). The viscosity in the capillaries is determined predominantly by the deformability of the erythrocytes. In capillaries connected in series the erythrocyte content (and hence the viscosity) is lower in the longer capillary loops (Chien 1982).

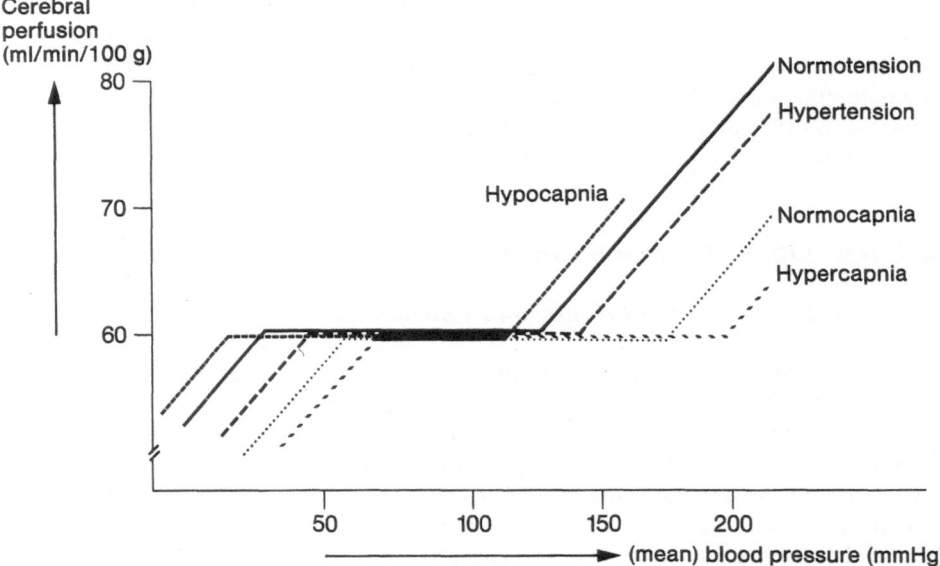

Fig. 2.4. Diagram illustrating autoregulation and how it is influenced by arterial CO_2 pressure and by chronic hypertension

2.3.2 Autoregulation

Over a wide physiologic range of mean arterial pressures (50 and 150 mmHg) the cerebral circulation is independent of the blood pressure. This is the result of a physiologic process known as autoregulation: the cerebral vessels contract with rising systemic blood pressure and dilate with falling pressure, thus keeping the cerebral perfusion constant (Harper 1986). Outside the above limits as well as under particular pathologic conditions, for example, in infarcted tissue and its vicinity, autoregulation is lost, and the circulation passively follows the blood pressure changes. The same values also apply to the conditions for a normal pCO_2 (see Sect. 2.3.3.1); with chronically elevated blood pressure the limits are displaced upward (Fig. 2.4; Strandgaard 1976). The physiology of autoregulation is not yet completely clear. It is convenient to adduce the Bayliss effect as an explanation, thus postulating the function of the smooth muscle cells of the vessel wall as the source of regulation.

2.3.3 Functional Regulation

Under physiologic conditions the perfusion of the brain is closely linked with the tissue metabolic requirements. As functional activation of the brain is associated with an increase in metabolic activity, cerebral function and regional cerebral circulation are linked; however, the mechanisms of this linkage are so far incompletely understood. A number of mediators can play a role; the action of the blood gases, the influence of cations, and other regulatory mechanisms still not finally clarified are discussed below.

2.3.3.1 Blood Gas Influences

An increase in p_aCO_2 leads to vasodilatation and a decrease to vasoconstriction. This regulation takes place in a p_aCO_2 range from 25 mmHg to about 60 mmHg; above 60 mmHg the cerebral circulation no longer increases, and vasodilatation is then maximal. The relationship between brain perfusion and p_aCO_2 concentration is presented in Fig. 2.5. Within the range noted this relationship may be taken as linear, with a 4% increase in perfusion associated with an elevation in p_aCO_2 of 1 mmHg (Harper and Glass 1965). CO_2 regulation is dependent on blood pressure. With low blood pressure the blood vessels are already primarily dilated, so that the influence of p_aCO_2 is less. When the vessels are maximally dilated at the lower limit of pressure-conditioned autoregulation, the CO_2 regulation is abolished. With strong functional activation the cerebral perfusion may rise before accumulation of CO_2 and tissue acidosis development. Hence functional regulation cannot be explained by the mechanism of CO_2 reactivity alone.

The p_aO_2 also has a regulatory influence on cerebral circulation. A fall in p_aO_2 below 50 mmHg leads to a rapid increase in perfusion. It is assumed that the mechanism of

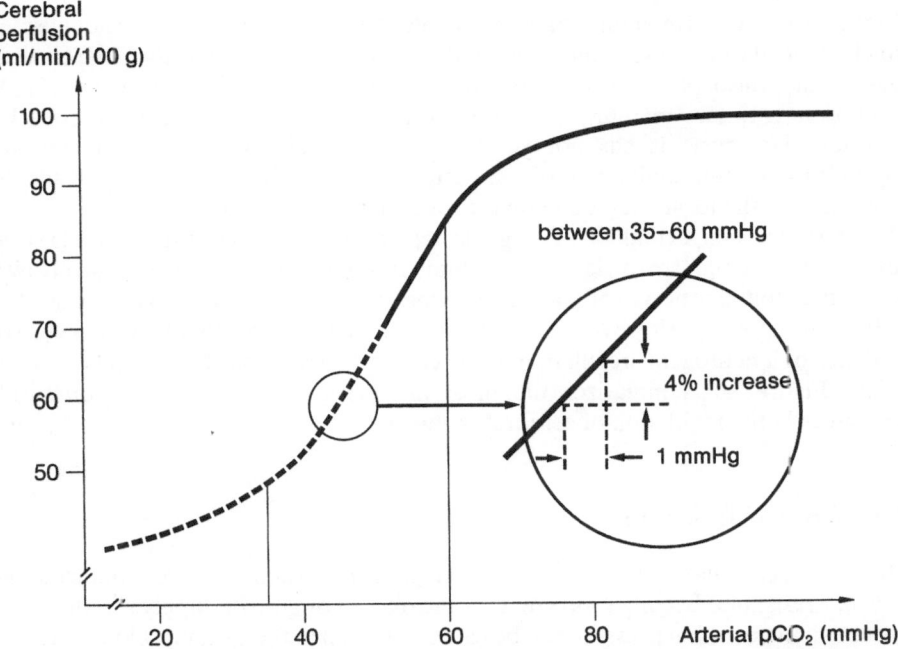

Fig. 2.5. CO_2 reactivity of cerebral perfusion: in the range between 25 and 60 mmHg there is a linear relationship between p_aCO_2 and cerebral perfusion, expressed as a 4% increase per mmHg

regulation by p_aO_2 is associated with changes in cellular metabolism (acidosis) in hypoxia. However, under physiologic conditions this regulatory pathway plays hardly any role (MacDowall 1965).

2.3.3.2 Ionic Influences

Whether the acid content (pH value, concentration of H^+ ions) can be regarded as a decisive factor in the regulation of local circulation in the brain is a matter of controversy. The immediate increase in cerebral circulation upon cortical activation and the delayed increase in cortical H^+ concentration have been adduced as an argument against an important role for H^+ in the early phase of functional hyperemia. Special importance seems to attach to potassium reactivity (Somjen 1979). K^+ is liberated into the extracellular space during cortical activation. This can reach the vascular musculature by diffusion and may be responsible for the increase in regional perfusion occurring simultaneously with the increase in K^+. After a short period the K^+ concentration falls again, but the circulation remains elevated. Hence it has been argued that the K^+ concentration has a carrier function in the initial rapid activation of the increase in perfusion, whereas regulation by p_aCO_2 could be responsible for the more permanent maintenance of the circulation.

2.3.3.3 Other Possible Regulatory Principles

On the basis of experimental studies in animals, it has been suggested that adenosine, which can lead to a dose-dependent vasodilatation when applied locally to the cortical vessels, may also play a role in the regulation of function (Winn et al. 1981). Adenosine traverses membranes and can therefore reach the vascular muscle by diffusion. However, it has not yet been shown that the increased adenosine concentration after activation of the central nervous system actually leads to promotion of the local circulation by the mechanism described above.

The existence and extent of neurogenic regulatory mechanisms for the cerebral circulation is also controversial. The cerebral arteries are surrounded extensively by a plexus of autonomic nerve cells, and many types of receptors have been demonstrated in the arterial walls. However, it has not been possible so far to adduce conclusive evidence of a neurogenic regulation of the cerebral circulation (Nelson and Rennels 1970). Figure 2.6 summarizes the most important, if partly still hypothetical, mediators in the regulation of cerebral perfusion.

2.4 Cerebral Ischemia

The cerebral circulation becomes inadequate if the perfusion pressure is reduced, the vascular resistance becomes too great, or the oxygen or glucose supply is reduced. A reduction in perfusion pressure can be caused by a fall in the systemic blood pressure (shock, cardiac arrest) or by an increase in the intracranial pressure. These conditions often lead to a global ischemia, i. e., all parts of the brain being affected. In contrast to

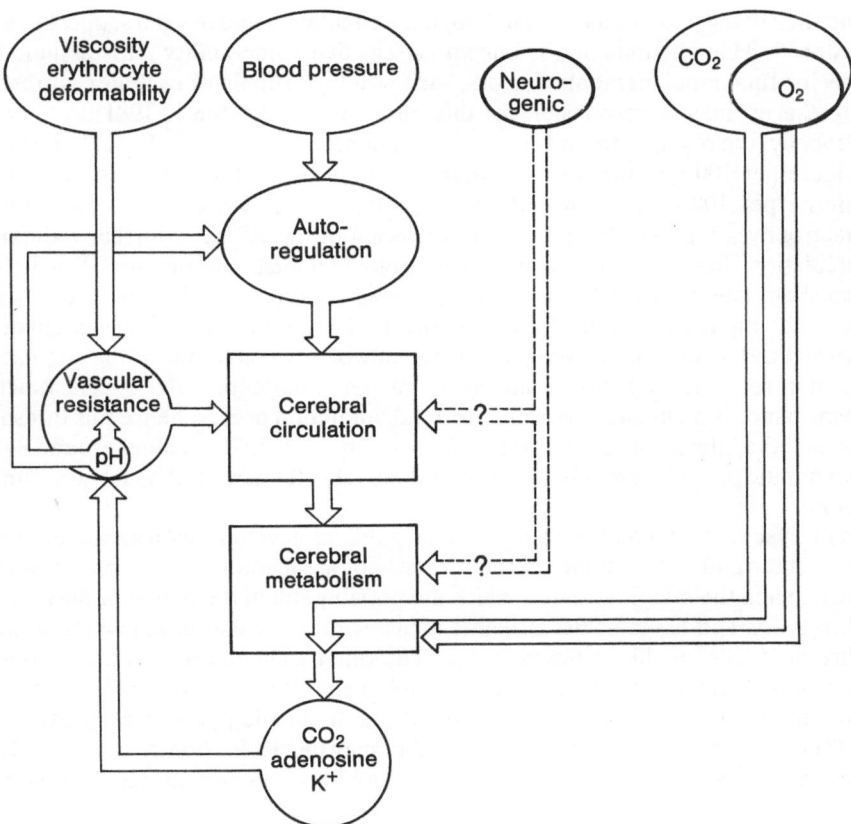

Fig. 2.6. Summary diagram of regulation of cerebral circulation

this is regional or focal ischemia, in which only particular regions of the brain become ischemic. This is caused by a series of different pathogenetic mechanisms (see Chap. 4).

2.4.1 Ischemic Thresholds and the Penumbra

Whatever the causes of local or global ischemia may be, they eventually lead to a focal or general reduction of perfusion in the central nervous system and hence to a reduced supply of O_2 and glucose. As has already been noted in connection with brain cell metabolism, and in contrast to other cells, the activity of brain cells is very rapidly impaired by disturbed energy supply. This is due to the virtually total dependence of the brain on glucose metabolism. Experimental studies have indicated the threshold values below which functional disorders appear as well as the fact that different parts of the brain and even different types of cells react to anoxia with varying sensitivity. Thus, particular hippocampal neurones react in a distinctive temporal pattern to impaired oxygen supply, with many cells seeming to withstand hypoxic phases longer and then dying within 3 days even though the circulation and oxygen supply have been restored. This phenomenon is known as selective vulnerability. It is assumed that specific functional metabolic factors, such as a high supply of excitatory transmitter substances, may be responsible for this variable reaction (Siesjö 1981).

Globally, the resting cerebral circulation amounts on average to about 50–60 ml each minute per 100 g of brain tissue. A reduction in the circulation to some 20 ml per minute per 100 g may not lead to observable consequences, although even here electrophysiologic studies may show a slowing of the EEG. A further reduction in circulation then leads to features of neurologic deficit, the functional or ischemic threshold (the terms are synonymous) having been passed. The evoked potentials may be impaired (see p. 166), and the EEG flattens out. If the circulation is normalized again, the neurologic deficits may be reversible, but if the circulation is further reduced to below some 8–10 ml per minute per 100 g, the functional disturbance is no longer reversible. Instead, infarction occurs; hence this threshold is termed the infarction threshold (Fig. 2.7; Astrup et al. 1979). Values around 8–10 ml per minute per 100 g are tolerated for markedly shorter periods than those around 12–14 ml.

In occlusion of a blood vessel an ischemic gradient develops, with severe ischemia in the center and – depending on the presence of a collateral circulation – less severe ischemia in the marginal zones, which are possibly still in the region of the functional threshold. The tissue at the ischemic focus, with a circulation below the infarction threshold, dies within a few minutes. The other ischemic tissues lie between the functional and infarction thresholds, and their fate depends on local perfusion conditions. This region has been termed the "ischemic penumbra" (Astrup et al. 1981). It has been shown that the penumbra may persist for hours, and possibly even for days. This is particularly relevant from the clinical standpoint since it provides the

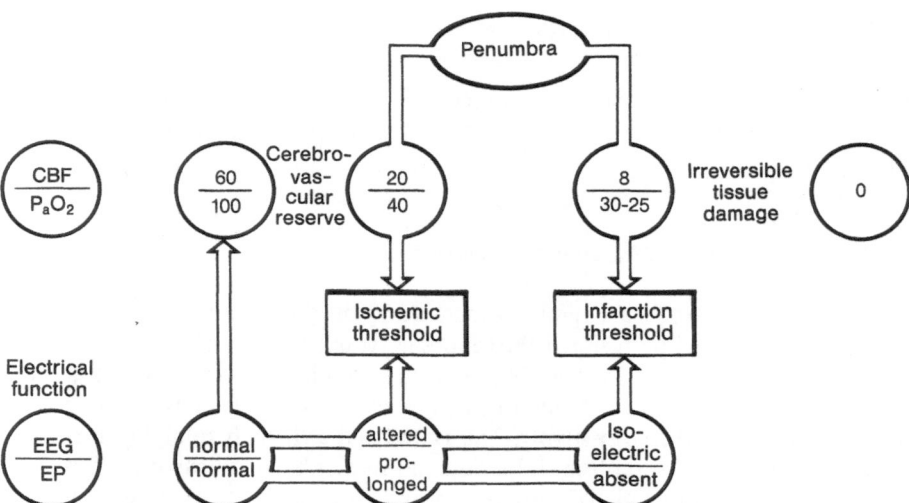

Fig. 2.7. Thresholds for defective cerebral perfusion (functional and infarction thresholds) and the critical oxygenation, showing the associated EEG and evoked potentials (*EP*) changes and the disturbances of membrane function which underlie the tissue damage

theoretical basis for therapeutic measures. The tissue is greatly at risk, and its restricted function leads to signs of neurologic deficit, but the damage at this point is not yet irreversible. Moreover, the circulatory conditions in the penumbra also show a temporal-dynamic mechanism. Initially, the vessels are maximally dilated due to the reduced perfusion pressure. There is then an accumulation of CO_2 with the acidosis. However, no further reactivity of the vessels occurs, and the result is vasoparalysis (vasoparalytic luxury perfusion; Lassen 1961). In contrast, the blood vessels outside the ischemic zone retain their normal physiologic tonus and can still react to changes in blood pressure and CO_2. If the pCO_2 now rises, the blood vessels in the healthy brain tissue also dilate, whereas the vessels in the penumbra no longer show any ability to react. There may be a redistribution of the blood supply at the expense of the ischemic penumbra, i.e., the penumbra is less well perfused, and there is a danger of transition from hitherto only functionally disturbed cells into areas of ischemic damage.

This vascular reaction is known as the cerebral "steal phenomenon" (Lassen and Palvölgyi 1968). There is also the opposite phenomenon which results in an initially more intense perfusion of the penumbra, known as the "counter-steal" or "Robin Hood" phenomenon. Although the significance of these pathologic vascular reactions is not quite clear, they emerge repeatedly in the discussion of pharmacologic measures against ischemic disorders of cerebral circulation.

In the zone of the penumbra, where there is maximal vasodilatation, the vascular resistance is determined mainly by the blood viscosity. Because of adhesion of leukocytes in the capillaries and because of accumulation of corpuscular blood components behind such leukocytes, or even spontaneously, the small vessels may become obstructed and are then not perfused again even if there is reperfusion of the main vessel. This is known as the "no reflow phenomenon" and applies to the only partial reperfusion in the infarcted tissue.

2.4.2 The Course of an Ischemic Lesion

If the perfusion falls below the ischemic threshold, breakdown of the stand-by turnover develops quite soon, and the ion pumps cease to function. The membrane potential also breaks down: K^+ ions flow into the extracellullar space while Na^+ and Ca^{2+} ions accumulate within the cell in exchange. This leads to the cell surface becoming negative and to extinction of the electrical irritability of the membranes (terminal depolarization). Initially, the depolarization of the cell membrane is potentially reversible, but if it persists, structural lesions develop which lead to infarction. This takes place rapidly once the perfusion falls below the infarction threshold (Fig. 2.7). Besides a disturbed perfusion, other factors such as hypoxia and hypoglycemia also have pathologic consequences. Because of oxygen lack, the energy-producing citric acid cycle with predominant production of ATP fails. Accompanying the decreased ATP formation from glycolysis, there develops a marked acidosis which, among other effects, impairs enzyme function via a raised H^+ ion concentration.

Moreover, the acidosis provokes a cerebral edema (see Sect. 2.5), which is characterized by cellular swelling, especially in the glial tissue, and has a mechanical

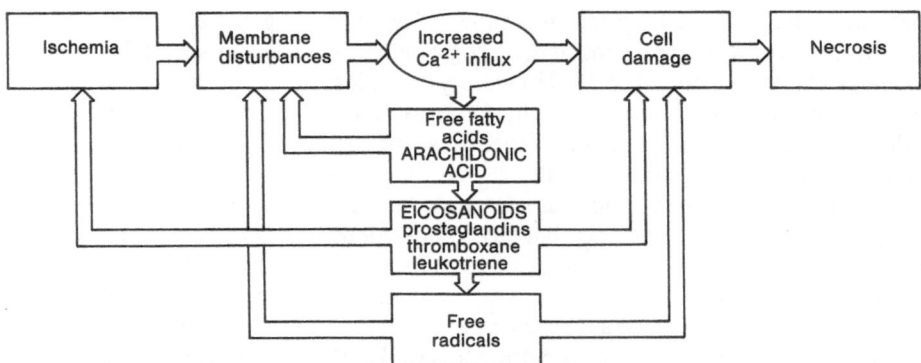

Fig. 2.8. The cascade of reactions in the course of an ischemic lesion, leading to metabolic derangement (see also Fig. 2.7)

influence on the microcirculation. The consequences are an increased vascular resistance and a further fall in perfusion pressure, with resulting extension of the ischemic area. The further course of an ischemic lesion is characterized by a cascade of reactions which finally lead to metabolic derangement and structural intracellular damage (Fig. 2.8; Hass 1981).

The involvement of Ca^{2+} ions in numerous intra- and extracellular processes and the reciprocal linkage of these systems is striking. This is also the theoretical basis of the attempt to limit the extent of the ischemia by a regulating influence of Ca^{2+} ions (Farber et al. 1981). The high, uncontrolled intracellular concentration of Ca^{2+} ions leads to excessive liberation of excitatory neurotransmitters and hence to an unnecessary and additionally energy-consuming hyperactivity in the ischemia-threatened tissue.

2.5 Ischemic Cerebral Edema

A further complication of cerebral ischemia is cerebral edema. This process involves the production of increased fluid content within the cerebral tissue as the outcome of locally or systemically damaging influences. Very soon after the appearance of ischemia there develops a cytotoxic cerebral edema. Due to osmosis the cell withdraws water from the extracellular space by virtue of its high macromolecular content. This mechanism is counteracted by the Na^+/K^+ pump in the cell membrane, which transports Na^+ and water back again into the extracellular space. In ischemia this pump mechanism fails, and the neurones swell. Hence cytotoxic edema is an intracellular edema.

If the ischemia persists over a longer period, a vasogenic edema may be added to the cytotoxic edema. This appears to be accompanied by damage to the blood-brain barrier, which certainly resists ischemia longer (probably because not only glucose but also fatty acids can be used as a substrate for energy metabolism) but is itself damaged after a latent period depending on the extent of the ischemia. Plasma constituents then flow into the brain tissue and travel in the extracellular space along the nerve fibers in the white matter, where they accumulate. Hence the vasogenic cerebral edema is an extracellular edema. The failure of the blood-brain barrier can be confirmed by isotope scintigraphy and CT with contrast medium. In the late stage, vasogenic cerebral edema appears as a fingerlike pattern of extension in the white matter. At least in the early stage of cytotoxic cerebral edema one finds a diffuse swelling in the territory of the affected artery. It is interesting that the disturbance of the blood-brain barrier is also associated with an increased risk of secondary hemorrhages after recanalization (so-called reperfusion trauma).

Extensive cerebral edema after ischemia can act like a space-occupying lesion. There is a gradual and accelerating rise in intracranial pressure, which initially makes demands on the buffer capacity (compression of the ventricular system, emptying of the CSF space). This rise has a further effect on the circulation since the perfusion pressure falls (Langfitt et al. 1965). With extensive space-occupying supra- or infratentorial lesions there may be upper or lower herniation and the development of an obstructive hydrocephalus. Finally, the process can lead to global ischemia and brain death. But even if the rise in intracranial pressure does not attain such global extent, the local effect with compression of the small vessels in the vicinity of the infarct and the penumbra is responsible for an increase in the ultimately infarcted tissue.

References

Astrup J, Symon L, Branston NM (1979) Cortical evoked potentials in brain ischemia. Stroke 8:51

Astrup J, Siesjö BK, Symon L (1981) Thresholds in cerebral ischemia. The ischemic penumbra. Stroke 12:723

Carafoli E, Crompton M (1978) The regulation of intracellular calcium. Curr Top Membr Transp 10:151

Chien S (1982) Rheology in the microcirculation in normal and low flow states. Adv Shock Res 8:71

Demopoulos HB, Flamm ES, Pietronigro DD (1980) The free radical pathology and the microcirculation in the major central nervous system disorders. Acta Physiol Scand [Suppl] 492:91

Farber JL, Chien KR, Mittnacht S Jr (1981) The pathogenesis of irreversible cell injury in ischemia. Am J Pathol 102:271

Harper AM (1966) Autoregulation of the cerebral blood flow: influence of the arterial blood pressure on the blood flow through the cerebral cortex. J Neurol Neurosurg Psychiatry 29:398

Harper AM, Glass HI (1965) Effect of alterations in the arterial carbon dioxide tension on the blood flow through the cerebral cortex at normal and low arterial blood pressure. J Neurol Neurosurg Psychiatry 28:449

Hass WK (1981) Beyond cerebral blood flow, metabolism and ischemic thresholds. An examination of the role of calcium in the initiation of cerebral infarction. In: Meyer JS, Lechner H, Reivich M, Ott EO, Arabinar A (eds) Cerebral vascular disease, vol 3. Excerpta Medica, Amsterdam, p 3

Katzmann R, Pappius HM (1973) Brain electrolytes and fluid metabolism. Williams and Wilkins, Baltimore

Langfitt TW, Weinstein JD, Kassell NF (1965) Cerebral vasomotor paralysis produced by intracranial hypertension. Neurology 15:622

Lassen NA (1961) The luxury perfusion syndrome and its possible relation to acute metabolic acidosis localised within the brain. Lancet II:1113

Lassen NA, Palvölgyi R (1968) Cerebral steal during hypercapnia and inverse reaction during hypocapnia observed by the 133-xenon technique in man. Scand J Clin Lab Invest 30:113

Lund-Anderson M (1979) Transport of glucose from blood to brain. Physiol Rev 59:305

MacDowall DG (1966) Interrelationships between blood oxygen tensions and cerebral blood flow. In: Payne, Hill (eds) Oxygen measurements in blood flow and tissues. Churchill, London, p 205

Nayler WG, Horowitz JD (1983) Calcium antagonists: a new class of drugs. Pharmacol Ther 20:203

Nelson E, Rennels M (1970) Innervation of intracranial arteries. Brain 93:475

Schweitzer ES, Blaustein MP (1980) Calcium buffering in presynaptic nerve terminals: free calcium levels measured with arsenazo III. Biochim Biophys Acta 600:912

Siesjö BK (1981) Cell damage in the brain: a speculative hypothesis. J Cereb Blood Flow Metab 1:155

Siesjö BK (1984) Cerebral circulation and metabolism. J Neurosurg 60:883

Somjen GG (1979) Extracellular potassium in the mammalian central nervous system. Annu Rev Physiol 41:159

Strandgaard S (1976) Autoregulation of cerebral blood flow in hypertensive patients. Circulation 53:720

Winn HR, Rubio GR, Berne RM (1981) The role of adenosine in the regulation of cerebral blood flow. J Cereb Blood Flow Metab 1:239

3 Epidemiology and Classification of Strokes

3.1 Epidemiology

3.1.1 Definitions

Epidemiology concerns the occurrence and distribution of diseases in the population. By *prevalence* is meant the number of cases of the disease at a particular moment in a given group of persons, for example, in the entire population of a certain territory or in a clearly demarcated population group. *Incidence* refers to the number of *new* cases of the disease occurring in a population in a particular period of time. Figures on prevalence and incidence are meaningful only if the given disease is unequivocally defined. If the definition is too specific, many cases are not included (false-negative cases), whereas too broad a definition leads to many false-positive identifications (Table 3.1). Disease *mortality* indicates the number of patients who die of the disease in a particular period of time (e. g., within a year). Since only a proportion of patients with cerebrovascular diseases die in the short term (early mortality), mortality data represent only an approximate estimate of incidence.

The sources of epidemiologic data include mortality statistics obtained at the national level as well as long-term observations on population groups. The determination of frequency figures, incidence, and prevalence forms the basis for analytic epidemiology, which concerns the causal factors of a disease. Thus, if the incidence for a particular population group has been established, this figure constitutes the absolute risk for a comparable group expressed in terms of probability. Events or determinants which influence the absolute risk are termed risk factors; these are mathematic abstractions which make no assertions as to the cause or pathogenesis of a disease.

Earlier epidemiologic studies did not take into account of the different etiopathogenetic subgroups. The distinction was made between cerebral infarction, cerebral hemorrhage – subarachnoid hemorrhage being considered separately – and a residual

Table 3.1. Epidemiologic parameters

Prevalence	Total number of persons in a population diseased at a particular moment
Incidence	Number of new disease cases annually
Mortality	Number of deaths annually

Prevalence = approximately the incidence × mean disease duration.

group including vasculitis, sinus thrombosis, and other uncommon vascular disorders. Special attention was also given to transient ischemic attacks (TIAs), which were likewise regarded as ischemic cerebral disorders. Nevertheless, the epidemiologic literature has managed to get by, using this classification, up to the present time.

3.1.2 Descriptive Epidemiology

3.1.2.1 Prevalence

Prevalence figures for cerebrovascular diseases are scant. Only few surveys have been conducted, and the reported mortality statistics must be interpreted with caution. Cerebrovascular diseases are the third most common disease group after heart and liver diseases. This is the case in all major industrial countries. Regular calculations are made in the United States, the latest dating from July 1, 1976 ("prevalence day"). This count established that there were 1.7 million individuals with cerebrovascular diseases in a population of 215 millions, an overall prevalence of 794 patients per 100000 inhabitants (Baum 1981); this figure varies with age (Table 3.2). Data from the Federal Republic of Germany (FRG) correspond largely to these figures.

Table 3.2. Prevalence figures (per 100000) for cerebrovascular diseases. (Data: US National Stroke Survey 1976; from Baum 1981)

Under 45 years	71
45–64 years	1067
Over 65 years	5411
Total	794

3.1.2.2 Mortality and Incidence

In Western industrialized countries cerebrovascular diseases likewise occupy third place in mortality statistics after cardiovascular and malignant diseases. In general there are approximately 100 deaths per 100000 inhabitants annually, but one finds important geographic differences in the mortality figures (Table 3.3; Fratiglioni et al. 1983). These are partly attributable to artifacts (national and regional differences in the completion of death certificates, variations in diagnostic accuracy). Environmental factors probably also play an important role, even more important than genetic predisposition. Thus, a study of Japanese emigrants in Hawaii and California showed that mortality and incidence among them was much less than in Japanese living in Japan (Takeya et al. 1984). Obvious racial differences exist in mortality and incidence; these emerge most clearly in the American studies showing that incidence is attributable to demographic conditions in the given country. This also applies to the FRG, where the death rate for cerebrovascular diseases in 1970 – 194 per 100000 inhabitants – was approximately double that in 1938. It is relevant here that the

Table 3.3. Geographic differences in mortality (per 100000) from cerebrovascular diseases. (From Fratiglioni et al. 1983)

Sweden	63.9	England	97.9
Denmark	65.9	Italy	99.0
Canada	68.1	New Zealand	100.0
Netherlands	72.7	Belgium	100.0
USA (white pop.)	72.9	Ireland	109.4
Switzerland	74.7	Federal Republic of Germany	110.5
Iceland	79.7	Australia	110.9
France	85.0	Finland	121.4
Norway	91.9	Scotland	128.7

Mean value 90.7

population pyramid of the FRG has become relatively broader; the average age of the population has also increased.

Mortality statistics in most Western industrialized countries have been declining over the past 20 years. Between 1957 and 1976 this decline occurred not only in the percentage of deaths from cerebrovascular disease in comparison with all other causes of death but also in the mortality rates for the entire population (Whisnant 1984).

Improved diagnosis undoubtedly also contributes to this tendency. The possibilities afforded by CT are of great importance, especially in view of the fact that at least 5% of cases clinically diagnosed as cerebrovascular diseases can be demonstrated to be based etiologically on quite different diseases, such as neoplasms or subdural hematomas. Further, the distinction between hemorrhage and infarction is now considerably easier.

Figures from the United States show that mortality due to cardiovascular diseases has also declined since 1950, by 30%, and with a marked acceleration in the past 10 years (Fig. 3.1). Mortality rates from cerebrovascular diseases show a similar and even more marked tendency. Similar observations have been made in various European countries. The incidence of cerebrovascular disorders in Western industrialized countries is between 150 and 250 per 100000 inhabitants per year (Garraway et al. 1979; Matsumoto et al. 1973). About one-fourth of cases are recurrent events. Incidence rises with age. The ratio of men to women is approximately 1:1.3 (Kurtzke 1985; Table 3.4). Reliable incidence rates have been provided by population studies in Rochester, Minnesota, from which it emerges that the incidence since 1950 declined by 1% every 5 years, then gradually increased again somewhat, and has fallen by 5% annually since 1972 (Fig. 3.2; Whisnant 1984). Observations in Japan and Sweden over a shorter period are consistent with this. Currently, however, this decline in stroke incidence has come to an end. One reason for this may be the increased detection of minor strokes by improved diagnostic techniques (Broderick et al. 1989). Although it is generally assumed that improvements in medical care and more efficient management of the risk factors, especially hypertension (Klag et al. 1989), are the most important explanation for the decline in incidence, this cannot be the sole explanation. This tendency was already apparent before there was any question of adequate management of hypertension.

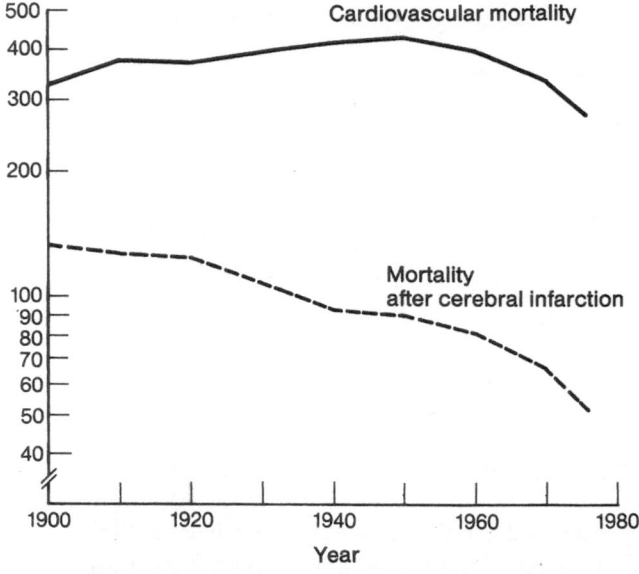

Fig. 3.1. Annual mortality (per 100000) for cardiovascular and cerebrovascular diseases. (From Whisnant 1983)

Table 3.4. Incidence figures for cerebrovascular diseases. (From Matsumoto et al. 1973; Garraway et al. 1979)

	1955–1969		1970–1974	
	Men	Women	Men	Women
Under 45 years	43	35	21	30
45–54 years	160	70	100	60
55–64 years	510	260	300	190
65–74 years	1080	600	720	520
Over 75 years	2500	1900	3350	2760
Total	214	136	153	119

When interpreting prevalence figures for the various types of cerebrovascular disease, it is of the greatest importance to consider the source of the data. In many countries, for example, data originating in hospitals show a greater number of younger and severely ill patients as well as patients presenting diagnostic problems. Data from pathologic studies involve the more fatal types of cerebrovascular diseases, especially cerebral hemorrhages. Calculations in the general population are without an adequate diagnostic basis; the most representative data appear to be those of the Framingham study, summarized in Fig. 3.3 (Wolf et al. 1983).

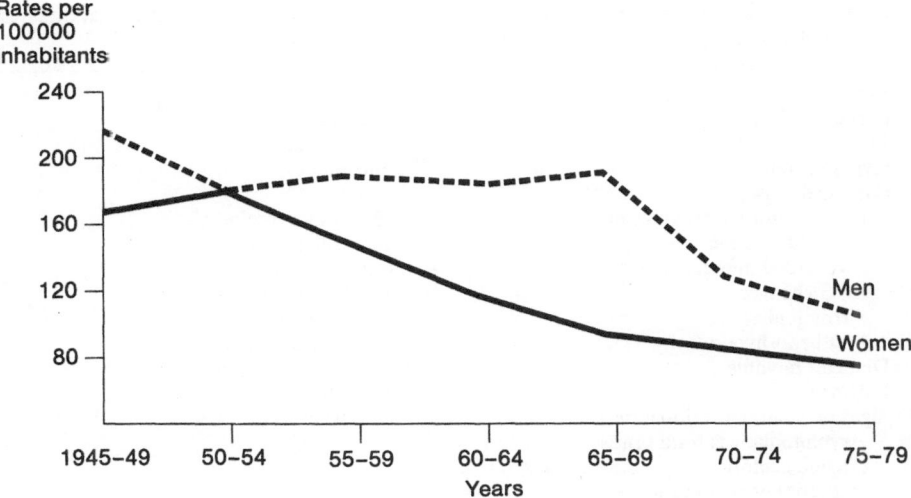

Fig. 3.2. Mean annual incidence of all first stroke episodes in Rochester, Minnesota, at 5-year intervals per 100000 inhabitants. (From Whisnant 1983)

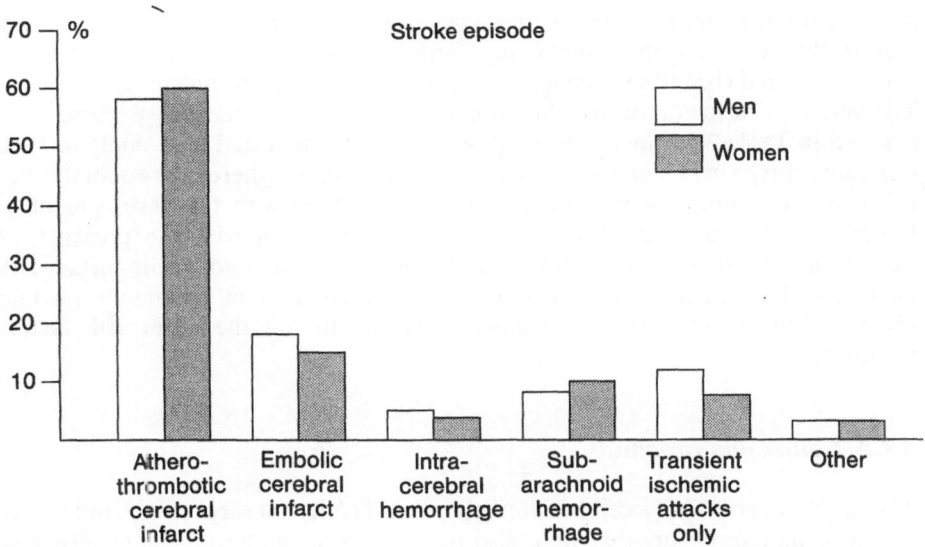

Fig. 3.3. Frequency of various cerebrovascular diseases by type. (From Wolf et al. 1983)

3.1.3 Risk Factors

Since an atherosclerosis of the blood vessel wall has been postulated for at least a proportion of both cerebral and myocardial infarctions, one might expect the same risk factors to apply to both these clinical diseases. However, for reasons that are not

Table 3.5. Risk factors postulated in the literature for the development of cerebrovascular diseases. (From Millikan et al. 1987)

Strong	Weak
– Earlier strokes	– Exogenous factors
– TIAs	– Life-style and habits
– Hypertension	Nicotine
– Cardiac diseases	Coffee
Inflammatory heart valve diseases	Hyperlipoproteinemia
Atrial fibrillation	Physical inactivity
Myocardial infarct	– Iatrogenic factors
ECG changes	Ovulation inhibitors
Arrhythmias	Cardiac surgery
Left heart hypertrophy	Kidney transplantation
– Diabetes mellitus	– Environmental factors
– Polycythemia	Climate
– Signs of general arteriosclerosis	Soft water
Asymptomatic carotid bruits	
Angina pectoris	
Intermittent claudication	

completely clear, this is not the case. Although the risk of developing a cerebrovascular disease is five times higher in patients with atheromatous changes in the coronary vessels, the risk factors important in myocardial infarction – blood cholesterol level, overweight, and cigarette smoking – are far less relevant to cerebrovascular disease. The various risk factors in the development of cerebrovascular diseases are summarized in Table 3.5. Not all of the possible risk factors listed here apply to each different subtype of ischemic cerebral disease. For example, there is no doubt that the existence of manifest hypertension is highly correlated with the development of lacunar cerebral infarcts. There is much less correlation with the presence of extracranial vascular lesions, while hypertension is certainly not an important risk factor for the incidence of embolic cerebral infarcts after inflammatory valvular disease. Similar circumstances can be construed for all the other risk factors mentioned here.

3.1.4 Course and Prognosis

The further course after a cerebral infarction or a TIA is, not surprisingly, influenced by the same risk factors that were also responsible for its development. Principal among these are advanced age, arterial hypertension, diseases of the heart and blood, diabetes mellitus, and dyslipoproteinemia. Apart from age, arterial hypertension is the most important prognostic factor leading to further cerebral ischemias and a higher mortality. A high correlation has been demonstrated between the level of blood pressure and the incidence of a cerebral infarct after previous TIAs or a poor prognosis of a completed infarct.

The prognosis is markedly worse when cerebral infarction and severe heart disease coincide (Fig. 3.4); this is rarely followed by survival. Cardiac failure or simply ECG changes indicative of left heart failure or coronary heart disease markedly reduce the

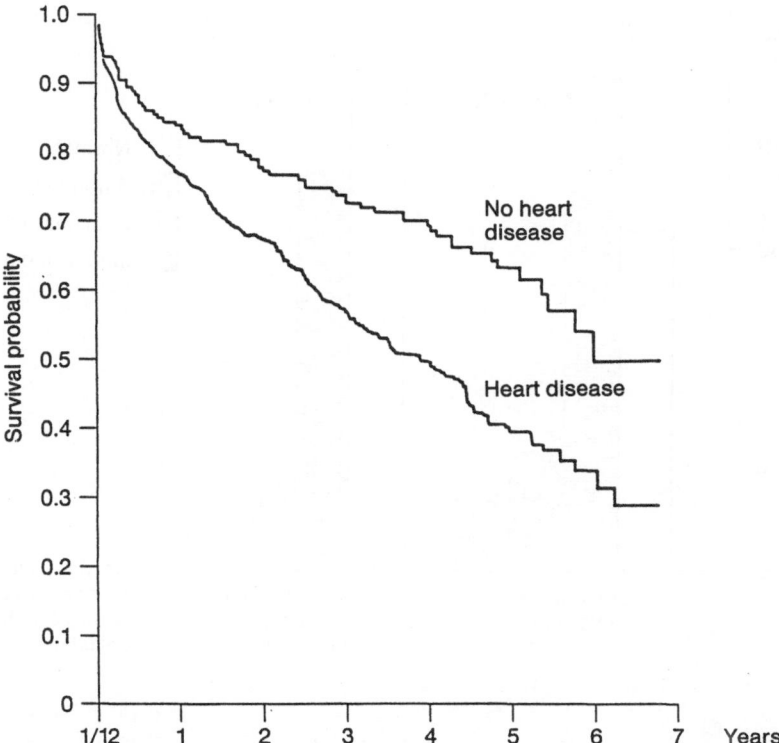

Fig. 3.4. Influence of cardiac diseases on survival rates after cerebral infarction. (From Chambers et al. 1987)

chances of survival. The more favorable prognosis of TIAs in the vertebrobasilar circulation compared with the carotid territory is probably based on the better collateralization.

After cerebral infarction, the prognosis for hemispheric lesions is on average somewhat more unfavorable as regards both survival probability and survival quality (Fig. 3.5).

Early mortality from thrombotic cerebral infarction (death in the first 4 weeks) is between 10% and 25% in hospitalized patients. In the 1st week primarily cerebral causes predominate (massive space occupation with transtentorial herniation), whereas in the 2nd–4th weeks cardiovascular complications (heart failure, pulmonary embolism, pneumonia) are most often the cause of death. Early mortality after cerebral embolism is higher and is estimated as high as 25%–30%.

Fatal outcome after the acute phase is due mainly to intercurrent infections or myocardial infarcts. As a rule there is a cumulative mortality of 40%–50% 5 years after a cerebral infarction, the death rate being highest within the first months after the infarction if the acute phase has been overcome, and the early mortality is disregarded. The risk subsequently stabilizes up to the end of the 1st year. After cerebral embolism about one-half of the patients die within 6 months.

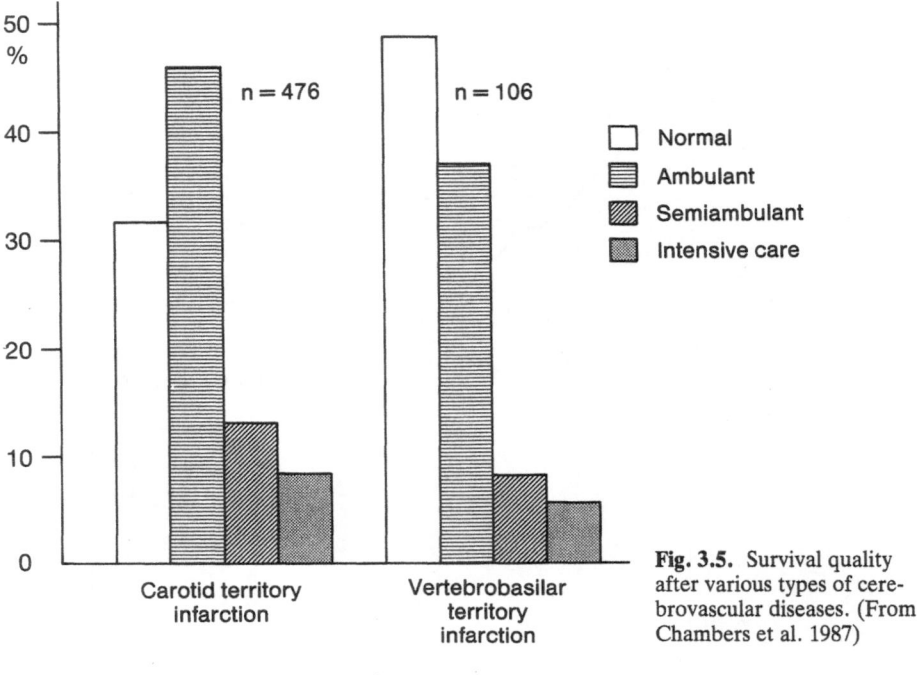

Fig. 3.5. Survival quality after various types of cerebrovascular diseases. (From Chambers et al. 1987)

A very striking and so far unexplained finding of some previous surveys on the long-term prognosis of cerebral infarcts is a marked sex difference. At least after survival of the acute phase, women seem to have a better prognosis than men and a smaller risk of death. The risk of suffering a further cerebral infarction, which is between 15% and 35% within the first 5 years, is also less in women.

Ensuring a thoroughly independent life is almost as important as the question of survival itself. Some two-thirds to three-fourths of surviving patients are able to walk again without support. Approximately this number of patients can also look after themselves completely (washing, dressing, etc.). However, only 25%–50% are able to resume work. The most intensive and earliest possible rehabilitation of both motor and neuropsychological performance seems capable of improving the prognosis.

The spontaneous course of cerebral infarcts and the prognosis in affected patients depends obviously upon age. Because biologic age is more important than calendar age, it is not possible to distinguish specific age cohorts in this respect; however, the prognosis is generally worse in patients aged over 65 years. Most younger patients can once again care for themselves in the further course after a cerebral infarction, whereas this is possible in only a small proportion of older patients (Fig. 3.6). The size of the infarct is of course also relevant prognostically. The larger the ischemic lesion and the more severe the initial neurologic deficit, the worse and more unfavorable is the further prognosis as a rule. Of course, it should be noted that a large cortical infarct and a small subcortical lacunar infarct may initially resemble each other clinically and yet differ fundamentally in prognosis. Lacunar cerebral infarcts also exhibit a generally better course than territorial infarctions due to thromboembolism,

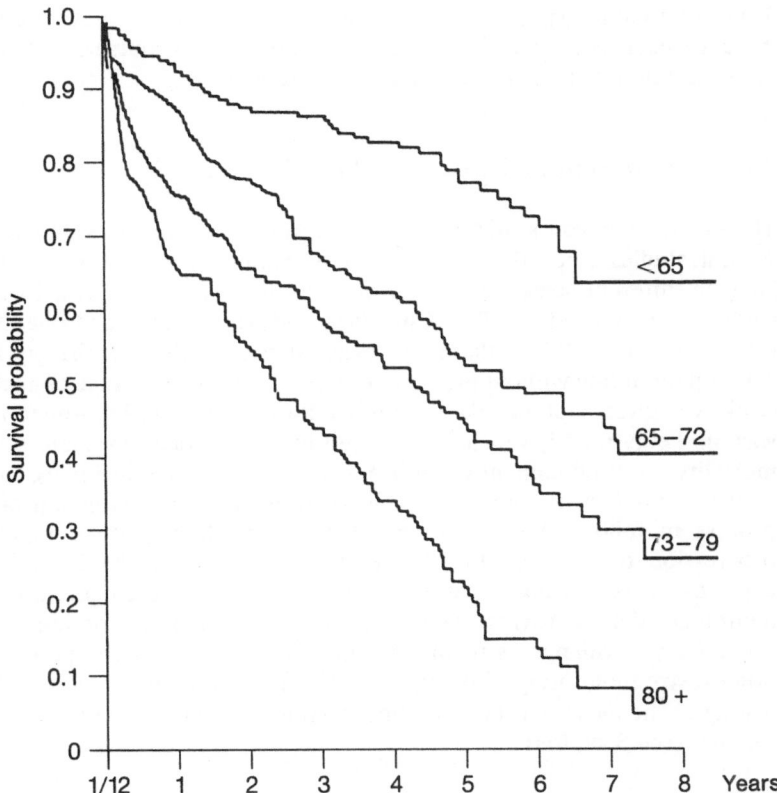

Fig. 3.6. Influence of age on survival rate after cerebral infarction. (From Chambers et al. 1987)

which necessarily follows from the anatomy with small subcortically located defects. Again, infarct size and site are related to the development of disturbances of consciousness. The various prognostic criteria must therefore always be considered in combination. In addition to disturbances of consciousness associated with gaze palsy, the presence of aphasia and visual field defects tend to be linked with an unfavorable course. With right-hemispheric cerebral infarcts, neglect of the left half of the body and anosognosia usually indicate a greater tendency to regression than hemianopic visual field disorders and hemipareses. With left-hemispheric infarcts or lesions of the speech-dominant hemisphere, Broca's and conduction aphasias have a better prognosis than Wernicke's aphasia; with severe global aphasia the further course is rather unfavorable.

The findings of the few studies published so far on the spontaneous course and prognosis of patients with TIA vary widely. The earlier findings by the Mayo Clinic of a 15-fold increase in infarct morbidity in the first 4 weeks after a TIA have not as yet been confirmed, whereas the majority of studies report a three- to fivefold infarct rate up to the end of a 2-year follow-up period with restoration of the initial risk. However, in connection with these figures it should be noted that all prospective studies have dealt with treatment populations using specific selection and study criteria. Up to now there has been no prospective series on the spontaneous course of patients with TIAs in the carotid territory with ipsilateral carotid stenosis.

3.1.4.1 Asymptomatic Extracranial Vascular Processes

The spontaneous course of asymptomatic extracranial processes has been observed in several studies since the introduction of noninvasive methods of investigation. Despite different selection criteria of controlled patients in two North American studies (Roederer et al. 1984; Chambers and Norris 1986) and one German study (Hennerici et al. 1987), there was concordance on the surprisingly low risk of a cerebral infarction without previous TIA (Fig. 3.7). The average annual incidence of stroke was given as about 1%. In contrast, the overall mortality – up to 7% annually – was markedly raised, which is explained by a coincident coronary sclerosis with a mortality of predominantly cardiac origin. While the incidence of permanent neurologic defects is therefore small, there is marked progression of the vascular process in follow-up observations. This is correlated with a rapid or uniform progression of the vasculopathy, with an increase in the individual risk of a cerebrovascular episode. However, as the majority of these patients remain without neurologic deficit, asymptomatic carotid lesions should not initially be treated operatively. Evidence as to the significance of a TIA to the patient himself and noninvasive monitoring of the vascular lesions permit an individual adaptation and testing of the most favorable treatment strategy in the event of deterioration in the findings (see Sect. 6.3).

3.2 Definitions and Classification of Strokes

3.2.1 Ischemia or Hemorrhage?

According to the epidemiologic definition of the World Health Organization, a stroke may result from a localized cerebral ischemia, an intracerebral hemorrhage, a subarachnoid hemorrhage, or a disturbance of cerebral venous outflow (sinus thrombosis). Each of these can lead to acute disorders of neurologic function which evoke the clinical picture of a stroke. Synonyms used for this include apoplexy or apoplectic attack; however, these terms should no longer be used as they do not determine the etiology that underlies the clinical syndrome. Determining this is not always possible with sufficient accuracy using clinical methods, as the differentiation between intracerebral hemorrhage and an ischemic episode and, in individual cases, the recognition of an encephalitis, a sinus thrombosis, a subarachnoid hemorrhage, or a hemorrhage into a tumor may be difficult.

Figure 3.8 shows that allocation to one of the etiologic groups of strokes is possible with the aid of imaging techniques. On the upper left side of the figure an ischemic infarct of a few days' duration in the territory of the middle cerebral artery is shown; next to this is the CT scan of a medium-sized intracerebral (basal ganglia) hemorrhage a few days old, and below is the CT scan in a patient with subarachnoid bleeding from

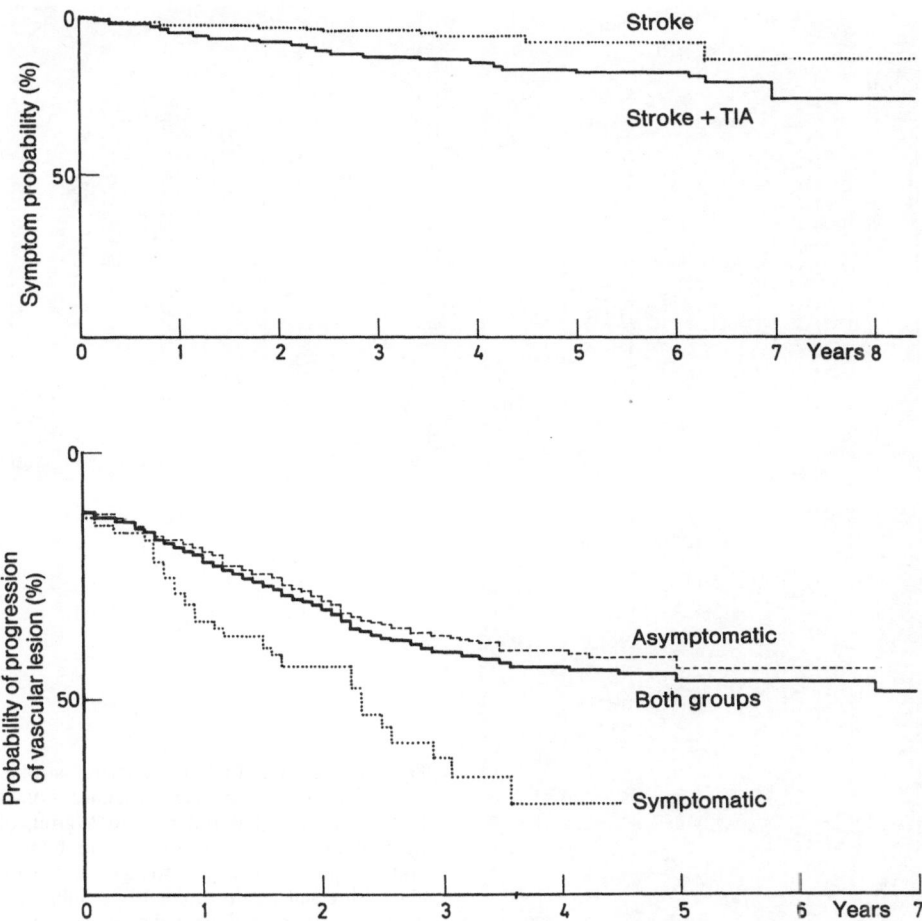

Fig. 3.7. Mortality and morbidity (TIA and cerebral infarction) in a series of 433 prospectively controlled, neurologically asymptomatic patients with extracranial vascular lesions. Annual mortality 6.8%, annual infarct rate (without previous TIA) 1.4%, combined TIA and infarct rate 2.9%

an aneurysm. Such patients may exhibit similar neurologic symptoms, with deteriorating hemiparesis and possibly also minor disturbance of consciousness.

The nature of the clinical syndrome and the severity of the stroke are determined by the extent of the ischemic zone (or hemorrhage) including its marginal zone and the site of the focus. In addition to the most common stroke pattern of a unilateral paresis affecting mainly the face and arm, there exists a range of other syndromes which are discussed in detail below.

The term stroke is used in the following chapters to describe a clinical state whose cause (ischemia, hemorrhage) is as yet unknown. If the etiology is that of ischemia, the functional disturbance is termed an ischemic *insult*. This ischemic insult may be based on a range of different causes: it may be produced by embolism, by local thrombosis, or hemodynamically. Independently of the pathogenesis, many focal

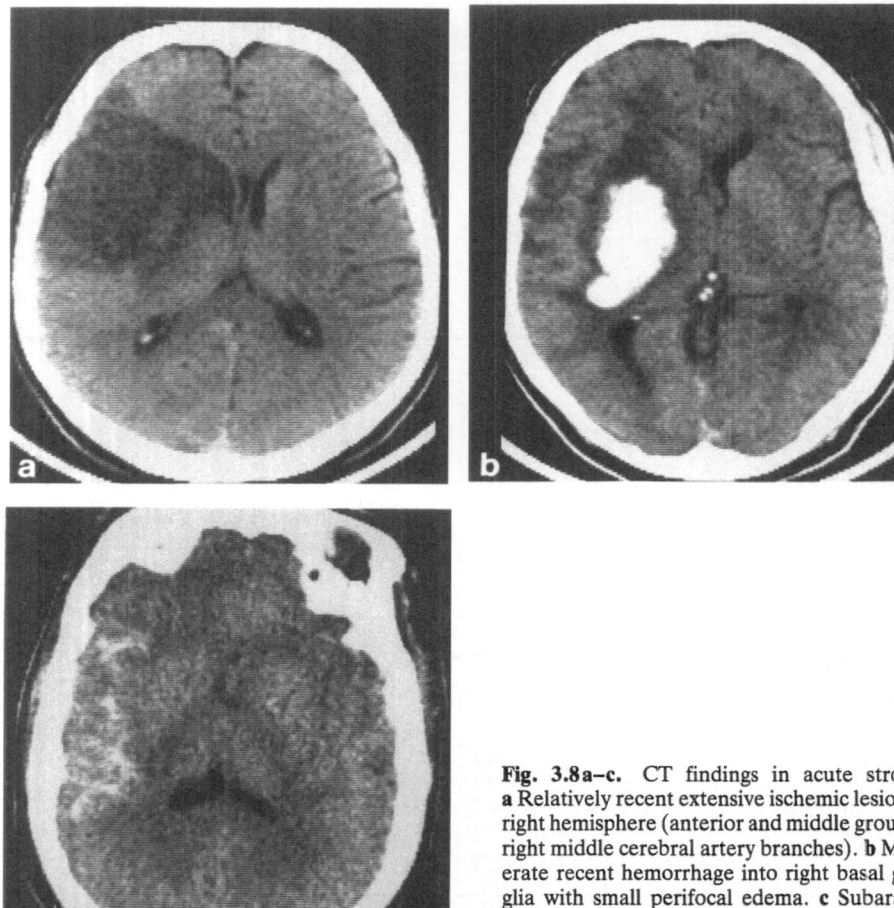

Fig. 3.8a–c. CT findings in acute stroke. **a** Relatively recent extensive ischemic lesion of right hemisphere (anterior and middle group of right middle cerebral artery branches). **b** Moderate recent hemorrhage into right basal ganglia with small perifocal edema. **c** Subarachnoid hemorrhage with special emphasis on the right insular cistern. "Stroke" was present in each case

ischemias may remain without morphologically demonstrable lesions. The clinical findings may then undergo rapid regression. If the ischemia persists, structural changes in the brain may result. This is described as an ischemic *infarct.* An ischemic insult therefore refers to the functional disturbance and an infarct to the structural substrate, as also demonstrated by imaging techniques. Figure 3.9 summarizes this nomenclature.

The ischemic cerebral infarct is primarily "white," i.e., bloodless. No further movement of blood takes place in its vessels, but at the periphery of the infarct congested hyperemic vessels are not uncommon (see Sect. 2.4.1). Secondarily, small petechial extravasations of blood may occur at the marginal zone of the infarct, the so-called hemorrhagic transformation of the infarct. Extensive secondary parenchymatous hemorrhages are rare in the natural course of ischemia; when they do appear, it is usually after cardiac emboli.

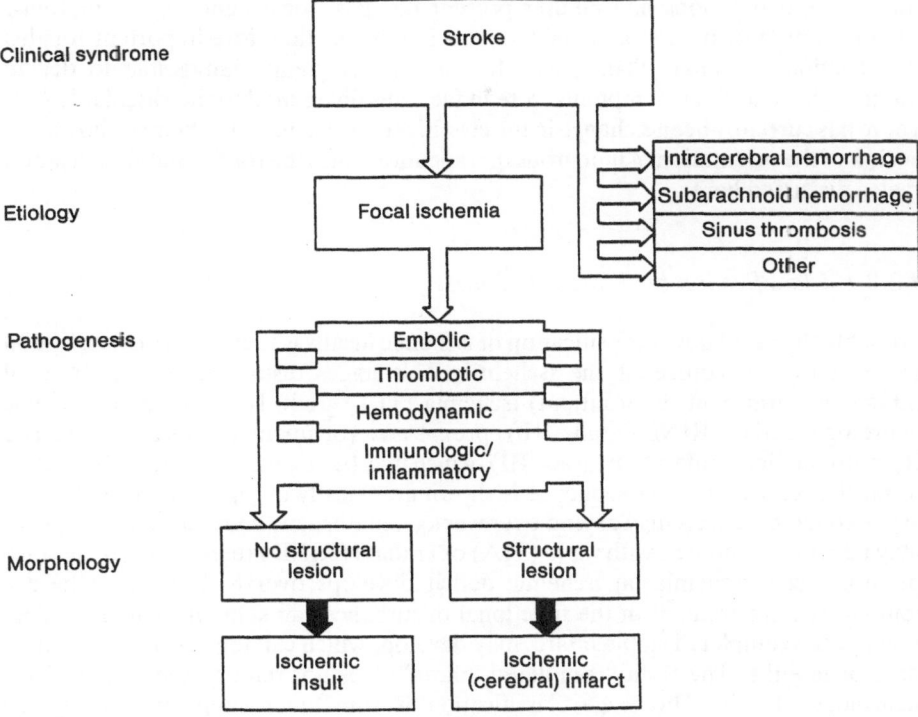

Fig. 3.9. Clinical syndrome, etiology, pathogenesis, and morphology

Global hypoxias (e. g., after CO poisoning or strangulation), loss of cerebral function after prolonged hypoglycemia, or global oligemic-hypotensive cerebral damage (after resuscitation, in protracted shock) lead to extensive barrier disturbances and secondary hemorrhagic infarcts, whose preferred sites are the subcortical medullary layer and the basal ganglia.

3.2.2 Classification of Ischemia
(see Caplan 1983; Hachinski and Norris 1985; Mohr and Barnett 1986)

The traditional principles for classifying ischemias are based on the temporal course of the stroke, the vascular territories affected, and the extent of the neurologic deficit (review by Courbier 1985). As one can see in the definitions listed in Fig. 3.9, an optimal classification would take into consideration the basic pathophysiologic mechanisms (Caplan 1983; Poeck 1986; Ringelstein et al. 1985). In the past this was hardly possible for lack of adequate diagnosis during life, and because of the conventional emphasis on hemodynamic factors it was not even intended. It is interesting in this context that earlier, surgically oriented systems of classification were based primarily on the state of the extracerebral vessels; these recognized an asymptomatic stage of cerebrovascular insufficiency in which a patient with extracranial vascular lesions had neither present nor past focal neurologic symptoms. Demonstration of the extracranial vascular lesion was therefore important for this classification (Vollmar 1980, 1985). It was also frequently impossible to decide whether the neurologic symptoms were in fact causally related to the vascular lesion. There has currently been a change in the classification of cerebral ischemias; however, in view of the orientation of numerous therapeutic studies the traditional classification is also discussed here.

3.2.2.1 Classification by Temporal Course

Probably the best known classification of ischemic insults is that based on description of the temporal course of the ischemia. The stages distinguished are those of threatened (transient, intermittent) ischemia (TIA; grade Ia), reversible ischemic neurologic deficit (RIND; grade IIb), progressive (or fluctuating) ischemia (grade II), and completed infarction (grade III), which may be associated with a stable deficit or partial regression. This sequence is shown graphically in Fig. 3.10. The phase of asymptomatic stenosis may extend over weeks, months, and sometimes years. There may be repeated attacks with rapid (TIA) or gradual (RIND) regression. In the stage of progressive ischemia an ischemic deficit develops over 6–48 h; even here a temporary improvement in the functional disturbance can sometimes be recorded. Finally, the completed stable infarct may develop, which can regress partially within days or months. The term "completed infarct" does not refer to the extent of the neurologic deficit. The stage classification is sometimes supplemented by the previously mentioned grade 0 of asymptomatic stenosis or embolism source.

Transient Ischemic Attacks

TIAs are localized disturbances of neurologic function which are completely reversible within 24 h. These last only a short time, at least 30 s and usually less than 1 h. Only 10% of attacks last longer than 6 h and one-half last less than 30 min (Levy 1988). The correct diagnostic allocation of the TIA to a vascular territory is therefore often hindered as the investigator no longer has objective findings as a basis but must depend on the patient's subjective account. Thus, it is often difficult retrospectively to distinguish an aphasic disorder from a dysarthria or hemianopsia from an amaurosis fugax. However, with the widespread application of imaging techniques to TIA patients it is possible to find corresponding lesions (20% with CT: Waxman and Toole 1983; Bogousslavski and Regli 1984; Awad et al. 1986; Salgado et al. 1986; Duke et al. 1986; and even more with MRI). Significant lesions can be demonstrated in patients after TIA by positron emission tomography (PET; Powers and Raichle 1985). The concept of TIA tells us nothing about the underlying pathogenesis. We now know that patients with small thalamic hemorrhages can present clinically with a TIA. A TIA can conceal small emboli, fluctuating hemodynamic disturbances, and lacunar infarcts. However, the majority of neurologists, specialists in internal diseases, and especially vascular surgeons associate the occurrence of TIAs with operatively accessible stenoses of arteries supplying the brain. TIAs and ischemic infarcts are variables in the temporal continuum of the different cerebral ischemias: they are

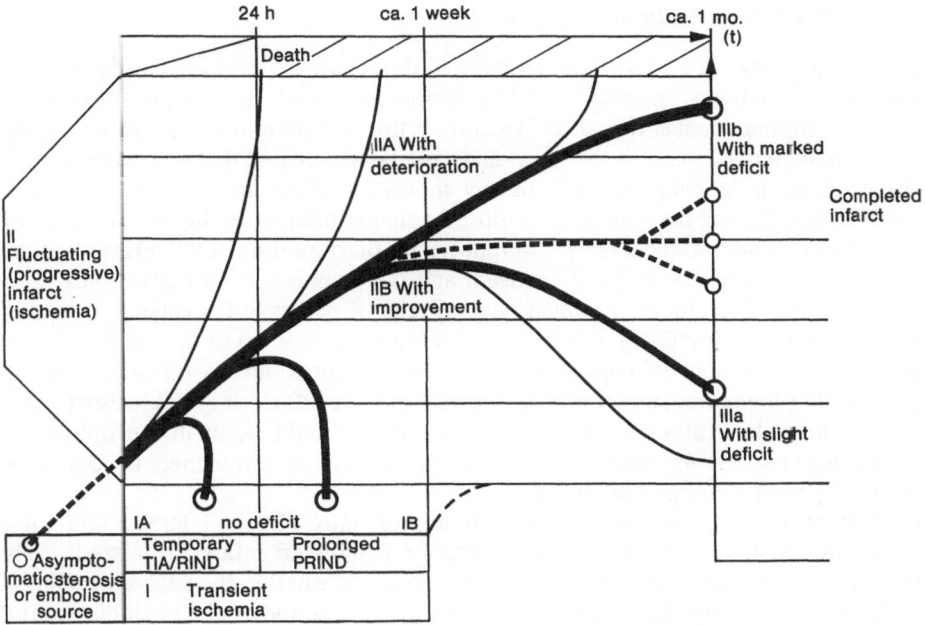

Fig. 3.10. Classification of ischemias by temporal course, reversibility, and resultant deficit. (From Courbier 1985)

symptoms and not disease states. It is not the TIA but its cause that must be established and treated. Also, as mentioned above, determining the temporal context is very arbitrary; by definition, the neurologic deficits should be capable of regression up to 24 h, but the majority regress in a much shorter time. It is fairly certain that a considerable ischemic deficit still continuing after some 4–6 h will no longer be reversible in the following 18–20 h. With slight limitations, this permits the early clinical diagnosis of a large infarct (Caplan 1988; Levy 1988).

If we nevertheless accept the definition of TIAs, another and not inconsiderable problem arises: Are "drop attacks" – some of these being forms of reflex syncope, atypical episodes of vertigo, or even common fainting – not also TIAs in the posterior circulation? These are also based on brief focal ischemic functional disturbances of the brainstem; they are completely reversible and may recur. Is the so-called intermittent basilar insufficiency (a "nondiagnosis" which should be rejected) therefore an accumulation of such TIAs?

Strictly speaking, in terms of the definition, these questions must be answered in the affirmative. At the same time, however, it must be conceded that these TIAs of the posterior circulation do not have the same warning function as TIAs of the anterior circulation and are much less frequently followed by manifest infarcts elsewhere (see Sect. 3.1.4). This view remains to be proven, however, and is based only on impressions. For various reasons, most traditional classifications do not regard these intermittent types of symptoms of the posterior circulation as TIAs; this is the approach followed here. Nevertheless, the problem should at least be addressed here as it does deserve attention.

Reversible Ischemic Neurologic Deficit

By definition, RIND is also completely reversible. However, it may persist for several days, and sometimes, as with the TIAs, lesions detectable by CT are found later despite complete clinical recovery. Because of this one sometimes speaks of a stage that is characterized mainly by extracranial vascular lesions and that is "symptomatic" only to imaging techniques, while having shown complete clinical regression. It is possible that this will become an even more frequent finding with the increased use of MRI after ischemic attacks. The period chosen for the definition of RIND is arbitrary. Here, only the concept of RIND is used, and the emphasis is on regression within about 3 days. Sometimes, however, one speaks of prolonged reversible ischemic neurologic deficit (PRIND), in which regression is possible up to the 7th day.

In contrast to a widely held opinion, a rapid clinical improvement with an only mildly persistent or fluctuating functional disturbance after an infarct does not justify a wait-and-see attitude. Rather, such transient ischemias should result in a prophylactic search for a treatable cause. Otherwise, the patient is threatened by death or incapacity after a completed infarct.

It must also be considered that the subdivision into TIA and RIND and their allocation to the categories of progressive or completed infarct is possible only retrospectively. At an early stage it cannot be assessed whether the neurologic deficit will prove to be completely reversible within a defined period or already indicates the final deficit of a later completed infarct. This naturally has important consequences for the introduction of early treatment: should one wait to see whether the symptoms undergo spontaneous regression or engage in early and aggressive treatment? Patients whose course would have progressed spontaneously with good prognosis may sometimes be given a treatment that unnecessarily entails risks.

Progressive Insult

The progressive insult constitutes a special diagnostic and therapeutic problem. Over a period of hours (even over days in the posterior circulation) the neurologic deficits increase progressively in severity and extent. Both clinical course with variable symptoms, possibly even including remission, and a course with continuously progressive deterioration of the neurologic deficit are possible. If an acute hemispheric ischemia coincides with an old contralateral infarct, topographic assignment of the neurologic symptoms can be extraordinarily difficult, both clinically and by imaging techniques (Fig. 3.11). A tissue lesion must not be present (hence an insult, not an infarct). Both forms may benefit from aggressive therapeutic procedures. Therefore, in both cases a rapid Doppler ultrasound and possibly also angiography should be performed to elucidate the pathogenesis of the insult. Taking the progressive insult as an example, it must again be pointed out that the various etiologic causes of ischemia (and of strokes as a whole) may be manifested as in this clinical picture. Hence a progressive insult is not necessarily to be equated with occlusion of a large vessel; it may equally well be the result of a lacune, a sinus thrombosis, or a vasospasm.

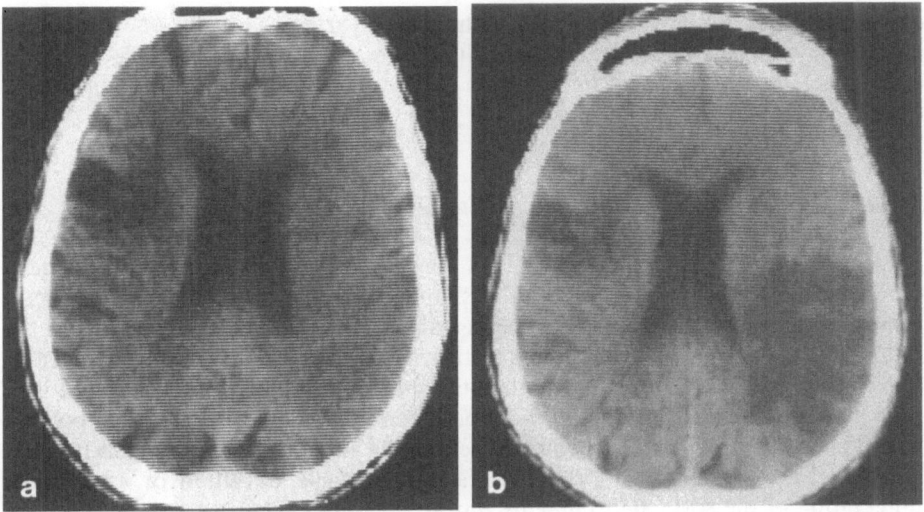

Fig. 3.11. a Left-hemispheric deficit in a patient with a preexisting right cerebral territorial infarct in the anterior middle cerebral artery territory. **b** Two days later the extensive left cerebral infarct in the middle and posterior branches of the MCA was detected

Completed Infarct

The characteristics of the completed infarct are neurologic deficits which have stabilized, and which persist for longer than 2–3 weeks. The concept of a completed infarct presupposes an ischemic tissue necrosis, which however may be morphologically incomplete and have a selective neuronal effect in rare cases. Then, and only then, CT demonstration may not be forthcoming. A completed infarct in the carotid territory becomes evident on CT after 12–24 h. In the vertebrobasilar territory an infarct may be clinically complete only after 72 h, and the phase of progressive insult may last even longer.

The term completed infarct does not imply any particular extent of the neurologic deficits. If only minor neurologic disturbances are found, it is referred to as a completed infarct with minor or moderate deficit. Thus, this may be expressed as a minor brachiofacial hemiparesis, a persistent intention tremor, or minor neuropsychological disturbances. A completed infarct with extensive functional disturbances (marked deficit) is evidenced, for example, by a severe aphasia, a persistent hemianopsia, and a high-grade hemiparesis developing to hemiplegia. Then the time is often past for prophylactic measures, and treatment is usually limited to conservative and rehabilitation procedures. However, if a patient with slight or moderate functional disturbance is threatened by further deficits in the same or an adjacent vascular territory due to a fresh infarction, prophylactic treatment is still reasonable after a completed infarct with stable deficit. Not uncommonly, completed infarcts with extensive functional disturbance have been preceded by TIAs, reversible insults, or completed infarcts with minor deficits in the same vascular territory. Sometimes the completed infarct with severe deficits occurs at the end of the progressive insult. Completed infarcts in different cerebral vascular territories lead one to suspect an embolizing disease or an inflammation in the cerebral arteries. Finally, one should not ignore the fact that many ischemic insults progress rapidly and uncontrollably to death, such as malignant infarction of the middle cerebral artery territory or basilar thrombosis.

3.2.2.2 Classification by Vascular Territories

Allocation of infarcts to the territories of the great vessels also forms part of many classifications. This seems theoretically simple, but may create some problems if brainstem lesions do not lead to the classical crossed syndromes familiar from the literature (cranial nerve involvement with contralateral paresis or sensory disturbance, see p. 71). Many monosymptomatic, fluctuating strokes with pure motor or pure sensory pareses can originate from both hemispheric and medullary or pontine lesions. In the early phase of hemispheric infarcts a (contralateral) paresis in areas supplied by the cranial motor nerves (such as tongue deviation or asymmetric innervation of the soft palate) may be repeatedly found. This is not necessarily the result of a paresis, in view of the bilaterally innervated cranial nerve nuclei but may be due to a central difference in tonus. Even the corneal reflex may be weakened unilaterally. Dysarthria occurs in both hemispheric (left as well as right) and brainstem lesions.

Another problem lies in correlating functional disturbances in the distribution of the posterior cerebral artery, which actually supplies supratentorial parts of the brain although in most cases it arises from the vertebrobasilar system. A transient hemianopsia or a quadrantanopsia is therefore clinically a hemispheric symptom, although in terms of vascular territory it signals the posterior circulation. Hence the distinction between an amaurosis fugax and a hemianopsia as carotid and vertebrobasilar warning signs, respectively, is very important, even if the patient sometimes cannot give a very clear history. This is complicated when, in many patients, the posterior cerebral artery is supplied mainly or in great part from the internal carotid via a large posterior communicating artery.

3.2.2.3 Further Approaches to Classification

Some classifications take into account the further pathogenesis of the ischemic insult, including data from regional blood flow measurements, cerebral blood volume measurements, operative indications, and data obtained from PET (review by Courbier 1985). In terms of metabolic parameters, three stages of ischemic lesions can be distinguished (see p. 26). In the first stage the perfusion pressure is impaired: ischemic symptoms occur through impairment of functional metabolism while structural metabolism is preserved. This state is reversible. In the stage of dysmetabolism, in addition to the change in regional perfusion and cerebral blood volume, the oxygen reserve capacity is diminished and structural metabolism endangered. The third phase is infarction, and here structural metabolism is deranged. Oxygen utilization, oxygen extraction, and cerebral blood volume are pathologically altered.

The three-stage classification set out in Fig. 3.10, whose main groups are transient, fluctuating, and completed ischemic insults, is based on a proposal presented at a symposium held in Marseilles in 1984 (Courbier 1985). These main groups are subject to descriptive modifications: the transient symptoms of an insult may, for instance, be short or prolonged, and the fluctuating insult may be associated with intermittent improvement or continuous deterioration. Finally, the completed infarct may show minor or severe deficits and can be seen in terms of a percentage scale. A comprehensive description of this stage can be obtained by incorporating the vascular territory affected and the findings of the angiographic and imaging studies. A patient with a high-grade stenosis of the internal carotid and transient ischemic attacks would be described as: "grade I a, left carotid, 95% stenosis, symptomatic, normal CT." A patient with completed stroke and increasing deficit based on a carotid occlusion would be classed as: "grade III b, left carotid occlusion, extensive territorial infarct of the middle and posterior middle cerebral branches, pronounced deficit." Unfortunately, this very differentiated grading is only poorly applicable to the microangiopathies, and in general the pathogenetic aspect of strokes is not sufficiently represented in this otherwise very clear classification.

3.2.3 A Suggested Pathogenetic Classification of Infarcts Based on CT and Angiographic Findings

The excellent collateralization of the arterial supply to the brain is discussed in Chap. 1. In addition to the basal collateral formation at the circle of Willis and the anastomoses between the extra- and intracranial vessels, there also exist extensive meningeal anastomoses between the large cerebral vessels. Weak points in this system are the long penetrating medullary arteries and the arteries to the basal ganglia, which correspond to functional end-arteries and are poorly collateralized. The pathologic, anatomic, angiologic, and CT morphologic findings often provide evidence as to the mechanism of development of an ischemic infarct (Ringelstein et al. 1985; Rodda and Path 1986; Zeumer and Hacke 1988). In particular, the morphologic description of an infarct zone based on the intravital CT and MRI findings, taken together with the results of ultrasound and angiographic studies, makes it possible to postulate the various pathogeneses of infarcts with a high degree of probability. The grade and extent of the individual infarct regions are thereby defined not only in terms of the site of the lesion or the degree of narrowing of a supply vessel but also by the grade and quality of the anastomoses (Zülch 1985; Hacke et al. 1987). The CT findings of the various infarct patterns are discussed in more detail in Sect. 5.3.1. Figure 1.11 on the arterial anatomy of the brain presents examples of various infarct patterns in which the essential information is whether the lesions are to be attributed predominantly to disease of the noncollateralized, penetrating, intracerebral small vessels (microangiopathies) or of the large cerebral arteries (macroangiopathies). We discuss in Chap. 1 the distinction between those infarcts situated in the distribution zone of a short or long circumferential artery (territorial infarcts) and those in the borderzone between two anastomosing vascular territories (extraterritorial infarcts). In these often hemodynamically caused infarcts, it is possible to distinguish low-flow infarcts (in the distal distribution zone of the noncollateralized middle cerebral branches) and borderzone infarcts between the territories of two or three large vessels. Examples of such patterns are presented in Sect. 5.3.1. Territorial infarcts arise from embolic or local thrombotic occlusion of large superficial cerebral arteries and are often wedge shaped and limited to the supply zone of an affected artery. Multiple territorial infarcts, however, are suggestive of cardiac emboli but also of vasculitis, especially when they involve the posterior and anterior territories in younger patients. Here, too, the morphologic findings offer a clue to the possible pathogenesis.

A special place is occupied here by occlusion of the lenticulostriate arteries in an obstruction of the proximal middle cerebral artery; this certainly corresponds to an infarct in the region of the long penetrating end-branches, but on the other hand, it to some extent affects a territory through the common involvement of a whole bundle of such penetrating arteries, i.e., that of the lenticulostriate arteries.

Microangiopathies arise when the small thin arteries penetrating deeply into the brain tissue undergo isolated or multiple disseminated thromboses. The corresponding infarct pattern is that of lacunes, which are an expression of a systemic disease of the small cerebral vessels with the prominent risk factor of hypertension. Subcortical arteriosclerotic encephalopathy probably constitutes a special form of this systemic disease of the small vessels in which lacunar infarcts are added to the diffuse hypodensity of the medullary layer. These can be demonstrated by CT and even better by MRI. However, it is still problematic here whether a whole range of these zones of abnormal signal intensity in the medullary layer found at MRI in older patients really correspond to a normal aging process in the brain, or whether they are evidence of a cerebrovascular disease (see p. 95; Awad et al. 1986).

If these indications are grouped with the description of the temporal course of the immediate or evolving crisis, the vascular area affected, and the extent of the neurologic deficits, we arrive at a classification which also considers the pathogenesis. For example, one patient might be spoken of as having fluctuating brainstem symptoms with rapid regression, normal Doppler ultrasound, and multiple supratentorial lacunar lesions, while another might have an extensive territorial infarct of the middle group of middle cerebral branches on the right side with dysarthria and severe sensorimotor hemiparesis without any tendency to regression, and with normal Doppler ultrasound findings and absolute arrhythmia. It is obvious that these two patients, with such different descriptions, require different therapeutic approaches.

References

Awad IA, Johnson PC, Spetzler RF, Hodak JA (1986) Incidental subcortical lesions identified on magnetic resonance imaging in the elderly. II. Postmortem pathological correlations. Stroke 17:1090

Baum HM (1981) The national survey of stroke. Stroke 12:59

Bogousslavsky J, Regli F (1984) Cerebral infarction with transient signs (CITS): do TIAs correspond to small deep infarcts in internal carotid artery occlusion? Stroke 15:536

Broderick JP, Phillips SJ, Whisnant JP, O'Fallon M, Bergstrahl EJ (1989) Incidence rates of stroke in the eighties: the end of the decline in stroke? Stroke 20:577

Caplan LR (1983) Are terms such as completed stroke or RIND of continued usefulness? Stroke 14:431

Caplan LR (1988) TIAs: we need to return to the question, "what is wrong with Mr. Jones?" Neurology 38:791

Chambers BR, Norris JW (1986) Outcome in patients with asymptomatic neck bruits. N Engl J Med 315:860

Chambers BR, Norris JW, Shurwell BL, Hachinski V (1987) Prognosis of acute stroke. Neurology 37:221

Courbier R (1985) Basis for a classification of cerebral arterial diseases. Excerpta Medica, Amsterdam, p 308

Duke RS, Bloch RF, Turpie AG (1986) Intravenous heparin for the prevention of stroke progression in acute partial stable stroke: a randomized controlled trial. Ann Intern Med 105:825

Fratiglioni L, Mattey EW, Schoenberg AG, Schoenberg BS (1983) Mortality from cerebrovascular disease. International comparisons and temporal trends. Neuroepidemiology 2:101

Garraway WM, Whisnant JP, Furlan AJ (1979) The declining incidence of stroke. N Engl J Med 300:449

Gautier JC (1985) Stroke in progression. Stroke 16:729

Hachinski V, Norris JW (1985) The acute stroke. Davis, Philadelphia

Hacke W, del Zoppo GJ, Harker LA (1987) Thrombosis and cerebro-vascular disease. In: Poeck K, Ringelstein EB, Hacke W (eds) Recent advances in diagnosis and management of stroke. Springer, Berlin Heidelberg New York, p 59

Hennerici M, Rautenberg W, Mohr S (1982) Stroke risk from symptomless extracranial arterial disease. Lancet II:1180

Hennerici M, Hülsbömer HB, Hefter H, Lammerts D, Rautenberg W (1987) Natural history of asymptomatic extracranial artery disease – results of a long-term prospective study. Brain 110:777

Klag MJ, Kelton PK, Seidler AJ (1989) Decline in US stroke mortality. Demographic trends and antihypertensive treatment. Stroke 20:14

Kurtzke JF (1985) Epidemiology of cerebrovascular disease. In: McDowell FH, Caplan LR (eds) Cerebrovascular survey report. National Institute of Neurology and Communicative Disorders and Stroke, Bethesda, p 1

Levy DE (1988) How transient are transient ischemic attacks? Neurology 38:674

Matsumoto N, Whisnant JP, Kurland LT (1973) Natural history of stroke in Rochester, Minnesota 1955 through 1969: an extension of a previous study, 1945 through 1954. Stroke 4:20

Millikan CH, McDowell F, Easton JD (1987) Stroke. Lea and Febiger, Philadelphia

Mohr JP, Barnett HJM (1986) Classification of ischemic stroke. In: Barnett HJM, Mohr JP, Stein BM, Yatsu FM (eds) Stroke – pathophysiology, diagnosis and management. Churchill Livingstone, New York, p 281

Poeck K (1986) Moderne Diagnostik und Therapie beim Schlaganfall. Dtsch Med Wochenschr 111:1369

Powers WJ, Raichle ME (1985) Positron emission tomography and its application to the study of cerebrovascular disease in man. Stroke 16:361

Ringelstein EB, Zeumer H, Schneider R (1985) Der Beitrag der zerebralen Computertomographie zur Differentialtypologie und Differentialtherapie des ischämischen Großhirninfarktes. Fortschr Neurol Pychiatr 53:315

Rodda RA, Path FRC (1986) The arterial patterns associated with internal carotid infarcts. Stroke 17:69

Roederer GO, Langlois YE, Jager KA, Primozich JF, Beach KW, Phillips DJ, Strandness DWE (1984) The natural history of carotid arterial disease in symptomatic patients with cervical bruits. Stroke 15:605

Salgado ED, Weinstein M, Furlan AJ, Modic MT, Beck GS, Estes M, Awad I, Little JR (1986) Proton magnetic resonance imaging in ischemic cerebrovascular disease. Ann Neurol 20:502–507

Takeya Y, Popper JS, Shimizu Y (1984) Epidemiologic studies of coronary heart disease and stroke in Japanese men living in Japan, Hawaii and California: incidence of stroke in Japan and Hawaii. Stroke 15:15

Vollmar JF (1980) Rekonstruktive Chirurgie der Arterien, 3rd edn. Thieme, Stuttgart

Vollmar JF (1985) Classification for surgery of cerebrovascular insufficiency. In: Courbier R (ed) Basis for classification of cerebral arterial diseases. Excerpta Medica, Amsterdam

Waxman SG, Toole JF (1983) Temporal profile resembling TIA in the setting of cerebral infarction. Stroke 14:433

Weisberg LA (1982) Lacunar infarcts: clinical and computed tomographic correlations. Arch Neurol 39:37

Whisnant JP (1983) The role of the neurologist in the decline of stroke. Ann Neurol 14:1

Whisnant JP (1984) The decline of stroke. Stroke 15:160

Wodarz R (1980) Watershed infarctions and computed tomography. A topographical study in cases with stenosis or occlusion of the carotid artery. Neuroradiology 19:245

Wolf PA, Kannel WB, Verter J (1983) Current status of risk factors for stroke. Neurol Clin 1:317

Zeumer H, Hacke W (1988) Ischämische Insulte. In: Hacke W (ed) Neurologische Intensivmedizin, 2nd edn. Perimed, Erlangen, p 89

Zülch KJ (1985) The cerebral infarct. Pathology, pathogenesis, and computed tomography. Springer, Berlin Heidelberg New York

4 Clinical Syndromes, Pathogenesis, and Differential Diagnosis

4.1 Symptoms and Syndromes – Temporal and Topical Aspects

The temporal sequence of signs and symptoms in patients with cerebral ischemia provides important information for the analysis of underlying pathophysiologic mechanisms and in the search for a major hemodynamic or embolic cause. The signs reported and symptoms assessed are useful for localization of the ischemic region of the brain and identification of the affected vascular territories. Even in the case of a typical clinical picture the clinical findings alone are often insufficient for unequivocal anatomic and pathologic identification, however important they may be in the choice of diagnostic and therapeutic measures. In the first few hours after cerebral ischemia, determining the prognosis is extremely difficult, and it is usually impossible to decide whether complete remission may be expected, or whether progressive development of a severe deficit is taking place. There is currently a debate as to whether cerebral ischemia due to thromboembolism should be treated in the acute phase by thrombolysis, in the same way as recent myocardial infarcts (Zeumer 1985; del Zoppo et al. 1986; del Zoppo and Hacke 1987; Hacke et al. 1988); these prognostic aspects are therefore particularly important, as only those patients in whom no rapid spontaneous remission is to be expected should be exposed to the risk of treatment-associated hemorrhage.

Determining the topical anatomic source of a focal neurologic deficit is therefore difficult, particularly in the absence of objective clinical findings, for we now know that supposedly characteristic clinical disturbances may be allocated to quite different cerebral regions on the basis of CT or MRI studies. The extent and site of the responsible structural defect can sometimes not be anticipated from the clinical picture. This is particularly important in aphasic disorders, with syndromes characteristic of defects in the Broca or Wernicke regions perhaps involving atypically situated lesions. It is also possible, as in the well-known disconnection syndromes, for secondary functional disturbances in metabolism to exist in the corresponding cortical regions which are in afferent or efferent linkage with the structures damaged by the primary ischemia: the lesion should not be related only to a subcortical structure if the functional deficit is considerably greater.

The temporal classification of individual types of cerebrovascular disease and the pathogenetic allocation of the infarcts on the basis of the CT and angiographic findings are dealt with in Chap. 3. Here we discuss the typical symptoms and syndromes that can be allocated to the carotid or vertebrobasilar territory on the grounds of their clinical features and their most common causes. We also consider the special types of neurologically asymptomatic severe cerebral angiopathies, concentrating on chronic multifocal conditions. Special attention is given to TIAs as warning symptoms of a threatened irreversible cerebral ischemia and to clues regarding the relevant pathologic mechanisms. Since in most cases these are not correlated with any objective neurologic or instrumental findings, the history as given by the patient and a careful clinical examination are particularly important. The recognition of a risk patient with hitherto neurologically asymptomatic carotid stenosis by means of the typical features of a TIA is very useful; it has been shown in several prospective studies that TIAs precede a cerebral infarct much more often than retrospective studies would suggest. At the time of a TIA, appropriate methods of investigation should clarify the differential diagnosis and possibly allow for prophylactic treatment, and TIAs should therefore not be trivialized through ignorance or lack of concern. It is also wrong to ascribe what is by definition the regression of symptoms to "successful nonspecific treatment" or carelessly to explain transient weakness and tingling in the arm as due to overexertion or disease of the cervical spine. Only a knowledge of the numerous possibilities even of rare features of focal neurologic deficits and their connection with possibly causal pathologic mechanisms allows a reasonable medical history. This is the basis for any continuing instrumental diagnosis and eventual treatment.

4.1.1 Carotid Artery Territory

Cerebral ischemia most often involves the territory of the carotid artery with its most important branches, the middle (MCA) and anterior (ACA) cerebral arteries. With a proximal localization of the vascular lesion in the extracranial portion of the carotid, the features of neurologic deficit vary greatly – the more distal the arterial lesion leading to an ischemia, the smaller are the possibilities of compensation through collateral circulation and the more uniform the clinical signs of deficit. We therefore discuss the different parts of the carotid artery and its branches and the corresponding typical clinical patterns.

4.1.1.1 Carotid Artery

In vascular lesions affecting the origin of the internal carotid artery (ICA; Table 4.1) there are often hemispheric TIAs of variable but short duration (30 s to 15 min), whereas symptoms persisting over 2 h may already be associated with parenchymatous defects an CT or MRI (see p. 133ff.).

The opposite upper limb and the face are usually clinically affected (unilateral brachiofacial symptoms); pareses and sensory disturbances may be distributed proximally or distally. Occasionally, only individual functions are affected, for example, those of the ulnar fingers of the hands. When the parts of the brain supplied by the ACA are affected, there are sensory or motor functional disorders of the contralateral leg. Mixed presentations are not uncommon in high-grade carotid obstructions in the neck. Series of reversible ischemic attacks occur more often in these cases than in low-grade stenoses, while longer lasting separate attacks associ-

Table 4.1. Lesions of the extra- and intracranial ICA, MCA, and ACA with types of clinical course. (From Caplan 1988)

Lesional site	Clinical course			Common pathogenic mechanisms
	TIA frequency	Recurrence	TIA/stroke insult ratio	
Bifurcation ICA in neck	+++	Often	3.27	Emboli from stenoses, *initially* usually complete lesion. Flow watershed infarcts, *initially* fluctuating
ICA siphon	+	Often	0.76	Unclear since rare, *initially* fluctuating
ICA carotid T	?	?		Very rare, usually not arterio-sclerotic
Ophthalmic artery	+++	Often	> 5.0	Emboli from plaques
MCA				
Caucasians	++	Rare		Emboli, territorial infarcts, *initially* usually complete
Asians and blacks	+	?	0.27	*Initially* usually fluctuating
ACA	++			Emboli from stenoses

ated with pronounced neurologic deficits are less common. Both types may result from hemodynamically or embolically produced ischemias due to high-grade stenoses or occlusions. Both types of pathogenesis can also be responsible for progressive insults, for example, recurrent emboli or anterograde thrombosis extension in the distal portions of vessels with occlusion of the ramifying collateral arteries.

Extracranial carotid lesions are often asymptomatic and also show an extremely low incidence of strokes in prospective studies. A marked increase in the incidence of cerebral ischemia, mainly TIAs, is often found in follow-up studies parallel to rapid progression of the vascular lesion (see p. 41); the annual stroke incidence is around 1% while the cardiac-associated mortality in this patient group is around 6%–8%. This is explained by a simultaneous coronary atherosclerosis in the context of a generalized arteriopathy (Hennerici et al. 1987). The collateralization of the some-times high-grade carotid stenoses or occlusions via the circle of Willis can be noninvasively studied using Doppler ultrasound techniques, and this provides information as to the hemodynamic aspects (Fig. 4.1).

This is another important prognostic parameter, since even cervical carotid lesions with pronounced hemodynamic effects often remain asymptomatic when good collateralization exists. TIAs are probably the expression of structural changes in such vascular lesions; as new sources of emboli, these usually produce short repeated attacks, less often persistent focal deficit (Mohr et al. 1978; Ringelstein et al. 1983). Cases with a progressive course or with fluctuating neurologic symptoms are very uncommon in comparison with infarcts involving occlusions of the distal parts of the

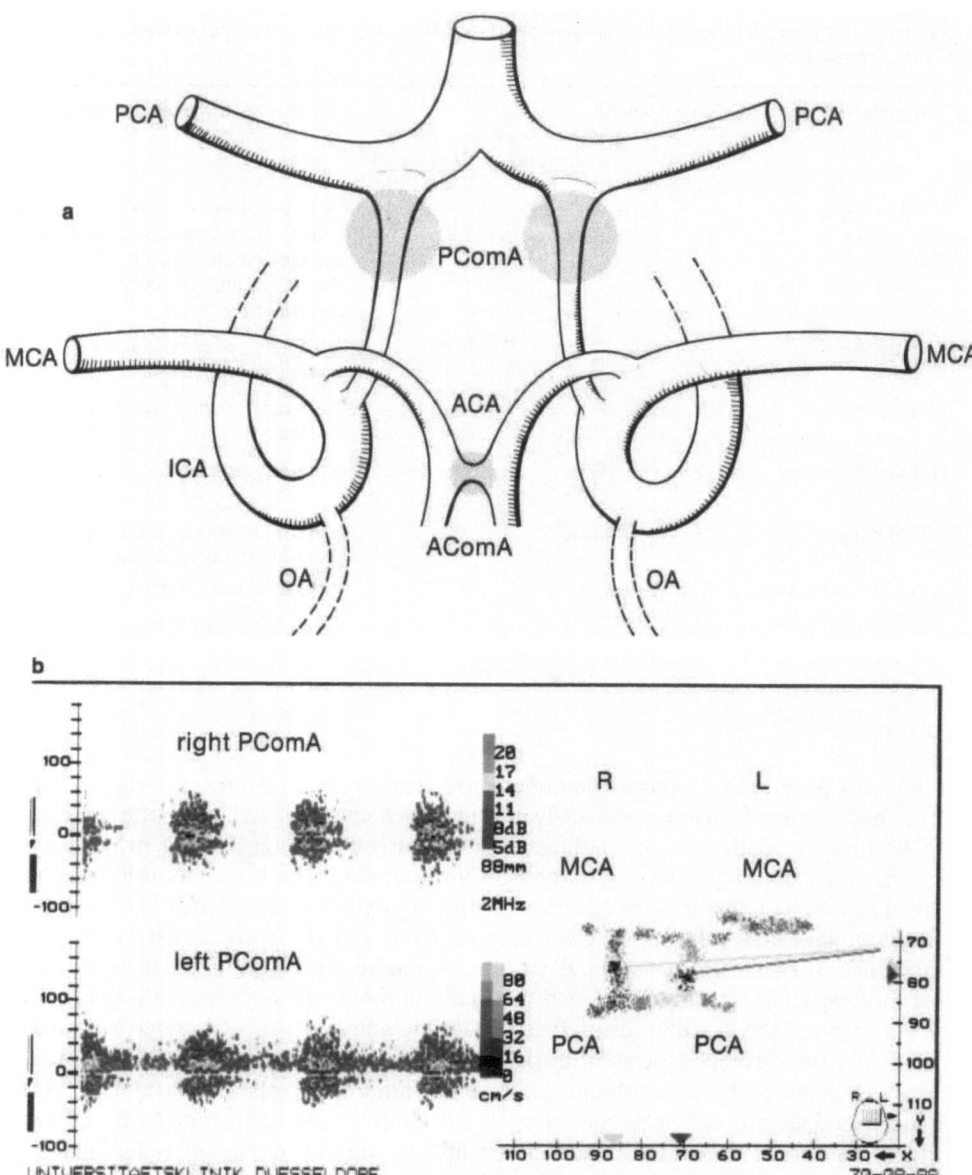

Fig. 4.1. Diagram (**a**) and transcranial Doppler sonogram (**b**) showing the collaterals in extracranial hemodynamically acting vascular lesions. **a** The ophthalmic arteries (*OA*) and the anterior and posterior parts of circle of Willis as collaterals of the opposite carotid or vertebrobasilar system in high-grade extracranial vascular lesions can be investigated using Doppler ultrasound. **b** Depiction of the circle of Willis and Fourier-transformed Doppler spectra of the posterior communicating artery on both sides in a patient with bilateral extracranial internal carotid occlusion. Evidence of "functional" stenosis in both posterior communicating arteries (*PComA*) as expression of effective collateralization. *ACA,* Anterior cerebral artery; *AComA,* anterior communicating artery; *ICA,* internal carotid artery; *PCA,* posterior cerebral artery; *MCA,* middle cerebral artery; *R,* right; *L,* left

vessels. This is also an argument in favor of an embolic mechanism in the great majority of cases (artery-to-artery embolism).

Vascular lesions affecting the carotid siphon either alone or predominantly have been much less studied (Table 4.1). Transient warning symptoms, for example, temporary visual disorders, are uncommon. Pareses of the contralateral facial and leg muscles without involvement of the upper limb have been reported as fluctuating initial features, but well-documented CT studies of infarcts do not exist, and the pathophysiologic mechanisms are obscure.

Lesions of the intracranial bifurcation of the ICA seldom lead to cerebral ischemias and are likely due to nonarteriosclerotic vascular processes, such as dissection, cardiac embolism, thrombosis in coagulopathies, or inflammatory vascular disease. If ischemia develops, and the collaterals are not functionally effective, hemiplegia may occur with early disturbance of consciousness and a risk of uncontrollable development of edema in the hemispheres or middle cerebral artery territory (malignant infarction; Spitzer et al. 1988).

4.1.1.2 Branches from the Carotid Siphon

The ophthalmic artery, as an anatomic, physiologic, and embryonic connection between the intracranial and extracranial circulation, arises from the carotid siphon (see p. 6). It traverses the dura and the optic canal into the orbit beneath the optic nerve and may be mechanically constricted at this site, with possible involvement of the nerve. In either case there are sometimes possibilities for operative decompression (Unsöld and Seeger 1984). Its course takes it around the optic nerve on the medial side under the superior oblique muscle, where it divides into a series of very variable end-branches, among them the central retinal artery, the lacrimal artery (laterally) which forms the important anastomosis with the middle meningeal artery, the anterior and posterior ethmoidal branches (medially), and the supratrochlear and supraorbital arteries (rostrally) which anastomose with the facial and superficial temporal arteries and are important landmark arteries in Doppler sonography.

After partial or total attacks of amaurosis fugax (Fig. 4.2) there is usually complete recovery. Retinal infarcts are very uncommon. There may be as many as 100 attacks per day. Typically this leads to a brief visual loss in one eye, usually extending vertically, less often horizontally. Sometimes only one part of the visual field is affected. Frequently there is total monocular loss of vision, and if visual function is preserved in the other eye, this may lead to uncharacteristic anamnestic data: monocular obscurations and clouded or hazy vision have the effect that the patient does not carry out visual checks of one eye against the other during the attack by closing one eye at a time. On the other hand, there may also be positive irritations arising from the neighborhood of ischemic areas such as colored scotomas, flashes of light, or fortification patterns, which are nearly always and erroneously diagnosed as due to migraine attacks (Goodwin et al. 1987). In acute central retinal artery occlusion there is sudden painless loss of vision; unlike an acute glaucoma attack, there is also no pain in the eyeball. Although proximal carotid lesions in the neck often produce both hemispheric and retinal ischemia, depending on the size of the embolized particles, it is uncommon for both to appear simultaneously. The prognosis after retinal TIAs is

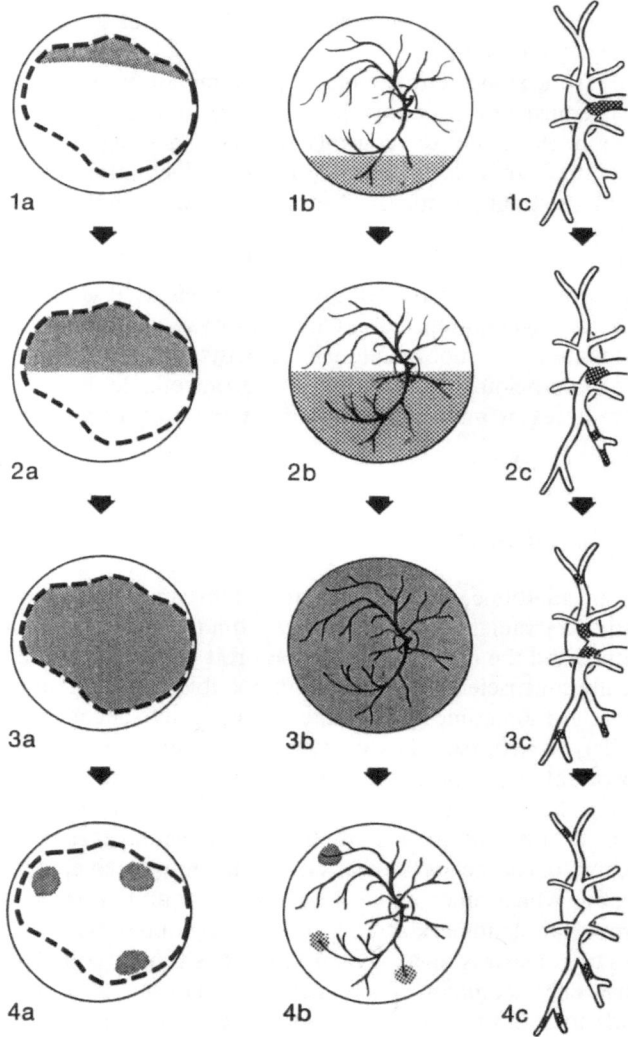

Fig. 4.2. Diagram of the dynamics of visual field alterations (*a*), retinal ischemic territories (*b*), and vascular lesions in the retinal arteries (*c*) in amaurosis fugax. The symptoms change with different positions of the vascular occlusion (*1–4*), corresponding to the ischemic territory. (From Toole 1984)

much more favorable than after retinal infarction or hemispheric TIAs since they are less often followed by cerebral insults (Table 4.1).

Attacks of amaurosis fugax occur much more commonly than hemispheric TIAs without demonstrable wall changes in the carotids. Gaul et al. (1986) noted pathologic Doppler/B-mode ultrasound findings in 77.2% of 500 patients with visual disorders and in 79% of the 171 classical amaurosis fugax attacks among them; of these only 16% and 21.6%, respectively, were hemodynamically relevant. Local stenotic lesions of the ophthalmic artery are extremely rare, whereas cardiac emboli lead to retinal ischemia probably more often than was earlier thought (Bogousslavsky et al. 1985). Much less common are severe residual defects after retinal ischemia with intraretinal hemorrhages, formation of microaneurysms, and dilatation of the large veins, which were formerly reported in the literature as present in up to 5% of patients with high-grade carotid stenoses and which may lead to permanent loss of vision (Tour and Hoyt 1959). Amaurosis fugax attacks should lead to search for an embolism source or a hemodynamically relevant arteriopathy.

The posterior communicating artery (PCA) also arises from the carotid siphon between the ophthalmic and anterior choroidal arteries. It gives rise to numerous branches to the diencephalon, thalamus, and caudate nucleus, among them the anterior thalamoperforating arteries (Fig. 4.3). These form a dense collateral network with the other thalamic arteries, usually supplied by the vertebrobasilar system (Table 4.2). Vascular variants are common, and the lack of uniformity makes difficult the allocation of vessel occlusions to clinical signs of deficit and infarcts demonstrable by CT or MRI.

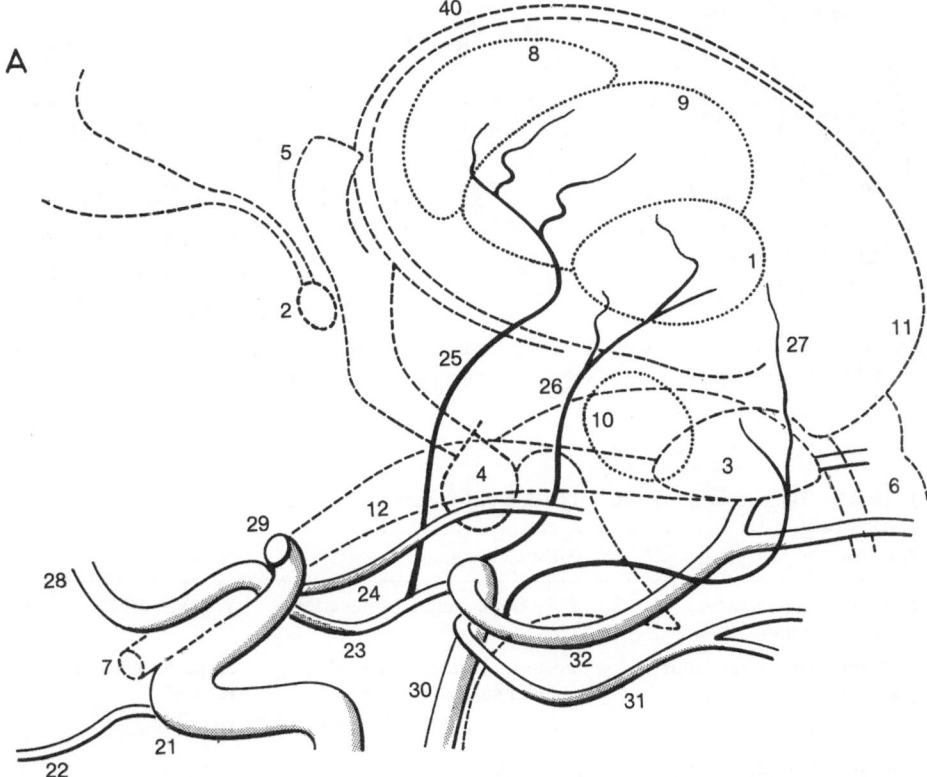

Fig. 4.3. Diagram of the arterial supply to the thalamus (**A**; modified from Schlesinger 1976) and CT sectional images showing thalamic infarcts in four regions (**B**; from Bogousslavsky et al. 1988). **A** *1,* Centrum medianum; *2,* anterior commissure; *3,* lateral geniculate body; *4,* mammillary body; *5,* fornix; *6,* lamina quadrigemina; *7,* optic nerve; *8,* anterior thalamic nuclei; *9,* medial thalamic nuclei; *10,* nucleus ruber; *11,* pulvinar; *12,* optic tract; *21,* internal carotid artery; *22,* ophthalmic artery; *23,* posterior communicating artery; *24,* anterior choroidal artery; *25,* anterior thalamoperforating arteries; *26,* posterior thalamoperforating arteries; *27,* posterior choroidal artery; *28,* anterior cerebral artery; *29,* middle cerebral artery; *30,* basilar artery; *31,* cerebellar artery; *32,* posterior cerebral artery

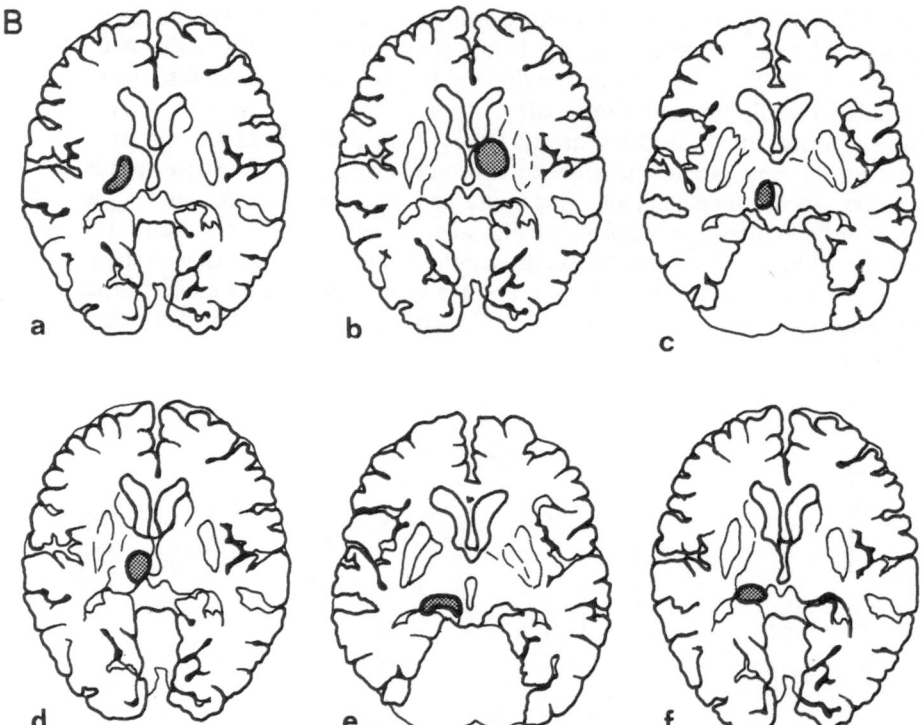

Fig. 4.3 B. *a,* Thalamogeniculate arterial territory; *b,* anterior thalamoperforating territory; *c, d,* posterior choroidal territory; *e, f,* posterior thalamoperforating territory

Table 4.2. Thalamic arteries with origin and distribution areas in the thalamus

Arteries	Most common origin	Area supplied
Anterior thalamoperforating (tuberothalamic)	Posterior communicating artery	VA, VL, DM
Posterior thalamoperforating (paramedian branches)	Posterior cerebral artery (P1) (basilar communicating)	Rostral brain stem IL, DM
Thalamogeniculate	Posterior cerebral artery (P2)	VL, VP
Posterior choroidal (inferolateral branches)	Posterior cerebral artery (P2)	P, LGB

VA, Ventroanterior nucleus; VL, ventrolateral nucleus; DM, dorsomedial nucleus; IL, intralaminar nucleus; VP, ventroposterior nucleus; P, pulvinar; LGB, lateral geniculate body.

However, it is possible to distinguish four quite characteristic syndromes (Bogous-slavsky et al. 1988):

1. Infarcts in the territory of the anterior thalamoperforating (tuberothalamic) arteries lead to no or only moderate contralateral, mainly brachiofacial, sensorimotor hemiparesis. Behavioral deficits are prominent, with apathy, disorientation, and lack of spontaneity, as well as occasional transcortical aphasia.
2. Infarcts in the territory of the thalamogeniculate arteries (P2 segment of the PCA) are the most common and typically lead to contralateral dysesthesiae, occasionally associated with hemineglect and hemiataxia as well as transcortical aphasic disorders in left-hemispheric lesions.
3. Infarcts in the territory of the posterior choroidal artery (inferolateral branches), which also arises from the P2 segment of the PCA, are extremely rare and cause a horizontal, homonymous sectoranopia, probably due to selective ischemia in the lateral geniculate body.
4. Bilateral infarcts in the territory of the posterior thalamoperforating arteries, which may arise from a common basilar communicating arterial trunk, lead to disorders of consciousness and memory, supranuclear pareses of gaze, and oculomotor nucleus/nerve damage due to ischemia in the rostral brainstem.

Ischemias in the zone supplied by the anterior choroidal artery are rare; these have recently been summarized by Helgason et al. (1986) in a review. The classical triad consists of a severe contralateral hemiparesis, unilateral sensory disorder, and homonymous hemianopia.

4.1.1.3 Middle Cerebral Artery

Ischemic infarcts are most commonly found in the territory of the MCA. The distribution of infarcts as shown by CT is presented in Fig. 1.10. Cortical territorial and borderzone infarcts are distinguished from subcortical ischemias in borderzones and lacunar syndromes on the basis of their localization and underlying pathogenic mechanisms.

In cortical ischemia in individual branches or in the entire MCA territory, a variety of deficits may be found according to the structures affected: sensory, motor, or sensorimotor features of varying severity on the contralateral side, gaze motor function, neuropsychological symptoms such as aphasias or apraxias, difficulty in reading or calculating, speech impairment, or impairment of the notion of performance, etc. The pathogenetic basis of (partial) middle cerebral infarction of predominantly territorial distribution is either embolism or atheromatous changes with thrombosis in the pial arteries (Table 4.1). In the Western industrialized countries of Europe and North America, arteriosclerotic lesions of the MCA are substantially more common in whites than in blacks; they are also much more common in these whites than in Asians. Cerebral ischemias in whites are more commonly caused by emboli, which may be very rapidly recanalized and hence no longer angiographically demonstrable even after a few hours. The varying pathomechanisms corresponding to different populations are shown in Japanese or American studies indicating a low TIA insult rate in a high proportion of black patients, whereas TIAs were more common in a London series (Corston et al. 1984). It is uncommon for the clinical picture to be fully expressed from the outset, and the course generally fluctuates over several hours or days. In the series of Caplan et al. (1986) the deficit was not fully established until after 1 week. This is interpreted as the expression of a hemodynamic obstruction, whereas another series in the United States (Shinar et al. 1985) showed a mostly embolic pathogenesis from cardiac or proximal extracranial sources with little fluctuation.

Subcortical ischemias, like infarction of the lentiform nucleus, may develop hemo-dynamically as borderzone or watershed infarcts (the basal part of the lentiform nucleus is supplied by the recurrent Heubner's artery from the ACA, the upper part by the lenticulostriate arteries from the MCA), may similarly take the form of "lacunar infarcts" (e. g., small, deep infarcts), or may be due to lipohyalinosis of end-arteries or embolically conditioned territorial occlusion of the origins of the perforating arteries. Clinically, there is usually a slight or moderate degree of hemiparesis, sometimes with superimposed dystonias and athetoid movements; not uncommonly there is also an increase in muscle tone. Obstructions of the lenticulostriate arteries lead to so-called "lacunar syndromes" (Soria et al. 1987; Fig. 4.4). In infarcts of the internal capsule there is often a pure motor hemiparesis of the opposite side of the body with marked spasticity, usually including the face; in more caudally located lesions of the pyramidal tract due to lacunar brainstem ischemia the face is often spared, and spasticity may be absent. Quite often the patients report dysesthesia for all sensory modalities, but without demonstrable deficit on sensory testing. Relatively rare, but characteristic, is the dysarthria/clumsy hand syndrome described by Fisher, with a distally emphasized paresis of the opposite hand, dysarthria, dysphagia, and facial weakness. This syndrome also occurs in lacunar brainstem infarcts. Many small subcortical lesions remain asymptomatic and are found incidentally upon CT or MRI. It should be noted that small, deep, "lacunar" infarcts with "lacunar symptoms" are not due exclusively to small vessel diseases (e.g., lipohyalinosis of penetrating terminal arteries) but may be indistinguishable both clinically and on CT and MRI scans from hemodynamically induced borderzone infarctions (e. g., in the *letzte Wiese* of MCA branches) or watershed infarctions (between MCA and ACA; Waterston et al. 1990).

Extensive subcortical ischemia (so-called end-flow infarcts) can also develop in occlusions of the MCA proximal to the origins of the lenticulostriate arteries when the convexity is supplied by collaterals. However, depending on the capacity of these anastomoses, wedge-shaped infarcts may also result in the watershed of the ACA or in the borderzone of the PCA (Fig. 4.5; see also p. 137ff.). The pareses affect the contralateral side of the body, and large series show that the arm is affected more commonly than the leg and the leg more than the face, the motor deficits being not uncommonly accompanied by sensory disturbances. Neuropsychological deficits are extremely variable, according to whether the dominant or nondominant hemisphere or both are affected (see Chap. 5).

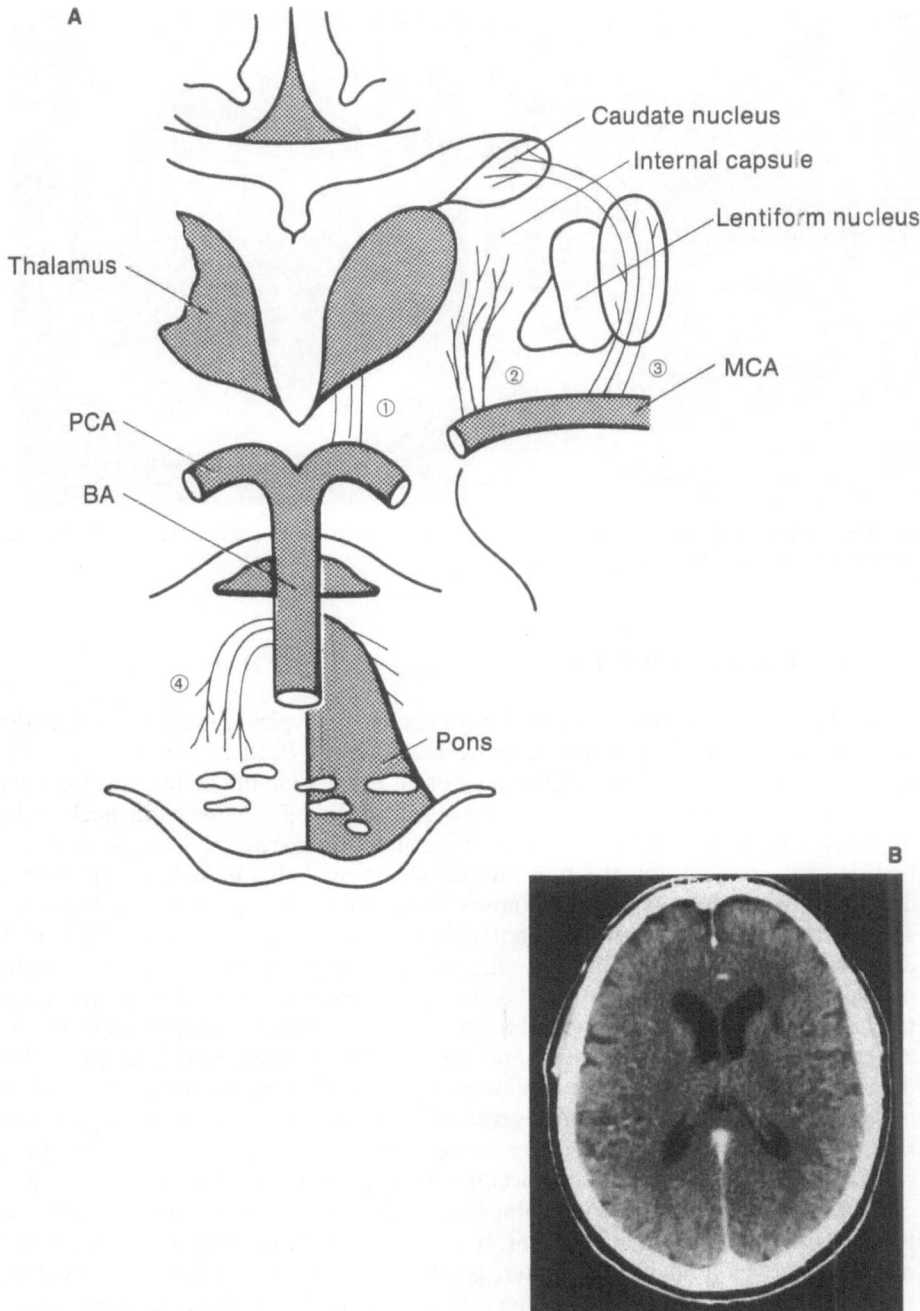

Fig. 4.4. A Preferential sites of lacunar infarcts in the vascular territories of the thalamoperforating arteries (*1*), the medial lenticulostriate arteries (*2*), the lateral lenticulostriate arteries (*3*), and the paramedian pontine arteries (*4*; modified from Soria et al. 1987). **B** CT of a typical lacune in the left anterior capsular region (territory of the lateral lenticulostriate arteries)

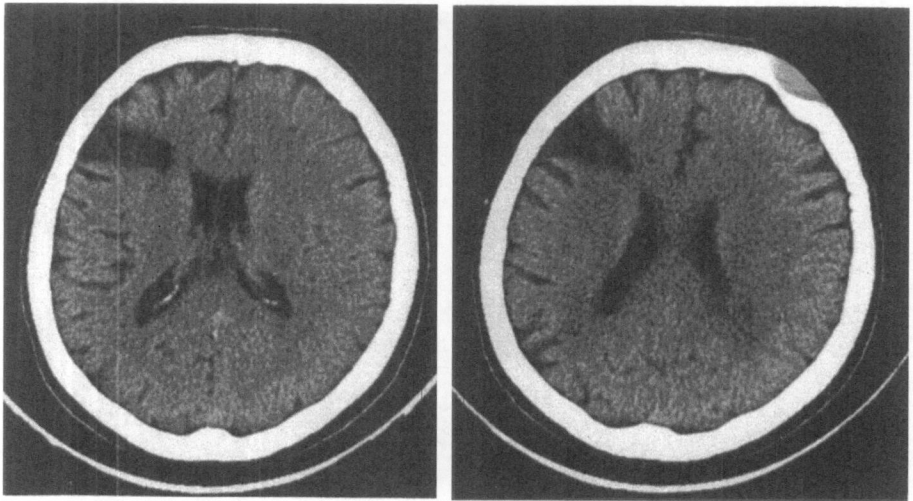

Fig. 4.5. Typical wedge-shaped watershed infarct between the territories of the ACA and MCA in an ipsilateral ICA occlusion

4.1.1.4 Anterior Cerebral Artery

Isolated occlusions or stenoses of the ACA are rare; the typical clinical features of the resulting deficit were summarized in a now classic paper by Critchley in 1930. Usually, infarcts in the territory of the ACA do not occur in isolation but include the territory of the MCA, since the underlying lesion is at the carotid bifurcation in the neck or the siphon, or usually both. Clinically, a distally pronounced paresis of the opposite lower limb is characteristic, but the hips and shoulders may also be affected if there is damage to the supplementary motor area with sparing of the hand and face (Fig. 4.6). The sensory disorders are usually minor and normally affect the fine-touch ability with disturbed two-point discrimination, although stereotopic disorders are occasionally present. Signs of neuropsychological deficit appear particularly in bilateral infarcts in the anterior flow zone or if the limbic system and the anterior corpus callosum are affected. Disconnection syndromes are manifested as disorders of orientation and as dysgraphias and apraxias of the ipsilateral hand. In addition, there may be mutistic disorders, loss of speech, and perseveration tendencies in lesions of the supplementary motor area. Involuntary mirror movements of the opposite hand have been described. Autonomic dysfunction occurs particularly in bilateral infarcts. Occlusions of the main trunk of the ACA including Heubner's artery are to be distinguished from lesions distal to the origin of the latter. It is to be noted in this context that the signs of neurologic deficit remain minor if there is collateralization with the opposite ACA via a patent anterior communicating artery, in which case the resulting picture is almost identical to that of a distal obstruction with thrombosis of the recurrent Heubner's artery. With a proximal occlusion there develops a severe hemiparesis, especially of the lower limb, with marked sensory disturbances, apraxia (in right-sided hemiparesis), disorders of consciousness and aphasic disorders if the dominant

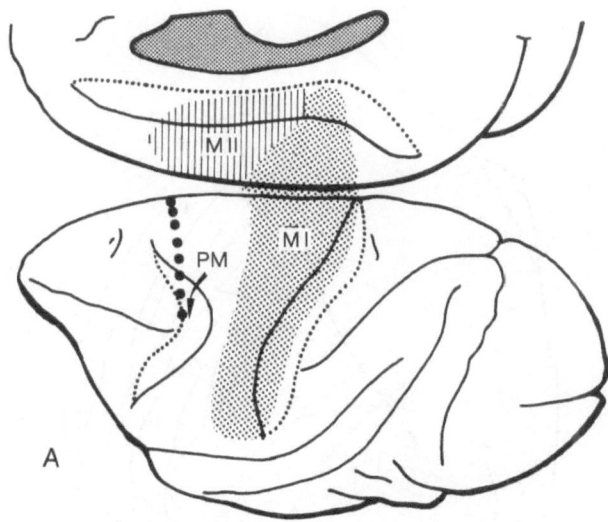

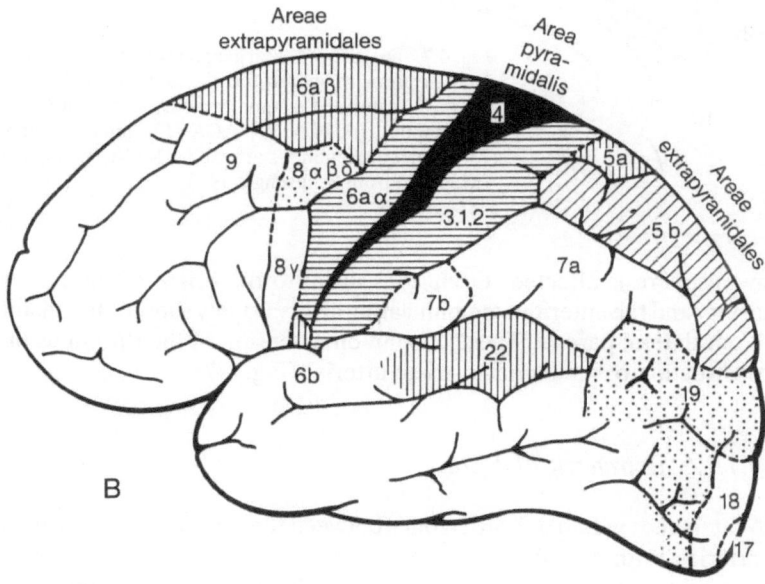

Fig. 4.6. **A** View of the left hemisphere of a primate showing the lateral (*below*) and medial (*above*) cerebral surfaces. *MI,* Primary motor cortex; *MII,* supplementary motor cortex (SMA); *PM,* premotor cortex. **B** View of a human brain (from Foerster 1936) with cytoarchitectonic regions as numbered by Vogt and Vogt (from Wise 1985). The primary motor cortex corresponds to area 4, the SMA and PM more or less to area 6 (from Freund 1987)

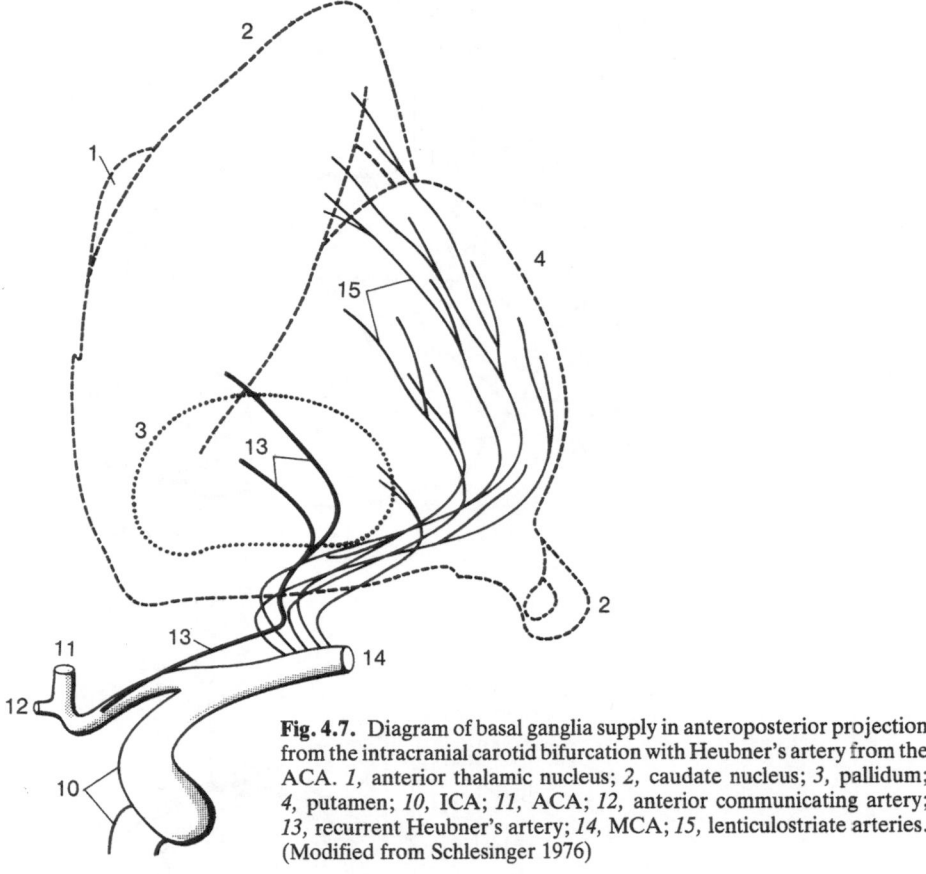

Fig. 4.7. Diagram of basal ganglia supply in anteroposterior projection from the intracranial carotid bifurcation with Heubner's artery from the ACA. *1*, anterior thalamic nucleus; *2*, caudate nucleus; *3*, pallidum; *4*, putamen; *10*, ICA; *11*, ACA; *12*, anterior communicating artery; *13*, recurrent Heubner's artery; *14*, MCA; *15*, lenticulostriate arteries. (Modified from Schlesinger 1976)

hemisphere is affected. Occlusions distal to the origin of the recurrent Heubner's artery and the anterior communicating artery usually show only a mainly brachiofacial contralateral paresis. These depend on extension of the thrombus in the MCA with obstruction of the lenticulostriate arteries (Fig. 4.7).

4.1.1.5 Extraterritorial Zones

Watersheds within or borderzones between the supply territories of the large cerebral arteries, with or without collateral networks, are particularly liable to ischemias for hemodynamic reasons. Phenomenologically, they are characterized by an extraordinary variability in the developing collateral circulation and the often remote topography of multiple foci over the entire hemisphere. Of pathogenetic importance is a marked fall in blood pressure, due to cardiocirculatory arrest or other causes, with high-grade impairment of carotid flow in the neck (cortical watershed infarcts or subcortical infarcts in the region of the lentiform nucleus) or impaired flow in the

MCA main trunk (subcortical infarcts). A watershed infarct between the anterior and middle cerebral territories (Fig. 4.5) is common, characterized by a proximally emphasized contralateral hemiparesis sparing the distal parts of the limbs if regions of the premotor and supplementary motor cortex are affected (Freund and Hummelsheim 1985).

In borderzone infarcts between the middle and posterior cerebral territories, and depending on whether the dominant or nondominant hemisphere is affected, extremely variable neuropsychological deficits may be combined with disturbed sensation on the opposite side of the body and homonymous visual field defects of varying degree. In occlusions of the MCA proximal to the origin of the lenticulostriate arteries extensive subcortical infarcts may develop, situated in the borderzone between the basal penetrating arteries and those of the convexity. Just as in lacunar infarcts in the middle cerebral territory, contralateral pure motor hemipareses may develop due to interruption of the descending motor tracts in the corona radiata, usually with limited improvement.

4.1.2 Vertebrobasilar Territory

The brainstem, occipital lobes, and mediobasal regions of the temporal lobes receive their blood supply from the vertebrobasilar circulation. Structures of the greatest functional importance are arranged in a confined space in this region. They include the nuclear areas for the organization of the motor functions of vision, swallowing, and speech, as well as the major connecting pathways between the two hemispheres, the cerebellum and spinal cord, the central structures of the autonomic nervous system, and the central regulation of respiratory and cardiocirculatory function. Because of the special anatomy of the vascular supply in this region with the formation of numerous individual variants and collateral networks, the allocation of the features of subjective and objective neurologic deficit in ischemia is far from easy. Surprisingly mild syndromes may be the product of largely intact collateral function even in high-grade vascular lesions affecting both vertebral arteries, but they may also result from segmental basilar occlusions. On the other hand, the obstruction of a small end-artery may lead to the most severe neurologic deficit, with permanent invalidism or death (e. g., in the classical Wallenberg's syndrome). Most of the classical syndromes named after those who first described them are seldom encountered any more; they involved a selection of individual cases with a fatal outcome and the most severe clinical deficits, whereas the overwhelming majority of features of neurologic deficit seen in disorders of the vertebrobasilar circulation are less severe. Nevertheless, the allocation of the clinical picture to anatomic structures still depends on an exact analysis of the neurophysiologic and neuroanatomic findings, as there are major restrictions on the value of imaging techniques – even including MRI – in the posterior cranial fossa. It is particularly difficult to assign the symptoms to the vertebrobasilar system when the only data available are from the history; disorders of the posterior circulation are far too often diagnosed on the basis of uncharacteristic symptoms. It is therefore desirable for at least two different typical signs to be reported before assuming the existence of a disturbance in the posterior circulation. This applies especially when uncharacteristic signs suggest an association between already recognized extracranial lesions and a cerebellopontine ischemia. A history of attacks of vertigo, which are very variably experienced and reported by individual patients, often leads to the erroneous diagnosis of a vertebrobasilar ischemia, extending from common complaints (vertigo on turning or lifting and lateral deviation of gait) through an irregular tendency to fall into "confusion," a feeling of "emptiness," "syncopal states," or "disorders of consciousness." On the other hand, variable disorders of speech and swallowing, double vision, bilateral perioral or acral tingling sensations, sensorimotor tetraparesis, tremor, or ataxia belong to the typical functional disorders of the brainstem and cerebellum. Not uncommonly features of deficit develop in ischemia in the territories of the PCA and cerebellar arteries which may lead to complex bilateral deficit patterns due to unpaired arrangement of individual ramifications or even of the main branches.

4.1.2.1 Branches Adjacent to the Aortic Arch and Extracranial Vertebral Artery

In addition to the carotid bifurcation in the neck, arteriosclerotic lesions particularly often affect the origins of the vertebral arteries, preferentially the proximal subclavian segments and the left more than the right. Less common are stenoses of the brachiocephalic trunk (under 1%; Hass et al. 1968). Both types of occlusive disease of arteries close to the aortic arch that supply the brain can lead to complex changes in hemodynamics with reversal of the circulation in the arteries connected with the carotid or vertebral system. The phenomenon termed subclavian steal syndrome, first described in 1961 by Reivich et al. on the basis of angiographic findings in two patients and by Fisher in an editorial in the same volume of the *New England Journal of Medicine,* is now diagnosed noninvasively using Doppler ultrasound techniques. Contrary to initial assumptions, it relates to a frequent type of manifestation of arteriosclerosis which occurs predominantly *without* disorders of cerebral function such as TIA or infarct as long as the vascular lesion is confined to the subclavian artery or the brachiocephalic trunk alone. In 324 cases of the subclavian steal phenomenon demonstrated using Doppler ultrasound, Hennerici et al. (1988a) observed the occurrence of stress-dependent pontine signs only four times. The patients were often symptom free for years. Therefore, the subclavian steal syndrome which is asymptomatic or associated with atypical symptoms is not an indication for surgery, which is required only occasionally for restriction of the use of the arm or distal emboli in the hand. However, as the course of the individual case cannot be predicted, and as the frequency of usually transient cerebral symptoms increases with the extent and severity of the extracranial vascular lesion, monitoring of the vascular process is necessary. This is also the case if lesions of the brachiocephalic trunk impair the hemodynamics in the carotid artery. The suspected diagnosis can be confirmed by palpation and comparative blood pressure measurement in both arms. With high-grade subclavian obstruction a hypertension requiring medication may be overlooked, or a drug-induced rise in blood pressure may even be produced if the blood pressure is measured only on one side. Occasionally vascular compression syndromes lead to stenosis of the subclavian artery and compression of the brachial plexus. This can also be diagnosed noninvasively using Doppler ultrasound and electroneurography. These forms of the disease constitute operative indications only in exceptional cases; it is generally sufficient to advise the patients which particular movements to avoid.

Rarely, in an aortic arch syndrome, the origins of all the proximal branches of the arteries supplying the brain are affected in their thoracic course; apart from congenital anomalies this is usually related to an inflammatory vascular process called Takayasu's syndrome, after the physician who first described it. This granulomatous arteritis occurs particularly often in women. Other inflammatory causes include endangiitis obliterans, sarcoidosis or tuberculosis, and mechanical factors (kinking, cervical ribs, mediastinal space-occupying lesions, or trauma). Aortic aneurysms and dissections (arteriosclerotic, syphilitic, traumatic, or spontaneous) or Erdheim-Gsell idiopathic medial necrosis may likewise produce an aortic arch syndrome. The symptoms depend on the individual territories of the affected arteries.

Arteriosclerotic vascular lesions most commonly affect the origin of the vertebral artery in its proximal extracranial portion. The intracranial and extracranial portions in the lateral part of the cervical vertebrae are affected with decreasing frequency. Hemodynamically induced ischemias due to confluence of the two vertebral arteries, which are often arranged asymmetrically, rarely occur since even with bilateral proximal vertebral occlusions the blood supply of the distal vertebral is often preserved via collaterals from the external carotid, the thyrocervical trunk, and muscular branches. Kinking in the proximal portion and at the origin itself are not uncommon; they are not hemodynamically relevant but constitute possible sources of emboli. Although the arteriosclerotic vascular lesions of the vertebral artery resemble those of the carotid from the epidemiologic aspect, they are persistently different in their clinical impact: TIAs in the vertebrobasilar territory are more common, shorter, and lead far less often to a subsequent infarct. The usual mechanisms are an acute thrombotic occlusion of the vertebral artery with inadequate collateralization or arterioarterial embolism (Caplan 1988).

4.1.2.2 Intracranial Vertebral Artery and Cerebellar Arteries

Intracranial vascular lesions of the vertebral artery are more serious than extracranial and lead more often to cerebral infarcts. They may clinically resemble basilar lesions if in structural anomalies the vertebral artery that alone is responsible for perfusion becomes stenosed. If both vertebral arteries are normal, occlusion of one vessel can lead to (a) a brainstem infarct (e. g., Wallenberg's syndrome), (b) a cerebellar infarct, (c) embolic occlusions of the distal basilar artery and its branches with rostral brainstem infarcts, or (d) cerebellopontine TIAs. It may also be tolerated asymptomatically.

The lateral brainstem syndrome described by Wallenberg in 1895 and attributed to occlusion of the posterior inferior cerebellar artery (PICA) is extremely rare in its classical constellation. The basis is usually an obstruction of the ipsilateral intracranial vertebral artery in the region of the PICA origin. The wedge-shaped infarct is situated in the territory of the dorsolateral penetrating brainstem branches (Fig. 4.8). With extension of the infarct dorsally, infarction of the PICA cerebellar territory often also occurs. Not infrequently, the infarct is preceded by TIAs with vertigo, nystagmus, numbness of the face, visual disorders, or transient gait disturbances. As in all

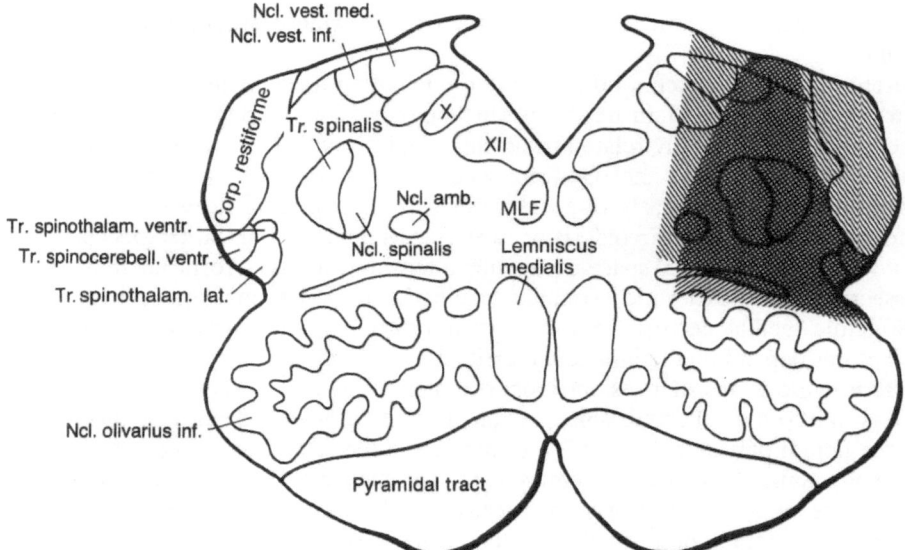

Fig. 4.8. Diagram of a lateral medullary infarct in the so-called Wallenberg's syndrome. *Hatched area,* most common extent of the infarct; *obliquely striped area,* larger infarcts. (From Currier et al. 1961)

vertebrobasilar circulatory disturbances, fluctuations over several days are common. More or less severe pain in the head or face are not uncommon and indicate involvement of the trigeminal nerve. Neck pain is common on the side of the occlusion. These prodromes are signs of disturbance of vestibular function or involvement of the connecting pathways to the cerebellum and the spinal afferents. The visual disorders are usually the expression of a lesion of the vestibulo-ocular system, while actual double vision with rostral extension of the ischemia to the supranuclear visual-motor centers and nuclear regions is not uncommon. Disturbance of swallowing is common and carries a risk of pneumonia; speech disorders and hoarseness indicate a lesion of the nucleus ambiguus with deeply extending infarcts. The characteristic signs of a crossed, dissociated impairment of sensation due to a lesion of the lateral spinothalamic tract are often absent or of only minor degree, whereas the ipsilateral half of the face is almost always involved. Ataxia of gait and pointing may be the expression of brainstem or cerebellar ischemia.

Trunk and positional ataxia, marked ataxia at extremities, and rebound phenomenon are important diagnostic signs of an additional cerebellar infarction. Increase of pressure in the posterior cranial fossa may lead to herniation with a fatal outcome unless decompression is achieved promptly by drugs or surgery. Supraventricular drainage alone is not sufficient. Since it is usually not possible to differentiate unequivocally between pontine and cerebellar ataxia, CT studies are essential in all cases with such marked disturbance. Careful attention must be paid to indirect signs such as compression of the fourth ventricle and enlargement of the temporal horns in the early stage, even if the cerebellar infarct is not yet demarcated. Clinically alarming symptoms include changes in the state of consciousness, hiccups, and vomiting.

Distal emboli in both superior cerebellar arteries (SCA), the posterior cerebral arteries, and the rostral basilar artery can lead to varied and extensive symptoms which, by themselves or together with the lateral medullary infarct, determine the clinical picture.

As in other vascular territories and with obstructive arteriopathies, however, only transient symptoms (TIAs) may occur, or if there is adequate collateralization even vascular occlusion may remain asymptomatic. Generally, isolated symptoms such as attacks of vertigo are seldom precursors of a brainstem infarct, especially if they persist for weeks. Even the so-called drop attacks, in which the patient reports a sudden loss of muscle tone with falling but without disturbance of consciousness, are seldom the expression of a vertebrobasilar ischemia despite the conventional view. They may have a variety of causes, even without the existence of any cerebrovascular or neurologic disease at all.

4.1.2.3 Basilar Artery and Branches

Obstructions of the branches arising from the basilar artery lead to a variety of rather similar clinical pictures, depending on their site and extent, which are sometimes named eponymously as separate syndromes (Table 4.3). The importance of these syndromes, which seldom occur in pure form, is minor as the distinction between them is of no therapeutic consequence. However, it is important to realize that in most lesions of arteriosclerotic origin in the middle and distal segments of the basilar artery thrombi may form which can ultimately occlude the vessel segmentally up to the next

Table 4.3. Examples of classical brainstem syndromes

Name	Site	Ipsilateral symptoms	Contralateral symptom
Parinaud	Corpora quadrigemina	Vertical gaze paresis (upward > downward) Convergence paresis, pupillomotor disorder	
Benedikt (upper ruber)	Midbrain Nucleus ruber	III nuclear paresis skew deviation	Hemiataxia Hyperkinesia Hemiparesis
Claude (lower ruber)	Midbrain Nucleus ruber	III nuclear paresis skew deviation	Hemiataxia Hemiparesis
Weber	Midbrain	Infranuclear III paresis, skew deviation	Motor hemisyndrome
Gasperini	Caudal pontine tegmentum	V, VI, VII, VIII lesion	Sensory hemisyndrome
Foville	Caudal pontine tegmentum	VI and VII lesion	Motor hemisyndrome
Wallenberg	Lateral medulla	Horner's syndrome, V, IX, and X lesion, hemiataxia	Dissociated cross sensory syndrome

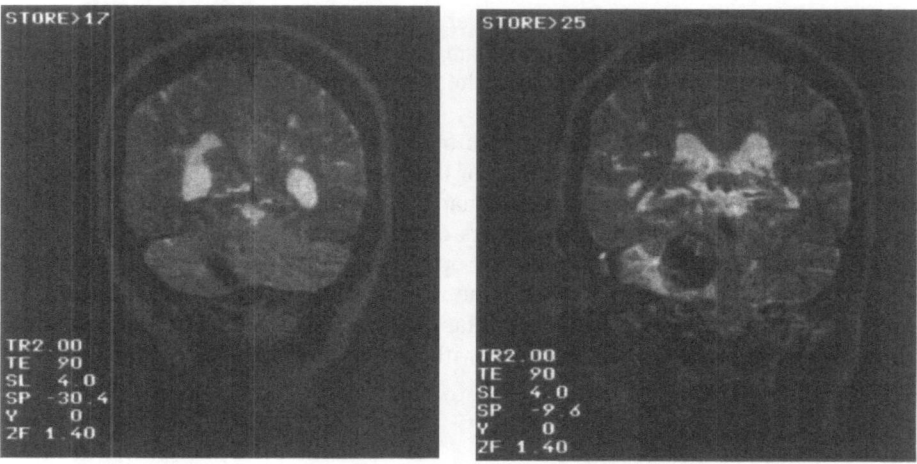

Fig. 4.9. MRI scans of posterior cranial fossa with dilative arteriopathy and aneurysm of basilar artery

circumferential branch (anterior inferior cerebellar artery, AICA; or SCA) or from the distal vertebral artery to the confluence or all together. Also frequent are dolichoectatic arteriopathies, which may lead in some cases to the formation of gigantic aneurysms (Fig. 4.9). In these usually older patients with multiple risk factors of an arteriosclerotic nature they can lead to numerous local and remote symptoms, possibly by obstruction of the aqueduct.

The picture of a thrombosis of the midportion of the basilar artery often develops after several TIAs and after days or weeks of a progressive course. The parts most

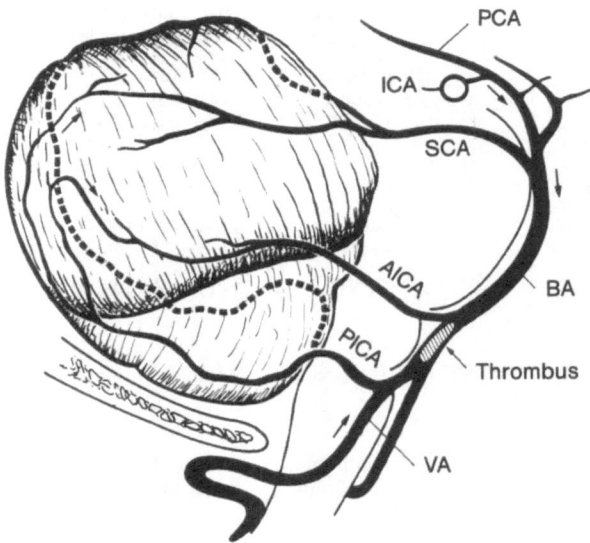

Fig. 4.10. Diagram of a segmental occlusion of the basilar artery with collateral circulation via the cerebellar arteries from the vertebral artery via the PICA to the AICA and SCA. In addition, collaterals exist via the ICA and the arterial circle to the rostral basilar artery. *BA,* Basilar artery; *VA,* vertebral artery; *PICA,* posterior inferior cerebellar artery; *AICA,* anterior inferior cerebellar artery; *SCA,* superior cerebellar artery; *ICA,* internal carotid; *PCA,* posterior cerebral artery. (From Caplan 1988)

commonly affected are the paramedian and basal portions of the mesencephalon and pons, provided the lateral and rostral portions of the region of the corpora quadrigemina can still be supplied by collaterals (PICA-AICA or PICA-SCA) via the cerebellum and from the circle of Willis by retrograde perfusion (Fig. 4.10), or when the medulla is adequately supplied with intact vertebral arteries or anastomoses (AICA-PICA or anterior corticospinal artery–vertebral artery). Severe neurologic functional disturbance regularly occurs because of the corticospinal and corticobulbar pathways traversing the region and the extensive localization of the so-called parapontine reticular formation (PPRF), the visual motor center. Unlike hemispheric lesions, compensatory mechanisms for the bilateral lesion are not feasible so that speech and swallowing disturbances as well as hoarseness are observed as bulbar symptoms together with a tetraparesis and oculomotor disorders. In 80% of basilar occlusions there are disorders of consciousness or of the sleeping-waking rhythm.

Signs of oculomotor dysfunction are:

1. Unilateral or bilateral paresis of horizontal gaze, usually with only minor subjective double vision in unilateral and bilateral PPRF lesions or nuclear abducens pareses
2. Unilateral or bilateral internuclear ophthalmoplegias in lesions of the medial longitudinal fascicle
3. Unilateral or bilateral peripheral facial paresis due to an intra-axial lesion of the facial nerve at the genu
4. A combination of a unilateral lesion of the PPRF and rostral visual motor center (rMRF) as an expression of the one-and-a-half syndrome

Vertical gaze is undisturbed, except for a limitation of saccadic movement and optokinetic nystagmus, if the mesencephalon and rMRF are intact. If the brainstem is deafferented from the cerebral hemispheres, there develops the so-called locked-in syndrome, where communication with completely tetraplegic patients in the waking state is possible only by slow vertical eye movements. Also characteristic of unilateral or bilateral pontine lesions are rapid spontaneous downward eye movements (bilateral with horizontal gaze palsy and coma; unilateral with increased ipsilateral horizontal eye movements): the so-called ocular bobbing. Pupillomotor function is also disturbed depending on the extent of the infarct or its associated edema. Likewise, myoclonias, flexion and extension synergisms, and changes in spontaneous respiration are extremely important as signs of progression or regression of symptoms and as precursors of a threatened herniation.

A thrombus in a vertebral artery which includes the ipsilateral PICA and the vertebral confluence leads to the picture of a caudal vertebrobasilar thrombosis (modified Wallenberg's syndrome). Here there is an extensive dorsolateral medullary infarct with involvement of the spinothalamic tract, the vestibular nuclei, and the connecting path to the ipsilateral cerebellum with rotational vertigo, nausea, crossed dissociated sensory disturbance, disorders of speech and swallowing, and ataxia. There is no disturbance of consciousness initially, but not uncommonly pain is reported at the back of the head and neck on the side of the vertebral-PICA occlusion, and sometimes there is a central Horner's syndrome. Central hearing disturbances are characteristic. Occlusion at the top of the basilar artery leads to bilateral infarction of the mesencephalon, thalamus, and occipital and medial temporal lobes (Caplan 1988). The usual cause is embolism from the heart or the proximal vertebrobasilar system. Depending on the extent, duration, and collateralization, there develop very varied clinical features, with disturbances of pupillomotor and oculomotor function and of consciousness, with disturbances of the sleeping-waking rhythm, somnolence, and stupor but also productive symptoms such as hallucinations, confabulation, and psychoses. Ischemia of the subthalamic nucleus can lead to involuntary movements with hemiballismus, as seen also in lesions of the thalamus and corpus striatum.

The different types of basilar thromboses can be distinguished clinically, pathogenetically, and neurophysiologically (Hacke 1986). Occlusions of the large circumferential arteries (PICA, AICA, SCA) due to atheroma or thrombi of the connected vertebral and basilar arteries are less common than infarcts due to lesions of the short penetrating arteries, but they are not clinically distinguishable. The symptoms are extremely variable because of the nonuniform collateralization. In the classical constellation the features of neurologic deficit in the territory of the AICA resemble those of lateral medullary infarction (territory of the PICA). Instead of the cranial nerves IX and X, the cranial nerves VII and VIII are affected because the ischemia extends further rostrally. The SCA shows anatomic variants less often than any other branch of the vertebrobasilar vascular territory. Isolated occlusions are less common than combinations with distal basilar embolisms. In the few cases reported in the literature (Adams 1943; Luhan and Pollock 1953) there is an emphasis on the absence of crossed dissociated sensory disturbances due to the position of the infarct above the spinal tract and the sensory trigeminal nucleus, and on the addition of involuntary ipsilateral arm movements and dysmetrias.

4.1.2.4 Penetrating End-Arteries

The lacunar infarcts already mentioned in connection with subcortical hemisphere infarcts are also very common in the brainstem. They arise as the consequence of embolic occlusions of small end-arteries and are usually multiple. They are also found in pathologic examinations without a history suggestive of cerebrovascular symptoms. Other preferential sites outside the brainstem are the thalamus and lentiform nucleus. Various clinical syndromes, most of them described by Fisher, are characteristic and are summarized in Table 4.4. These can occasionally be demonstrated by CT or MRI, but small parenchymatous defects escape detection even using these methods. Demonstration and topographic analysis can be achieved to an increased extent by

Table 4.4. Important types of lacunar infarction

Name of syndrome	Site
Pure motor stroke	Internal capsule, brainstem
Pure sensory stroke	Thalamus, brainstem
Sensorimotor stroke	Internal capsule with thalamus
Dysarthria/clumsy hand syndrome	Brainstem (rarely lentiform nucleus)
Ataxic motor syndrome	Brainstem (with brachium conjunctivum)

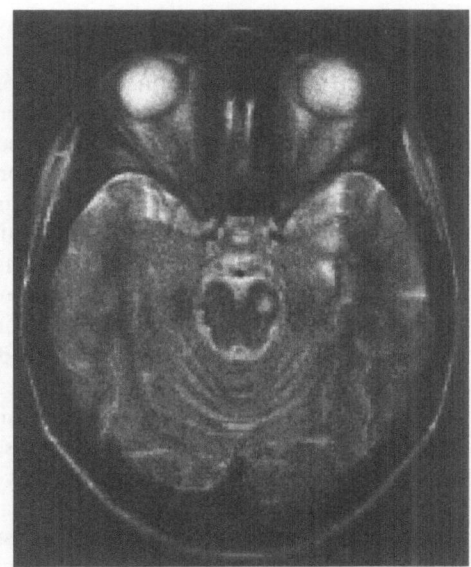

Fig. 4.11. Lacunar lesion in brainstem close to left crus cerebri in a pure motor stroke

selecting the investigational parameters in MRI appropriately and by using additional computer programs for three-dimensional reconstruction (Fig. 4.11). Clinically silent foci are often detected in this manner. On the other hand, characteristic clinical deficits are often not associated with corresponding features in the structural representation. A series of subcortical infarcts also constitutes a serious problem for the clinician, for they are often difficult to diagnose. In the pure sensory stroke dysesthesia and pain may dominate the clinical picture but without objective signs by formal testing of sensation. Abnormal findings with neurophysiologic techniques may be extremely helpful in these situations (see Sect. 5.4.2).

A series of unusual syndromes have been sporadically described in the literature, for example, pure dysarthrias.

Important factors in differential diagnosis include:

1. A preexisting hypertension
2. Usually, absence of TIAs before the stroke
3. Fluctuating development of the symptoms over several days without disorders of consciousness

Best known are the pure motor and pure sensory hemisyndromes, usually sparing the face, as well as the dysarthria/clumsy hand syndrome with minor dysarthria and disturbance of intrinsic motor function in the hand, homolateral ataxia with distal lower limb paresis, and Weber's or Claude's syndrome (see Table 4.3) in lesions of the paramedian mesencephalic arteries.

4.1.2.5 Posterior Cerebral Artery

Emboli are the most common cause of posterior infarcts. These are usually due to cardiac sources of emboli or proximal vascular lesions of the cerebral arteries, but in one-third of patients the cause remains obscure (Pessin et al. 1987). In addition to the occipital lobes and large parts of the temporal lobes, the PCA also supplies the rostral brainstem and the thalamus via a series of proximally originating arteries (Fig. 4.3). A characteristic syndrome of a posterior infarct is homonymous visual field defect, whose form and expression may be useful in localizing the lesion. In infarcts in the territory of the calcarine artery the exact extent of the visual field limitation (with or without a macular fissure) can be determined clinically with a white or red hatpin; however, there are usually no visual field defects in infarcts of the visual association areas (parietal and parietotemporal arteries). Sometimes these are not even reported by the patients, especially if the nondominant hemisphere is affected. A series of complex neuropsychological functional disorders are to be noted in this context and can be easily overlooked if not specifically sought (see p. 110 ff.).

Patients with calcarine infarcts experience a usually gray defect and restriction of their visual field; possibly via a primitive visual center, they develop compensatory mechanisms to reduce their spatial handicap. Optokinetic nystagmus is usually impaired to the contralateral; visual evoked potentials show asymmetries. In contrast, patients with visual neglect have no subjective visual field defect but do not recognize objects, writing, or pictures. Optokinetic nystagmus is often less markedly impaired. Visual hallucinations or illusions occur particularly in patients with infarcts in the nondominant hemisphere and may consist of amorphous bright-dark contrasts, colors, shapes, structures, and sometimes patterns and scenic experiences. These may result in agitated states which are misinterpreted as delirium or psychosis. Even if it is not possible to study the visual field in these patients using the latest refinements in technique, such misdiagnoses should always be avoided by considering the possibility of a homonymous hemianopia. Extremely helpful is the demonstration of a reduced optokinetic nystagmus, which can be examined even in patients with disturbed consciousness. Visual perseverations or metamorphopsias (bent or twisted objects) are less common. With lesions of the dominant hemisphere, uncommon disconnection syndromes are also described, such as pure alexia with retention of the ability to speak and write and with or without disorders of color naming when color discrimination is preserved. The thalamic branches may be affected, depending on the site of the thrombosis at the origin of the PCA, with resulting sensorimotor and ataxic disturbances (see Table 4.2).

Disorders of memory, amnesic and transcortical sensory aphasias, visual agnosias and apraxias, and prosopagnosias are uncommon and frequently indicative of bilateral cerebral infarcts; however, they occasionally also appear in extensive infarcts with damage to the hippocampal region, the thalamus, and subcortical connecting pathways. Involvement of the often unilaterally placed basilar communicating artery often leads to severe memory disorders (Sect. 4.1.1.2). Transient global amnesia (Feuer and Weinberger 1987) is a special form and is often ascribed to bilateral disorders of the hippocampal circulation; to what extent this is true and whether vascular changes in the carotid or vertebrobasilar circulation involving the PCA play a role is as yet undecided.

The interpretation of transient global amnesia as a local circulatory disturbance in the vertebrobasilar territory encounters considerable difficulties. Müller and Mase (1981) postulate a hypoplasia or occlusion of the anterior choroidal artery, which normally supplies the hippocampus together with the posterior choroidal artery. If a critical fall in pressure occurs in the latter, the anterior choroidal artery can substitute as an anastomosis if its anatomic disposition is normal. There are no appropriate angiographic-anatomic studies in the literature, but these authors published data from some of the patients whom they had carefully investigated which support their hypothesis. On the other hand, it is still undecided whether bilateral disturbance of hippocampal function is required for the development of transient global amnesia, or whether unilateral lesions may also account for the disturbance of verbal memory.

An analysis by Müller (1989) of eight representative studies on 122 patients calculated the risk of recurrence as 3.4% per year. Within a mean follow-up period of 5 years a further recurrence followed the first in one-fifth of the patients studied, and two or more episodes occurred in one-tenth of them. In contrast, the risk of stroke proved not to be raised in comparison with a population matched for age and sex, and life expectancy was not diminished. Verbal memory disorders may be observed as persistent deficits, even after a single episode of amnesia.

4.2 Pathogenetic Aspects

4.2.1 Arteriosclerosis

Arteriosclerotic lesions of the extra- and intracranial arteries of the brain constitute the most common cause of stroke. Epidemiologic studies have paid attention to the influence of risk factors in general and in cerebrovascular diseases in particular (Caplan et al. 1986; Yatsu 1986). These confirm the general experience of a usually multifactorial interaction of hypertension, diabetes mellitus, reduced serum levels of HDL cholesterol, nicotine abuse, and obesity in arteriosclerosis of the coronary arteries or coronary heart disease, but show only a loose association with vascular lesions of the cerebral arteries or with TIAs and insults. There is no definite knowledge of the pathogenetic mechanisms which might explain this difference. One important exception consists of the special form of chronic hypertension which leads to high-grade constrictions of the arterioles and very small arteries (50–200 µm in diameter). Not uncommonly there exist obscure or intensively treated severe renal diseases (dialysis, renal transplantation) which themselves promote the arteriosclerotic process.

Unlike arteriosclerosis of the large cerebral arteries, for whose development raised blood pressure seems of little significance, the vessel wall of the penetrating, small-caliber end-arteries is thickened by the long-term deposition of hyalin, amorphous lipid products, and fibrin (fibrinoid necrosis). In the territories supplied by such arteries lacunar infarcts develop which are of primary hemodynamic origin or are, occasionally, due to other mechanisms, such as secondary to embolic occlusion. Also, microaneurysms are often found at the sites of division of the small cerebral arteries and may cause subcortical hemorrhages which are difficult to separate from primary ischemic lesions by presently available brain imaging techniques. Other risk factors may also be related to cerebral ischemia with sufficient confidence; severe changes in lipid metabolism (e. g., in hetero- and homozygotic LDL receptor anomalies, which are now treatable by plasma separation and drug therapy) can lead to severe coronary arteriosclerosis and secondarily to cerebral emboli. Complication of coronary arteriosclerosis is also recognized with other heart diseases as a risk indicator of cerebral ischemia, with embolic mechanisms being more common than hemodynamic factors (e.g., arrhythmias, valve lesions, cardiomyopathy, cardiac surgery with air embolism or secondary hypoxia after resuscitation).

Still undecided is the pathogenetic relevance to cerebral ischemia of a number of other factors such as climatic changes, changes in the composition of drinking water, lack of mobility, and oral contraceptives. The significance of these in the development of venous circulatory disorders is now recognized, but the risk of arterial ischemia is markedly increased only in combination with nicotine abuse and before menopause. A number of still quite hypothetic mechanisms have been suggested as other factors. Some authors believe, for example that increased alcohol abuse has a damaging effect due to secondarily increased blood pressure. Acute intoxications are said to lead to changes in fibrinolysis, while stress factors may influence immunoregulatory cells (macrophage function) via autonomic and hormonal effectors and could lead to disturbances of lipid metabolism. The significance of obesity in the pathogenesis of cerebral ischemia is seen today as being an aspect only of secondary hypertension or diabetic metabolic disturbance.

Two theories have been proposed for the development of arteriosclerosis of the large cerebral arteries: the lipid theory favors a disorder of cholesterol metabolism (Brown et al. 1981; Yatsu and Loeb 1981), whereas Ross and Glomset (1976) underline the importance of initial endothelial damage, with the reparative mechanisms that follow determining the course of the disease. The two hypotheses appear to complement each other and probably emphasize temporarily differing aspects of a complex pathogenetic process.

Pathologic, angiographic, and – in recent years – various ultrasound studies have provided a range of important data about the frequency and distribution of extracranial arteriosclerotic vascular lesions in particular; the influence of numerous risk factors and indicators has been discussed, such as that of age and sex in the development of cerebrovascular events (Adams and van der Eecken 1953; Hutchinson and Yates 1957; Whisnant et al. 1961; Torvik and Jörgenson 1964; Fisher et al. 1965a, b; Hass et al. 1968; Blackwood et al. 1969; Toole et al. 1975; Hennerici et al. 1981; Kunitz et al. 1984). The following is a summary of the information obtained in these studies:

1. Arteriosclerosis affects the carotids in the neck sustantially more often than the vertebral arteries and the intracranial vessels. Local geometric and hemodynamic factors in addition to the general pathomechanisms already mentioned are probably responsible (Hennerici et al. 1986).
2. The extent and degree of the carotid lesions increase with age; men are affected in the 4th and 5th decades, women usually only toward the end of the 6th decade. Even now, surprisingly little is known about the dynamics and topography of these lesions; because of the lack of long-term noninvasive studies the frequency and importance of reparative mechanisms have been considerably underestimated. Experimental data and the findings in new prospective studies in man show that

regressive or healing phases occur spontaneously in arteriosclerosis of the carotid system in up to 20% of cases (DePalma et al. 1970; Malinow 1984; Hennerici et al. 1985; Norris and Bornstein 1986; Ehringer et al. 1987).

3. Carotid occlusions most frequently occur at the extracranial bifurcation, seldom more distally. If flow impairment exceeds 80%–90% of luminal narrowing, an anterograde thrombosis may develop that extends intracranially into the carotid siphon and further into the basal cerebral arteries to give the picture of a progressive stroke (Little et al. 1980), or emboli may be released into the large cerebral arteries (occlusio-supra-occlusionem, artery-to-artery embolism). Subtotal carotid occlusion (also known as pseudo-occlusion of the ICA) is not always demonstrable using Doppler sonography if a small signal originating from the remaining flow is missed. In such cases selective intra-arterial angiography is required (Countee and Vijayanathan 1979). Further imaging of the collateral carotid system is useful to display the collateralization, but supraocclusional embolism can also be studied. Sometimes retrograde filling of the proximal carotid siphon is demonstrable, which can be taken as a separate, exceptional indication for operation of an ICA occlusion. The question of systemic fibrinolysis is also relevant in this context and forms the basis of several ongoing studies. In these cases the caroticotympanic artery and a further branch of the ICA to the pterygoid canal remain patent (Paullus et al. 1977).

4. In about one-fourth of patients with carotid occlusion there are marked stenoses of another cervical artery, often on the opposite side (Fisher et al. 1965; Hennerici et al. 1981; Hutchinson and Yates 1957). The next most common preferential site, the carotid siphon, quite often shows relatively flat calcifications as early forms of arteriosclerosis, but high-grade stenoses are uncommon, possibly because of the more favorable hemodynamic situation. Only three studies have been published on the spontaneous course of siphon stenoses, the symptoms of which differ from those encountered in extracranial vascular lesions (Craig et al. 1982; Marzewski et al. 1982; Wechsler et al. 1986; see Table 4.1).

5. Carotid occlusions and stenoses are often asymptomatic. Diagnosis of such patients has been increasing, particularly since the introduction of noninvasive ultrasound techniques and in patients with previously recognized peripheral or coronary vascular disease. These patients are generally found to have well-preserved distal collaterals via the anterior or posterior circle of Willis, whereas the ophthalmic anastomosis plays only a subordinate role (Fisher et al. 1965a; Hennerici et al. 1982, 1987; Powers et al. 1987; Rautenberg and Hennerici 1988).

6. The frequency and clinical significance of a hemorrhage into a preformed arteriosclerotic bed have given rise to controversy in the literature. Imparato et al. (1979) found a high prevalance in symptomatic carotid lesions and therefore regarded such changes as reliable indicators of a threatened or actually completed cerebrovascular event; this had been disputed by several earlier authors (Fisher et al. 1965a; Bornstein et al. 1990). Up to now the imaging ultrasound techniques have not proven capable of distinguishing reliably between hemorrhages and other morphologic changes in the vessel wall (Hennerici 1987).

7. In advanced stages of arteriosclerosis the common and internal carotid arteries in the upper part of the neck may also be involved in the vascular process, but high-grade stenoses are rare.

8. Ulcerative lesions and irregular surface conditions of plaque formation are common throughout the carotid system (18% in an autopsy study by Fisher et al. 1965 a) but may heal spontaneously (Hennerici et al. 1985). Their significance as potential sources of emboli or residues of past embolization remain as obscure as their possible capacity to be influenced by drug treatment.

9. Epidemiologic investigations in the black and white populations of the United States by Caplan et al. (1986) have shown that supraclinoid lesions of the ICA occur significantly more often in blacks than in whites (Gorelick et al. 1984). These data confirm the gross pathologic studies of earlier years (McGill et al. 1968) and show similarities to findings from Japan and China which report a predilection for vascular lesions in the intracranial portion of the ICA and its end-branches (ACA and MCA) in Asian populations (Mitsuyama et al. 1979).

Several studies carried out on animal models have produced encouraging results regarding the regression of experimental arteriosclerosis after the return to a normal or hypocaloric diet either alone or in combination with various drugs (see Hennerici 1990). In contrast, pathoanatomic, epidemiologic, and clinical studies in man on this subject are by no means univocal. Those arguing in favor of regression in man note (a) the capacity of arteries to adapt and to recover from previous lesions, (b) the inflammatory rather than degenerative nature of arteriosclerosis, (c) the slow and variable course of the disease from its onset in early infancy to senescence, and (d) the encouraging results of animal experiments and recently of plasmapheresis in homo- and heterozygous patients with LDL receptor abnormalities. Pessimists stress (a) the inaccessibility of the lipid material and cell detritus in the core of the plaque to humoral and cellular recovery mechanisms, (b) the lack of methods to monitor adequately the course of the disease in vivo, as well as the limited usefulness of criteria to establish regression in man, and (c) the inadequacy of the transmission of results from animal studies to man.

Suggested mechanisms of regression of atherogenesis are summarized in Table 4.5. At present even positive reports tend to suggest a reduced progression of arteriosclerosis rather than a real regression of established plaques. Since there is no solid evidence that regression of human arteriosclerosis really takes place, it cannot be assessed or separated from other mechanisms leading to the restoration of intra-arterial circulation. On the other hand, regression of intimal lesions (even of advanced stages) is well documented in different animals and appears to be more frequent than "healing." Further detailed morphometric work is necessary to validate these findings. This is particularly true for studies performed in humans, the designs of which have hitherto been too limited to allow any definite conclusion. Research in this field has been greatly hampered by the difficulty in monitoring arteriosclerosis sequentially in prospective long-term follow-up series, qualitative rather than quantitative angiography being the only method for the investigation of the blood vessels. This method is also far from ideal because it provides no data on structural changes in the arterial wall. Since the risks associated even with digital subtraction techniques continue to restrict the performance of repeat angiograms to cases with significant clinical indications, noninvasive methods such as Doppler sonography, ultrasound echotomography, and in particular flow color-coded Doppler (Steinke et al. 1990 a, b) imaging may provide more significant results. These methods can easily be adapted

Table 4.5. Classification of atherogenesis and suggested mechanisms of regression

Stages	Pathology	Mechanisms
Initial phase	Fatty streaks	Cholesterol depletion Inhibition of immunomediated processes
	Lipid plaques	Endothelial recovery, reduction of macrophage/monocyte-generating toxic metabolites Lipid elimination from smooth muscle cells and macrophages
		Inhibition of platelet function
	Fibrous plaques	Smooth muscle cell atrophy and loss of proliferation Intimal thinning Cholesterol efflux and transport
		Restructuring with loss of foam cells
		Lipophagocytosis
Advanced phase	Soft plaques	Disintegration of cells Breakdown of extracellular space
		Resolution of cell necrosis Monocyte enzyme activity, lipolysis
		Loss of foam cells
	Hard plaques	Vessel ectasia and dilation
Complications	Thrombosis	Intraplaque hemorrhage resolution
		Plaque disrupture and reendothelialization
	Embolic occlusion	Eicosanoid activity and fibrinolysis

technically to monitor atherogenesis in general at the carotid bifurcation. Refined techniques are producing promising tools for future studies in humans on mechanisms involved in regression or reduced progression in vivo. The functional significance of these developments needs to be further illuminated before their clinical implications can be ascertained.

4.2.2 Arterial Dissection

In recent years, dissections of the extracranial carotid artery and to some extent those of the vertebral artery have been increasingly diagnosed as the cause of TIAs and strokes (Hart 1988). After the first description by Jentzer (1954) sporadic cases were reported in which a traumatic or spontaneous origin of the dissection was debated (Hart and Easton 1986). With improvements in angiographic technique, the introduction of noninvasive methods for the demonstration of extracranial vascular processes and especially by increased attention to the characteristic clinical signs, an increasing number of cases have been diagnosed in recent years. This has led to a marked change regarding the suspected prognosis of this clinical picture; in contrast to earlier assumptions of a high mortality, recent reports show that the majority of patients have a favorable prognosis and sometimes complete restoration of health (Marx et al. 1987). The exact prevalence of this disease state is still unknown, but estimates range up to 5% of all ischemic strokes in young adults (under 45 years); 70% of all patients collected by Hart and Easton (1986) were between 35 and 50, and there was no sex-related predisposition. Pathogenetically, following an as yet obscure triggering mechanism, there is a hemorrhage into the vessel wall, of which various types exist: with intimal dissection there is a marked narrowing of the vessel lumen, whereas with intramedial or subadventitial dissection there may be dilation with or without pseudoaneurysm formation and simultaneous irritation of the sympathetic plexus. While in many patients the time interval (hours or days) after a preceding trivial injury may be impressive, there have not as yet been any clear differential criteria between spontaneous dissection and the so-called traumatic form, especially as severe trauma is very uncommon. Suggested predisposing parameters are usually so-called textural disorders of the nature of Marfan's syndrome or fibromuscular dysplasia, which are present, however, in only up to 15% of patients with carotid dissection.

Still obscure with regard to etiopathogenesis are the cases reported in earlier literature which certainly resemble the clinical and angiographic picture after dissection of the carotid artery, but without intramural hemorrhage or other deficits in the pathologic-anatomic substrate found upon operation (an operation previously performed frequently). Especially when there is a history pointing to vasomotor headaches and migraine attacks, these cases arouse the suspicion that functional spasmodic mechanisms also play a role.

The diagnosis of a dissection is likely from the history and the clinical picture if there is unilateral pain at the back of the head and in the neck with or without Horner's syndrome (oculosympathetic form) or with delayed appearance of focal ischemic symptoms (focal form). The forms may overlap in individual patients, with the characteristic pain predominating in over 90% of patients (Mokri et al. 1986). The 146 cases collected by Hart and Easton from the literature often presented with unilateral pain in the back of the head and in the neck (79%), associated with a partial Horner's syndrome (49%), a TIA (45%), or a stroke (33%).

At Doppler sonography, the usual initial finding is that an extensive, abnormal "to-and-fro" phenomenon with an orthograde and retrograde late systolic flow component in the ICA after an early, systolic, cranially directed, low-flow signal (Fig. 4.12; Hennerici et al. 1989). This phenomenon, produced by the raised vascular resistance over a long extent, is observable in the entire region of a dissection of the carotid segment in the neck. If, in addition, the ultrasound examination shows the characteristic constriction with the appearance of a long "dunce cap" of the vessel lumen above the bifurcation and/or partially thrombosed blood in the vessel wall itself, the diagnosis can be made as reliably as by angiography. The combined use of angiography and MRI scans, allowing direct display of the wall hematoma, provides a safe and completely noninvasive access to the diagnosis in many cases. From the therapeutic aspect, angiography can then be postponed, with the particular aim of obtaining improved angiographic demonstration of pseudoaneurysmal changes after reopening

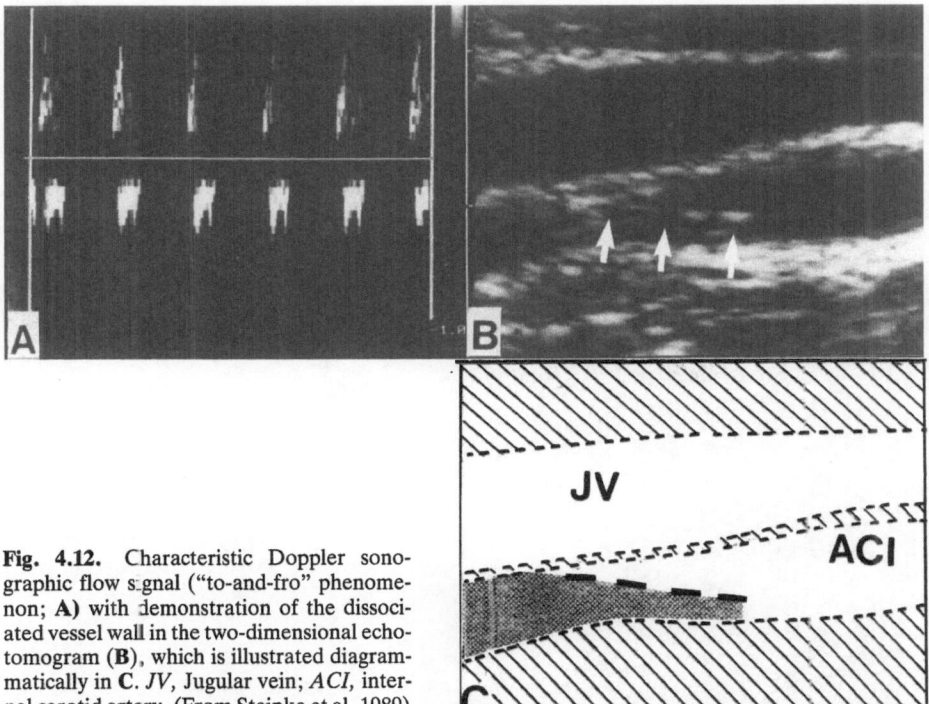

Fig. 4.12. Characteristic Doppler sono-graphic flow signal ("to-and-fro" phenome-non; **A)** with demonstration of the dissoci-ated vessel wall in the two-dimensional echo-tomogram (**B**), which is illustrated diagram-matically in **C**. *JV,* Jugular vein; *ACI,* inter-nal carotid artery. (From Steinke et al. 1989)

of the vessel lumen. These pseudoaneurysms, often in a submandibular position, can worsen the prognosis as sources for embolism and should therefore raise the question of operative treatment. The characteristic radiologic findings are shown in Fig. 4.13. Occlusions of the ICA were found in 17% of the series studied by Mokri et al. (1986) and in 38% of that studied by Biller et al. (1986). The rate of embolism was given as 14% and 18%, respectively.

Noninvasive methods of investigation also permit prospective studies of the treatment of this syndrome. In addition to surgical measures with removal of the hematoma, arterial resection, occlusion of the distal extracranial section of the ICA, and insertion of an extracranial-intracranial (EC-IC) bypass, conservative methods of treatment have been tried, initially by intravenous heparin and/or calcium antagonist infusion and subsequently by coumarin therapy or platelet-aggregation inhibitors. In particu-lar, the time interval between the beginning and the end of an anticoagulant regime could be better regulated by means of noninvasive monitoring techniques. However, any mode of treatment must take into account for the high rate of spontaneous recovery; Hart and Easton (1986) found 70% of patients with good regression, and 14% had only minor residues.

Vertebral artery dissections are less common but resemble carotid dissections clinically and angiographically; a review based on over 100 published cases was presented recently by Hart (1988). It is possible that these constitute a cause of disorders of the posterior circulation in young adults that is frequently overlooked or

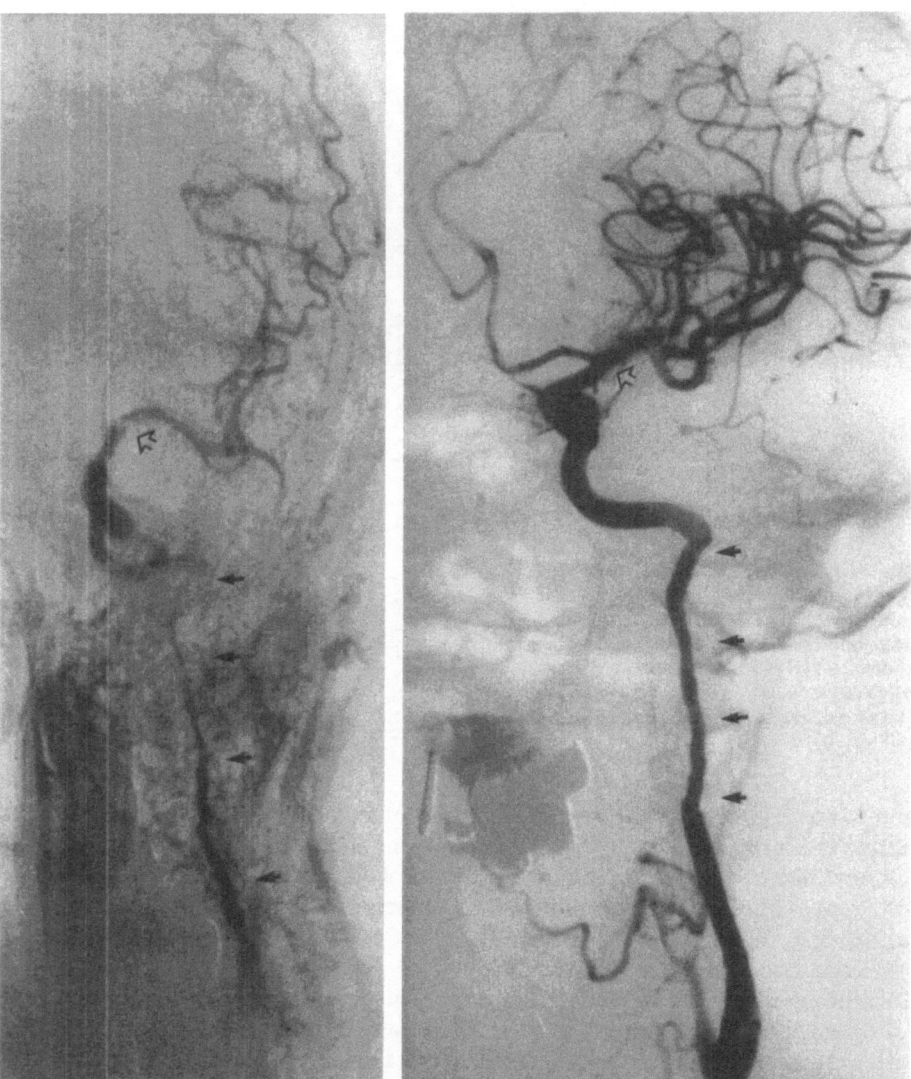

Fig. 4.13. Arteriogram of a carotid dissection in a 17-year-old with recurrent TIAs. The first study (*left*) shows a typical "dunce cap" tapering band of contrast up to the skull base (string sign). Control examination (*right*) after 3 weeks showed marked regression of the stenosis and considerable recanalization. Note the associated improvement in the intracranial hemodynamics; initially no contrast entered the anterior cerebral artery

not recognized in the angiogram. It is important to distinguish these from strokes in migraine patients and from thromboembolism, which constitute the chief causes of infarction in this age group. Not uncommonly they present with the picture of a lateral medullary infarct or an inferior brainstem syndrome. They frequently affect the proximal third of the vertebral artery and occur spontaneously or are produced traumatically in chiropractic maneuvers. They should also be considered in so-called whiplash injuries of the neck with brainstem symptoms; a free interval of some hours or days from the triggering mechanism is particularly striking, even if in the individual case the connection cannot be established beyond doubt, especially in trivial injuries. An accumulation of bilateral vertebral dissections in the context of fibromuscular dysplasia (FMD) has repeatedly been described.

In addition to hemodynamic mechanisms, thromboembolic complications must also play a role, as in pseudoaneurysms. As with carotid dissection, pain at the back of the head and neck occurs at the onset and determines the clinical picture; fluctuating symptoms over weeks and months up to the climax of the disorder are not uncommon. With intracranial extension and subadventitial hemorrhage there may be pressure symptoms and subarachnoid bleeding (10% of all cases). The spontaneous course is determined by the neurologic deficit; the frequently irregular and extensive stenoses with pseudoaneurysms can undergo spontaneous regression. The diagnosis is made by angiography. Some 85% regress spontaneously within 2–3 months, and recurrences are rare (less than 3%).

Intracranial arterial dissection appears to be much less common, and the clinical symptoms deviate from those of the extracranial form. The patients are generally younger (around 25 years), the dissection usually takes place in the subintimal layer of the vessel wall, and the prognosis is markedly worse because of the localization of these vascular lesions and the limited possibilities of collateralization. Traumatic mechanisms may play a greater role, although this may be purely a selection artifact due to the diagnosis being exclusively angiographic. MRI angiography may provide a new access to the diagnosis of this type of dissection.

4.2.3 Fibromuscular Dysplasia

In 1938 Leadbetter and Burkland reported a case of FMD with hypertension and renal artery stenosis in a boy aged 5 years. The first patient with this unusual vascular disease outside the renal arteries was a clinically asymptomatic woman with the characteristic angiographic signs of FMD of the extracranial ICA (Palubinskas and Ripley 1964). In 1965, Connett and Lanche attempted operative treatment for the first time, and Morris et al. in 1968 described arterial dilation as a principle of treatment. The pathogenesis and treatment of this disorder have as yet not been clarified beyond doubt (see review by Healton 1986). Basically, there is a structural anomaly of the vessel wall, particularly affecting the tunica media. This shows a connective tissue proliferation, with or without hyperplasia of the smooth muscle cells, which form concentric rings. This is the most common type of FMD (90%), and it can also occur in the intima or adventitia with an irregular dilation and multifocal stenoses in the adjacent arterial segments.

Rupture of the vessel wall may lead to arterial dissection; arteriovenous fistulae, aneurysms, or combinations of these may develop (Fig. 4.14). The incidence of FMD as evidenced by large angiographic studies is between 0.53% and 6.8%; bilateral manifestations occur in about 60%. The clinical presentation is inconclusive and may reflect ischemic stroke, intracranial hemorrhages, or an entirely asymptomatic course. In a series of 349 patients collected from the literature, Healton (1986)

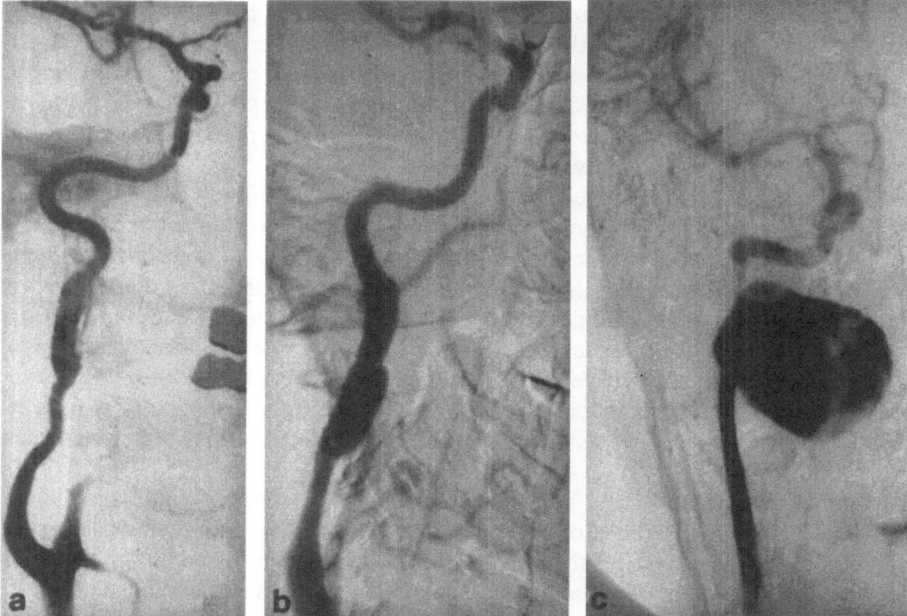

Fig. 4.14. Arteriograms of pseudoaneurysms in patients with spontaneous dissection of the carotid artery based on a fibromuscular dysplasia (**a**), with traumatic dissection (**b**), and in a mycotic aneurysm (**c**). All the patients were operated on for recurrent focal ischemias, and the preoperative diagnoses were histologically confirmed

reported cerebral infarct in 15%, TIA in 33%, and atypical symptoms and intracranial aneurysms in 13% each. In 24% of patients the diagnosis was made by chance during angiographic examination for other reasons. There is a clear predominance of the disease in women (87%) of middle age, although the reason for this is unknown. The spontaneous course of the disease is obscure, but its prognosis appears favorable even without treatment. The relatively low stroke rate argues for conservative management and against operative treatment – at least in the asymptomatic stage.

Special attention should be paid to meticulous control of blood pressure, and a search should always be made for coexisting renal artery stenosis. The indications for neurosurgical intervention with large intracranial aneurysms do not differ from those applying to other aneurysms.

4.2.4 Arteritis

The clinical picture of cerebral arteritis is extremely variable and depends on both the etiology and the affected vascular territories. Arteritis may occur in a connective tissue disease or in disease mediated by immune complexes, for instance, in panarteritis nodosa, systemic lupus erythematosus, dermatomyositis, Wegener's granulomatosis, allergic angiitis (e.g., Churg-Strauss syndrome), or Takayasu's arteritis (Berlit et al. 1983; Levine and Welch 1989; Hankey 1991). Less common are infective granulomatous arteritis in syphilis, tuberculosis, malaria, or fungal infections. The appearance of antiphospholipid antibodies (lupus coagulant and anticardiolipin antibodies) is associated with an immunologically mediated inflammatory vascular disease; in addition, however, hemostaseology is also affected. The occurrence of antiphospholipid antibodies is associated with an increased risk of thrombosis (Levine and Welch 1987, 1989).

Pararheumatic disorders (e. g., Reiter's syndrome, Sjögren's syndrome, Melkersson-Rosenthal syndrome) as well as etiologically quite different types of diseases such as thrombangitis obliterans, Sneddon's syndrome (see Sect. 4.2.6), or Moya-Moya disease may present with arteritis. Usually arterioles and capillaries are affected and the large arteries (carotid and vertebral system) spared. However, this does not apply to Takayasu's disease, giant cell arteritis, or Moya-Moya disease, which affect primarily the main extra- and intracranial arteries. Purely intracranial arteritis may evade even angiographic depiction of all the cerebral arteries; this diagnosis is suggested in the presence of multilocular and segmental vascular interruptions and segmental narrowings. Although the laboratory findings may provide important diagnostic tools (Table 4.6), cerebral artery biopsy may be necessary to establish the diagnosis in the pure cerebral forms.

Giant cell arteritis, also known as temporal or cranial arteritis, is an inflammatory vascular disease of older patients. A generalized vasculitis centered on the region of the extracranial carotid system is characteristic. Histologically, the disease process is evidenced by inflammatory infiltration and granuloma formation in the media with fibrosis and intimal proliferation, followed by vascular stenosis and thrombosis. The etiology remains unclear, but paraneoplastic and various immune-mediated mechanisms have been suggested. Clinically, there is headache with dysesthesia of the face and head, fever, loss of weight, and a tendency to apathy, fatigue, and loss of concentration at the onset of the disease. The temporal arteries are frequently swollen and pulseless; polymyalgia rheumatica may precede the disease by several years. Visual impairment occurs as the leading complication with a 40%–50% incidence in large series, without previous TIAs, due to thrombosis of the posterior ciliary arteries or the central retinal artery, which sometimes characterizes the beginning of the disease.

Moreover, other cerebral and spinal cord arteries may be included in the disease process and lead to severe neurologic deficits often with little tendency to regression. Even the carotid siphon is often markedly affected. Thromboses sometimes extend in retrograde fashion into the cervical segment of the carotid system and frequently lead to complication. The ESR is markedly increased in many patients but may also be normal. Even biopsy of the temporal artery may yield completely unremarkable results (one-third of cases), especially when steroid medication (a single low dose is sufficient) has already been started. The most important therapeutic measure is immunosuppressive treatment with corticosteroids and azathioprine in adequate dosage until normalization of the subjective clinical picture and the raised ESR, and this should be continued without interruption. Premature reduction of the steroid dose leads not uncommonly to fatal complications.

Moya-Moya disease was first observed by Takeuchi and Shimitsu in 1955. It was originally thought to be a disease limited to Japan, but clusters of the disease were

Table 4.6. Laboratory findings in the vasculitides. (Modified from Berlit et al. 1983)

	Pan-arteritis nodosa	Lupus erythematosus	Rheumatoid arthritis	Temporal arteritis	Allergic granulomatosis	Wegener's granulomatosis	Thromboangitis obliterans
Blood							
Increased ESR	++	++	++	+++	++	+++	∅−+
Eosinophilia	++	∅	∅	∅	+++	+	∅
C-reactive protein	++	+	++	+	+	++	++
Antinuclear factors	∅	+++	+++	∅−+	∅	∅	∅
Rheumatic factor	++	++	+++	∅	+	+	∅
Antielastin titer	∅−++	∅−++	∅	∅	∅	∅	+++
Circulating immune complexes	+	+	+		∅	+	+
Immunoglobulins							
IgA	↑↑↑	Normal	↑←←	Normal	Normal	↑↑	Normal
IgG	Normal	↑↑↑	←	←	Normal	→	Normal
IgM	Normal	Normal	Normal	←	Normal	↑↑	Normal
IgE	Normal	Normal	Normal	Normal	↑↑		↑↑
Complement							
C3	↓↓→	↓↓↓→	Normal	↑↑	Normal	Normal	Normal
C4	→		Normal	∅/++	Normal	Normal	↑↑
HBs antigen/anti-HBs	+++	∅	∅	∅	∅	∅	∅
DNA antibodies	∅	+	+	∅	∅	∅	∅
CSF							
Cell increase	++	+	∅	∅	+	∅−+	+
Protein increase	++	++	++	+	+	∅−+	+
Eosinophilia	∅−+	∅	∅	∅	+−++	∅	∅
Tissue							
Tissue antigens	?	HLA-DR3 HLA-DR4	?	HLA-B8 A10	?	HLA-DR2	HLA-B8 HLA-B12
Positive immunohistology	++	++	+	+++	+	++	++
Biopsy from:	Muscle Kidney	Skin	Skin Joints	Temporal Artery	Skin	Kidney Lung	Arteries

Explanation of symbols: +++ usually present; ++ often present; + seldom present; ∅ not present; ↑↑↑ usually raised; ↑↑ or ↓↓ often raised or lowered; ↑ or ↓ seldom raised or lowered.

later found in Europe and North America. Over 1000 cases have been analyzed in detail since its first description (Gotoh 1983). The cause is unknown, although constitutional genetic factors as well as inflammatory and immune-mediated processes have been suggested. Clinically, young patients develop cerebral ischemias (TIAs and strokes), while in most older patients the clinical picture is dominated by hemorrhages and epileptic attacks. Prevalence is somewhat more common in young women. The spontaneous course varies widely and is not individually predictable. Diagnosis is made by the angiographic demonstration of high-grade stenoses of the intracranial portions of the ICA, proximal segments of the ACA and MCA, and an abnormal vascular network (rete mirabile) in the region of the skull base (Fig. 5.48). Transdural anastomoses between arteries of the extra- and intracranial supply territories have also been described. The use of platelet-aggregation inhibitors in addition to steroids has been suggested, but this treatment has not as yet been validated. It also remains unclear whether the course is favorably influenced or the risk of cerebral ischemia or hemorrhage reduced by operative measures (e.g., an EC-IC bypass or an omental transplant).

4.2.5 Dilational Arteriopathy

Not uncommonly a diffuse dilation and elongation of the vessels is the cause of TIAs and cerebral strokes. Again, embolic mechanisms play a leading role. Loop formations (kinking and coiling) are due to diffuse loss of elasticity based on arteriosclerotic lesions. Dilational vascular lesions may affect not only the vertebrobasilar territory, where they have often been reported, but also the intra- and extracranial carotid system. In addition to the structural angiographic findings, there are characteristic low-flow velocities with abnormal flow signals in the extra- and intracranial Doppler sonograms. The ectatic vascular changes can sometimes lead to formation of aneurysms (Fig. 4.9) with secondary thrombosis. Headaches and pressure symptoms on cranial nerves and the brainstem are then demonstrable due to changes in the vicinity of these sometimes space-occupying vascular lesions. In addition, there may be thromboembolic complications and less often hemorrhages (subarachnoid or parenchymatous bleeding). Even less common are nonarteriosclerotic ectasias due to other systemic disorders, for example, the expression of systemic lupus erythematosus, Marfan's syndrome, or congenital metabolic diseases (homocystinuria and the mucopolysaccharidoses, etc.).

4.2.6 Nonarteriosclerotic Vasculopathies

In addition to the previously discussed inflammatory arteriopathies, arteriosclerotic vascular lesions, dissections, and FMD, the differential diagnosis of cerebral ischemia in young adults (under 45 years) must take into consideration other causes.
Cerebral ischemia often occurs in patients with a history of migraine attacks (especially, focal migraine) despite a still obscure pathomechanism (e. g., spreading depression). A reduction in cerebral blood flow, but also luxury perfusion has repeatedly been described. In addition, it has been shown that a series of changes

affecting hemostasis develop during migraine attacks, but it has not yet been possible to decide whether these are causal or merely epiphenomenal. Besides a liberation of various platelet and macrophage metabolites, an elevation of thromboxane and platelet factor IV levels promoting platelet aggregation has been observed. It remains unclear to what extent these patients are predisposed to spasmodic vascular reactions. This has given rise to controversy about an increased risk in cerebral angiography. It is interesting in this context that an increased prevalence of migraine has been noted in nearly all published studies of carotid and vertebral artery dissection.

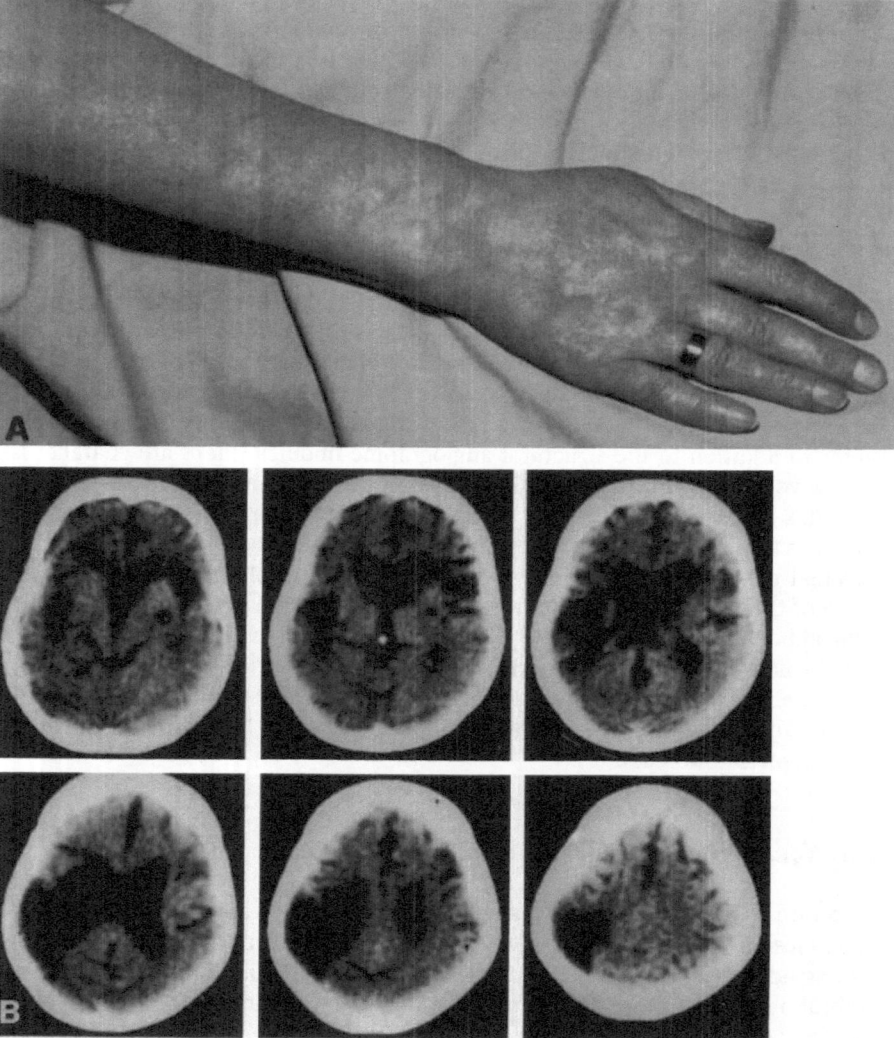

Fig. 4.15. A Typical example of Sneddon's syndrome with livedo reticularis of the skin. **B** Multiple infarcts in CT

Dermatologic disorders and their association with cerebral ischemias have been reported increasingly in recent years. The syndrome characterized by Sneddon as livedo reticularis (Fig. 4.15) with cerebral infarcts, mostly in young women, is etiologically unexplained (Burton 1988). There is a striking contrast between the often only minor neurologic deficits and the severe parenchymatous changes at CT. The only major angiographic finding is a rarefaction in the terminal flow pathway, and even very detailed laboratory studies have as yet given no clue to the pathogenesis. Skin biopsy specimens show focal intimal hyperplasias with proliferation of smooth muscle cells and isolated fibroblasts, as well as thrombotic vascular occlusions without signs of inflammation. A common disease with dermatologic manifestations is Fabry's angiokeratoma corporis diffusum (sphingolipidosis) with deposits of glycolipids in the endothelial cells of the arterioles. In addition to the vessels of the central and peripheral nervous system, the kidneys and heart are affected. Reddish brown papular lesions are found in the genital region, trunk, and thigh. The Kohlmeier-Degos syndrome also begins with a reddish papular rash on the trunk, the lesions later undergoing centrifugal white discoloration; this leads to cerebral infarction involving the small and medium arteries with hyalin formation and secondary thrombosis. Polyneuropathies and polyradiculopathies as well as gastrointestinal symptoms may also occur.

Cardiac diseases, as sources of emboli, less often via globally reduced perfusion, can lead to hypoxia and cerebral ischemia (see Sect. 5.1.5). After a myocardial infarction, and generally in the first 6 weeks, 2% of patients develop neurologic features on the basis of embolism. Patients who demonstrate an akinetic segment in the ventricular wall and those who develop an aneurysm of the heart wall have a greater permanent risk of embolism. Atrial myxoma is a rare tumor that manifests chiefly with cerebrovascular complications. Formerly, heart valve defects were the main sources of emboli, but the use of antibiotics has led to a marked decrease in defects of inflammatory origin. Thromboemboli frequently occur with advanced and often already recognized valvular disorders, whereas emboli from adhesive material in infective endocarditis may complicate the initial stage of the disease and even disguise the first clinical manifestation. Infective emboli also lead to such clinical pictures as meningitis and subarachnoid hemorrhage from septic aneurysms. Mitral valve defects and aortic stenosis, especially when associated with atrial fibrillation, constitute embolic sources and should be treated with anticoagulants. On the other hand, the significance of such conditions as mitral valve prolapse is still controversial. The initial assumption was that this is a harmless auscultatory finding with a late systolic murmur and a middiastolic click; however, data then accumulated to link ischemic cerebrovascular disorders with this condition (Barnett et al. 1980; Zenker et al. 1988). Mitral valve prolapse is based on a myxomatous degeneration of the chordae tendinae, which become overstretched and allow prolapse of the valve into the atrium during systole. Since such a prolapse can often remain asymptomatic, other pathogenetic mechanisms have been debated and investigated (Scharff et al. 1982). Besides the formation of platelet aggregates, cardiac arrhythmias probably also play an important role.

On the other hand, acute cerebral ischemia has effects on cardiac function. Disturbances due to excessive sympathetic activity with consequent ECG changes, arrhythmia, and even an increase in serum enzymes are often initially attributed to myocardial infarction and call for further differential diagnostic examinations.

Disorders of hemostasis and systemic immunologic diseases can lead to ischemia due to changes in the clotting mechanism of the blood as well as enzyme defect syndromes (deficiencies of antithrombin III, protein C, or protein S), paraproteinemias, changes in the complement system, and cryoglobulinemias. Important tests for differential diagnosis are listed in Table 5.2. Specific antibodies, circulating immunocomplexes, and activated lymphocytes can lead to endothelial lesions, as can mechanical, immunologic, chemical, or infectious noxae. Hyperlipidemia, homocystinemia, or hypoxia can produce epithelial denudation, and similar damage can be produced by bacterial or viral infections via endotoxins or immunologic mediators (Hacke et al. 1987). Many of the factors mentioned are potent stimulators of the coagulation mechanism (del Zoppo and Harker 1984). Changes in intrinsic thrombolysis based on activation of plasminogen to plasmin are also important in infarct formation and the course of the disease. Plasmin is responsible for fibrin breakdown. Plasminogen is converted into its active form by fibrin-bound tissue plasminogen activator (tPA) or by urokinase plasminogen activator (scuPA). For their part, the plasminogen activators are inhibited by a whole group of plasminogen-activator inhibitors. Thrombin catalyzes an increase in the activity of tissue plasminogen activator and a

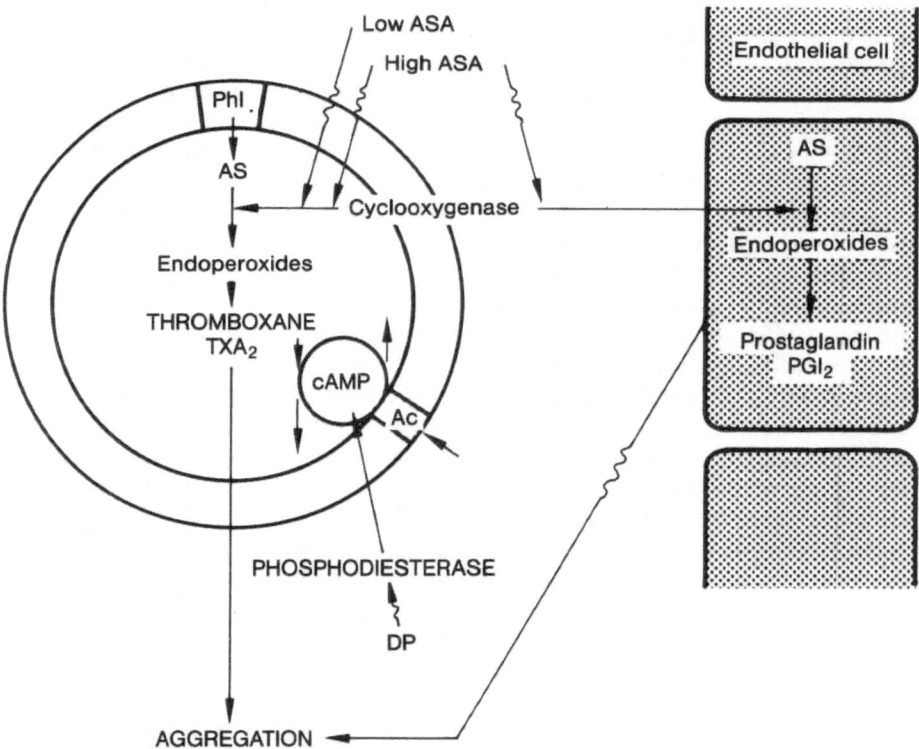

Fig. 4.16. Pharmacologic action of thrombocyte aggregation inhibitors. *ASA,* Acetylsalicylic acid; *Phl,* phospholipids; *As,* arachidonic acid; *Ac,* adenylcyclase; *cAMP,* cyclic AMP; *DP,* dipyramidol; ⌇⌇, inhibition

reduction of inhibitor activity. The molecular mechanisms of plasmin activation differ for the different thrombotic substances; to some extent, complexes are formed whose ultimate effect is stimulation of plasmin to release fibrin as fibrin breakdown products. Not only humoral clotting factors, but also cellular mechanisms play an important role. Their ability to be influenced via platelet-aggregation inhibitors constitutes an important therapeutic principle in the prophylaxis of both cerebral and cardiac ischemia. In this context special importance attaches to cyclo-oxygenase, an enzyme of the thrombocytes and endothelial cells (Fig. 4.16). Cyclo-oxygenase is inhibited by platelet-aggregation inhibitors. In the platelets cyclo-oxygenase is involved in the formation of thromboxane, which promotes aggregation, whereas the enzyme contributes to the formation of prostacyclin in the vessel wall and thus exerts inhibitory action on aggregation. Platelet aggregation can be inhibited by very low doses of acetylsalicylic acid (ASA) in vitro, whereas inhibition by the protective prostacyclin is of only short duration. This is the basis of the as yet theoretical supposition that very low doses of ASA have a potentially greater effect in inhibiting aggregation than currently administered doses for the prevention of stroke and TIA (300 mg/day). It is not clear whether prostacyclin is of functional importance in the regions in which atheromatous plaques replace the normal endothelium, or when platelet-aggregation inhibitors of the ASA type influence prostacyclin synthesis if thromboxane production is completely blocked. It is possible that ASA doses of around 30 mg are sufficient for such enzyme inhibition.

4.2.7 Drugs and Alcohol

There is an increased occurrence of ischemic infarcts in connection with the use of cocaine or crack (Levine et al. 1987). The pathogenesis is still unknown. Cerebral ischemia can likewise be precipitated via the secondary vasculitic processes after the intake of drugs, for example, amphetamine. Chronic alcohol abuse seems to be associated with an increased risk of strokes. Possible risk factors for this are the association with hypertension, reduced fibrinolytic activity, and increased factor VIII activity (Gorelick 1987). Finally, patients with alcoholic liver disease may develop coagulation disorders which account for the noted slightly increased frequency of primary cerebral hemorrhages in heavy drinkers. The induction of cardiac arrhythmias and reduction in cerebral blood flow due to vasoconstriction of the cerebral resistance vessels contribute to the development of ischemias.

4.2.8 Other, Rare Causes

Rare forms of cerebral ischemia include extra- and intracranial aneurysms, tumors growing from the vessel wall or adjacent structures, especially the vascular nerve supply, arteriovenous dural fistulae, irradiation vasopathies, and metabolically induced obstructive lesions. These are not discussed in detail here.

4.3 Special Types

4.3.1 Asymptomatic Vascular Processes

Asymptomatic lesions of the extracranial portions of the arteries supplying the brain were able to be reliably comprehended and prospectively observed only after the introduction of noninvasive ultrasound techniques. The demonstration by auscultation of a cervical murmur was formerly often taken as evidence of carotid stenosis; however, this is associated with up to 25% false-positive and 25% false-negative findings and is therefore of no reliable diagnostic value (Hennerici et al. 1981). Several prospective studies with Doppler ultrasound have consistently shown that there is a low morbidity and mortality from cerebral infarcts in neurologically asymptomatic patients with extracranial flow restrictions, whereas the cardiac mortality is significantly increased (Hennerici et al. 1982, 1987; Roederer et al. 1984; Chambers and Norris 1986). Pending a final analysis of these data, the latest data from the Düsseldorf series (as of June 1988) in 433 patients (262 men, 171 women, mean age 61.8 years, mean follow-up 50.2 months) confirm the earlier observations: 128 patients (29.6%) had died at the time of the last analysis, 74 (17%) from cardiac causes but only 11 (2.5%) from a cerebral infarct. Seventeen patients (3.9%) suffered a nonfatal infarct and 42 (9.7%) TIAs. This corresponds to an annual infarct rate (inclusive of deceased patients) of 1.4% and a TIA rate of 1.6%. The group of patients with initially high-grade impairment of carotid flow were particularly interesting as these were presumed to have an especially high risk of stroke. Of the 49 patients entering the study with over 80% carotid stenosis, two suffered an ipsilateral cerebral infarction without preceding TIA; the annual stroke rate in this group was only 1.1%. On the other hand, carotid occlusions show a worse prognosis, probably due to extension of the vascular lesions into other territories (opposite carotid and vertebrobasilar system) with reduction of the collateral capacity whereas intracranial disease is rare (Hennerici et al. 1986). In 167 neurologically asymptomatic patients transcranial Doppler examinations showed that the incidence of related subsequent flow impairment is very small – only two intracranial stenoses were found. At the same time a well-marked collateralization of the sometimes high-grade extracranial obstructions was demonstrable.

All the data so far available relating to the spontaneous course of asymptomatic extracranial arterial disease argue *against* early carotid endarterectomy, although the results of current studies comparing the use of surgery versus conservative treatment by platelet-aggregation inhibitors are still being awaited. Until then, the recommendations made in Chap. 6 remain open to debate.

4.3.2 Multi-infarct Syndromes

4.3.2.1 Subcortical Arteriosclerotic Encephalopathy

Subcortical arteriosclerotic encephalopathy, or Binswanger's disease, is characterized anatomically by a series of lacunar infarcts combined with demyelinization of the white matter layer. Corresponding clinical symptoms are gate apraxia, incontinence, and dementia associated with usually focal neurologic deficits and a history of chronic hypertension. CT and MRI support the clinical diagnosis if multiple small deep infarcts and diffuse white matter lesions are obvious (Zeumer et al. 1982; Babikian and Ropper 1987).

4.3.2.2 Multi-infarct Dementia

Following a suggestion of Hachinski, so-called multi-infarct dementia is characterized by a type of dementia developing in recurrent, bihemispheric, cerebral infarcts. Differentiation from presenile and senile dementia (Alzheimer's disease) as the most common type of demential disorder is obvious; however, it remains uncertain whether multi-infarct dementia is not merely a coincidence of Alzheimer's disease with cerebral infarction in at least part of the patients; overlapping with subcortical arteriosclerotic encephalopathy may also occur. As positron emission tomography studies of cerebral metabolism have shown, isolated disturbances of cerebral function directly due to subcortical infarcts may present clinically as disconnection syndromes, which may be confused with development of dementia. Reactive depressive moods based on focal disorders of cerebral performance should also be distinguished.

4.3.2.3 Corresponding Bihemispheric Lesions

Rare special types of bihemispheric lesions lead to impressive clinical pictures if corresponding regions of the brain are affected. The clinical picture of pseudobulbar paralysis presupposes bilateral interruption of the corticobulbar pathways to the caudal cranial nerves; it develops as a consequence of recurrent infarcts in the

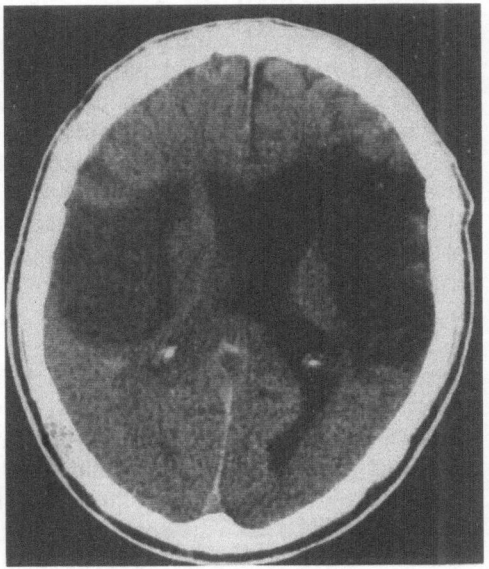

Fig. 4.17. Old and recent middle cerebral infarcts with severe dysarthria, swallowing paralysis, and tetraspasticity more marked on the left side with preexisting right-sided hemiparesis

region of the internal capsule of both lateral cerebral fissures, less often in the region of both cerebral peduncles. Occasionally, the history suggests a two-stage event, with an initially unilateral lesion and good remission. The second event then leads to a more severe clinical picture than would be expected from the extent of the infarct recurrence alone. At CT, the demonstration of recent and old bilateral symmetric ischemic lesions is important (Fig. 4.17). The clinical presentation combines dysarthria to anarthria, paralysis of the tongue and swallowing, and positive primitive reflexes (snout reflex) in a tetraparesis of variable degree with an exaggerated masseter reflex. Affective incontinence with compulsive laughing or crying is characteristic; signs of involvement of the second motor neurone with muscle wasting and fasciculation are absent.

4.3.2.4 Secondary Hemorrhagic Transformation

To some extent ischemic infarcts undergo hemorrhagic transformation in the first few days. The concept of secondary hemorrhages embraces uni- and multifocal, petechial, or confluent bleeding (imbibition of blood) as well as massive associated space-occupying hemorrhages (parenchymatous hemorrhages (Fig. 4.18; Hart and Easton 1986). The proportional incidence of secondary hemorrhagic transformation varies, depending on the pathogenesis of the primary ischemia. Pathologic studies estimate its incidence as 2%–21% after nonembolic infarcts and 51%–71% in embolic infarcts (Hart and Easton 1986; Okada et al. 1989). The estimated incidence varies so greatly because the boundary between "white" and "red" infarcts is ill defined. Virtually every infarct shows minute peripheral petechiae, but these are not considered by every pathologist as sufficient for the diagnosis of hemorrhagic infarct, and they cannot always be detected during lifetime even by MRI. The timing of the transformation is variable; it probably occurs most often between the 4th day and the 2nd week after the infarct. The higher frequency after embolic infarcts indicates that spontaneous recanalization of an occluded vessel seems to have an influence on the hemorrhagic transformation. Small petechial hemorrhages can develop through bleeding associated with diapedesis without the involvement of recanalized vessels. Large confluent hemorrhages are presumably due to the rupture of (ischemically damaged) vessel walls. Clinical manifestation of secondary hemorrhagic transformation is fortunately rare, and then usually only with large hematomas.

Moreover, it is not always possible to relate clinical deterioration to a hemorrhagic transformation, as the development of the cytotoxic edema attains a maximum at the same time and may hence itself be responsible for such deterioration. Progression of large hemorrhagic transformations can readily be demonstrated by CT and MRI studies. Hornig et al. (1987) were able to show by the routine CT monitoring of patients treated with low-dose heparin that the proportion of infarcts undergoing hemorrhagic transformation during 4 weeks was over 20%, although such transformation was associated with clinical deterioration in only three patients. There is significant evidence that the probability of hemorrhagic transformation is correlated with the size of the infarct: large territorial infarcts are more often transformed than smaller ones (Hart and Easton 1986). Moreover, older patients have hemorrhagic infarcts more often than do younger patients (Okada et al. 1989), even though more

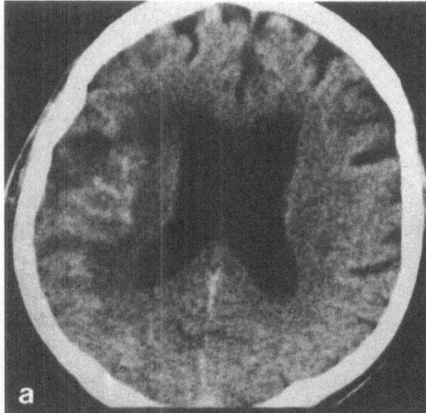 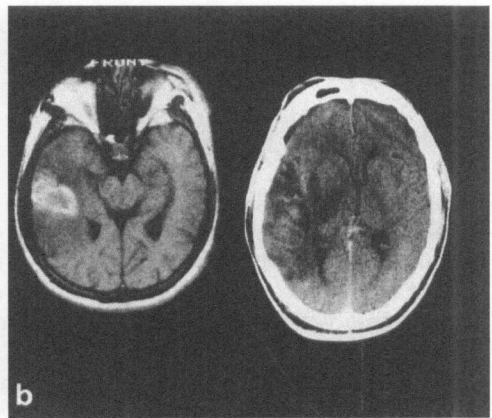

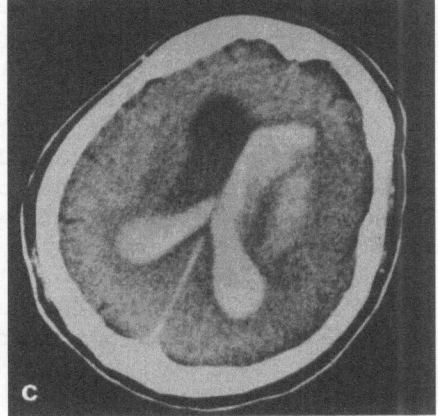

Fig. 4.18a–c. Different types of secondary hemorrhagic transformation after primary ischemic
infarct. All examples are taken from heparin-
treated patients. **a** Small blood imbibition in part
of the infarct zone in right middle cerebral territorial infarct. **b** Extensive blood imbibition without
space-occupying effect in MRI (*left,* T1-weighted
image; *right,* CT). The lesions in **a** and **b** usually
occur without clinical deterioration and are detected only during CT monitoring. **c** Parenchymatous
hemorrhage with secondary space occupation and
rupture into ventricle in completed left middle
cerebral infarct

patients with embolic infarcts are found in the younger patient group. Finally, the
time when (spontaneous) recanalization occurs may exert an influence on the
probability of the development of hemorrhagic transformation.

There is evidence that the incidence of hemorrhagic transformation is not influenced
by anticoagulation, although the extent of the transformation, if it occurs, seems to be
increased (Cerebral Embolism Study Group 1983; Cerebral Embolism Task Force
1989). The frequency and clinical importance of the hemorrhagic transformation of
ischemic infarcts is of special clinical and therapeutic interest in the context of the
controversy as to the indications for heparinization after various subtypes of acute
ischemic infarcts (Scheinberg 1989; Phillips 1989; Miller and Hart 1988, 1989; see also
Chap. 6). In one study (Ott et al. 1986), clinical deterioration did not occur even when
secondary hemorrhages had been demonstrated by CT and anticoagulation had been
continued. Yet the indications for thrombolytic therapy depend largely on the fear of
increased incidence and expression of hemorrhagic transformation rather than on
data from properly designed trials.

In our opinion, the clinical importance of hemorrhagic transformation has been
overestimated, and no increased incidence of secondary hemorrhages has been

observed during anticoagulant and thrombolytic treatment. It should be stressed once again that this is a subjective assessment.

4.4 Differential Diagnosis

Problems in differential diagnosis arise from the plurality of the clinical features, the variable vascular anatomy with nonuniform collateral circulations, and the different pathomechanisms which interact to produce the individual clinical picture. Diagnosis is made more difficult by lack of information about the onset and course of the illness, incomplete observation and defective recording of findings, as well as overlap with other diseases.

Exclusion or confirmation of a hemorrhage in the acute phase is possible only by CT or MRI studies. These techniques should be used in both daily clinical practice and in clinical studies as the most important measures for clarifying the differential diagnosis. Reabsorbed hemorrhagic foci can sometimes be distinguished from a healed ischemic zone only by additional MRI studies. As well as the familiar primary cerebral causes of a cerebral hemorrhage, differential diagnosis requires in particular the distinction of secondary types, for example, those resulting from hereditary or sporadic forms of clotting disorders (protein C, protein S, antithrombin III deficiency) and vascular amyloidoses. Two hereditary types can be distinguished, both with autosomal dominant inheritance. The "Icelandic type," without hypertension, leads to cerebral hemorrhages in family members aged 20–40 years and also to ischemia, since the amyloid deposition in the arterial wall leads to hyalinization of the arterioles. In the "Dutch type," recurrent hemorrhages occur between the ages of 40 and 60 years due to amyloid deposition in the arterioles of the cerebral and cerebellar arteries and the arachnoidal vessels. The sporadic types of the so-called congophilic amyloid angiopathy preferentially involve leptomeningeal and intracortical vessels and lead to hemorrhages (Fig. 4.19). Diagnosis is often possible against the background of a generalized primary or secondary amyloidosis (Glenner and Murphy 1989).

Subarachnoid hemorrhages produce the classical clinical picture of sudden-onset crushing headache, meningism with usually sparse evidence of focal neurologic deficit, so that there are little grounds for confusion. However, many patients are already comatose initially and no longer exhibit neck rigidity. Only rarely in subarachnoid hemorrhage is early CT study unremarkable; supplementary lumbar puncture then aids the differential diagnosis. Unruptured cerebral aneurysms may manifest with transient or permanent focal neurologic deficits (Fisher 1980). It has been suggested that intra-arterial emboli arising from partially thrombosed aneurysms are involved in the pathogenesis. Cranial CT, MRI, and angiography facilitate the diagnosis.

Arteriovenous malformations lead via an intracranial steal phenomenon to transient or persistent focal neurologic deficits (Bogousslavsky et al. 1985). Here too CT, MRI, and angiography permit correct diagnosis. Chronic subdural hematomas are evidenced in the majority of cases by headache, progressive disturbance of consciousness of varying extent, and only minor focal neurologic deficits. However, in individual cases they can also give the impression of ischemic events, so that diagnostic difficulties may arise when there is no history of trauma. This may well be the case in

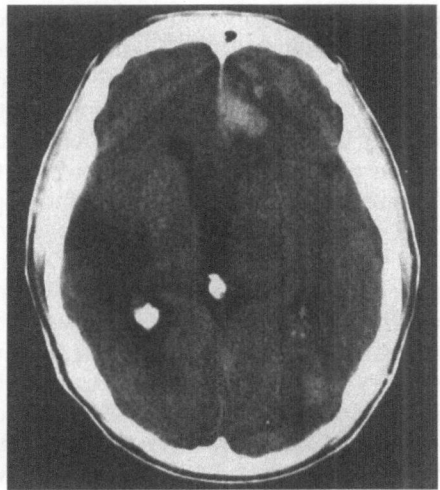

Fig. 4.19. CT image in congophilic amyloid angiopathy, demonstrating a residue of a right temporal hemorrhage, a recurrent left occipital hemorrhage of 2 weeks, and a fresh left frontal hemorrhage

30%–50% of patients with subdural hematomas (Cameron 1978). The symptoms may be those of TIAs in which aphasic disorders are particularly frequent (Moster et al. 1983), and the clinical picture may resemble that of an acute infarct (Luxon and Harrison 1979). In such cases CT may be relied on to clarify the diagnosis, although it should be borne in mind that there are also isodense subdural hematomas that can be detected only by the use of contrast medium or MRI.

Subdural empyemas can also cause confusing clinical features, especially if general signs of inflammation are absent. The diagnosis is then likewise made by CT (Luken and Whelan 1980).

Cerebral abscesses usually become manifest by a progressive disease course with headache, disturbed consciousness, papilledema, and increasing focal neurologic deficits. Fever occurs only in some 40%–60% of patients. However, in individual cases the acute onset of focal neurologic features may dominate the clinical picture lead and to confusion with ischemic infarction (Nielsen et al. 1982; Chun et al. 1986). With the aid of imaging techniques (CT and MRI) the distinction from an ischemia is usually straightforward, but differential diagnosis from tumors is difficult. Occasionally, angiography is required for further clarification.

Intracranial tumors can cause symptoms which mimic transient ischemic attacks or completed ischemic infarcts. The clinical picture of an acute infarct is often produced in such cases by hemorrhage into a previously asymptomatic tumor. Transient focal neurologic deficits as initial features may result from intermittent, increasing edema in the vicinity of the tumor. Symptoms related to the posterior territory can arise through compression of the posterior cerebral artery in the tentorial cleft when the intracranial pressure is raised.

As a rule, an intracranial tumor can be distinguished from a cerebral ischemia by means of CT or MRI, but if the earliest manifestations are due to hemorrhage into the tumor, this may conceal the true nature of the lesion and mimic a primary intracerebral hemorrhage. In such cases the situation can be clarified by serial CT and MRI examinations.

Encephalitic focal symptoms are occasionally difficult to distinguish in differential diagnosis from neurologic deficits of ischemic origin. Just as with cortical infarcts, the CSF may show a positive inflammatory reaction with pleocytosis and increased protein. On the other hand, a normal CSF does not completely exclude an encephalitis in its early stages. Herpes simplex encephalitis requires special mention as the therapeutically most important form. Acutely developing focal neurologic features may often dominate the clinical picture, sometimes but not always associated with confusion and disorientation which not uncommonly conceal a Wernicke's aphasia. Up to 40% of patients are afebrile (Koskiniemi 1981), and in 10%–20% the CSF is unremarkable (Kennard and Swash 1981). CT findings are usually unremarkable in the early days, but electroencephalographic slowing is found even in the initial stages of the disease, especially in the temporal region (Hacke and Zeumer 1986). Of course, focal electroencephalographic changes are also often present in cerebral ischemias. In recent years, MRI has proven very helpful in the diagnosis of herpes simplex encephalitis, as this allows demonstration of the encephalitic foci earlier than with CT. Because of the otherwise unfavorable prognosis, suspected cases should be treated as herpes simplex infections.

In patients with acquired immune deficiency syndrome (AIDS), focal lesions sometimes lead to clinical features that may be confused with cerebral ischemias. This includes opportunistic infections with *Toxoplasma gondii* (single or multiple contrast-enhanced lesions in CT), herpes simplex, cytomegalovirus, mycobacteria, *Candida*, and cryptococci, aspergilloma, the lesions of progressive multifocal leukencephalopathy, and primary cerebral lymphoma. Moreover, AIDS may lead to cerebrovascular complications that result in ischemic infarcts, sometimes associated with nonbacterial thrombotic endocarditis (Levy et al. 1985). The herpes zoster infection which often develops in AIDS patients can lead to an arteritis associated with ophthalmic zoster. Autoimmune thrombocytopenia can be the cause of cerebral hemorrhages. Usually, however, the previous course of the disease and the associated features are indicative of the underlying disease process in AIDS patients, with acutely developing focal neurologic features.

It is difficult in differential diagnosis to distinguish between TIAs and focal epileptic attacks. In such cases, the diagnosis may be facilitated by careful history taking, although this may of course encounter serious difficulties in focal sensory episodes. In primary motor attacks, tonic-clonic movements of the affected limbs precede a possible postictal paresis. It is true that abnormal movements have been described also in TIAs, and these may be difficult to differentiate in the history (Baquis et al. 1985). In pure sensory attacks, and in contrast to TIAs, the patients describe gradual progression of the relatively brief sensory disorders. The demonstration in the electroencephalogram of potentials characteristic of epilepsy may facilitate the diagnosis, and of course this is often made in the free intervals between attacks. Postictal pareses of the nature of Todd's paralysis frequently give rise to the misdiagnosis of an ischemic infarct and not uncommonly in vascular epilepsies direct suspicion toward a simple infarction. Earlier infarcts may be the cause of such focal, or primarily focal and secondarily generalized, attacks with associated transient focal neurologic deficits (vascular epilepsy). Since focal epileptic attacks may occur as early manifestations of an intracranial space-occupying lesion, CT or MRI clarification should always be obtained in doubtful cases, and these should be repeated from time to time if necessary when the initial findings are negative, but clinical suspicion persists.

Although epileptic attacks may be an initial feature in the context of cerebral venous sinus thromboses, their clinical features are not usually hyperacute. More often, on more detailed analysis, gradually increasing headaches are usually the first indication of increased intracranial pressure brought about by the disturbance of venous drainage. Hypoglycemia may become clinically manifest in rare cases as transient focal neurologic deficits. Most of the patients hitherto observed have been insulin-treated diabetics. The systemic features customarily associated with hypoglycemia may be absent. The neurologic deficits, with few exceptions, are rapidly and completely reversible after the administration of glucose. The mechanism underlying the focal neurologic deficits in hypoglycemia is unknown, but a selective neuronal vulnerability has been postulated (Wallis et al. 1985; Foster and Hart 1987).

Hypertensive crises may be associated with transient focal neurologic deficits which are rapidly reversible after regulation of the arterial blood pressure. If the deficits persist despite antihypertensive therapy, it must be assumed that the acute rise in blood pressure has given rise to a cerebral infarct (Healton et al. 1982). An intracerebral hemorrhage must be excluded by CT investigation.

In young patients with acute onset of unilateral clinical features, the first manifestation of multiple sclerosis comes in the differential diagnosis. In many cases MRI, immunologic biochemical investigations, and evoked potentials permit the diagnosis; however, these may be negative even in the presence of a demyelinating process in its initial stages (Matthews et al. 1982; Jacobs et al. 1986). On the other hand, very occasionally in cerebral ischemias false-positive results may be obtained that are suggestive of a demyelinating disease, including the demonstration of oligoclonal immunoglobulins (Rostrom and Link 1981). In these odd cases only the further course of the disease finally establishes the diagnosis.

Peripheral nerve lesions may mimic focal cerebral symptoms in quite exceptional cases. The differential diagnosis between a brachial plexus lesion and a central monoparesis is important in this context. Radial nerve paresis due to nocturnal pressure damage may also occasionally give rise to misinterpretation. On the other hand, closely circumscribed cortical parietal infarcts can lead to central pareses of an extremity which can be distinguished from a lesion of a peripheral nerve only by detailed testing of muscle function. In these cases, clinical examination almost always ultimately enables the correct diagnosis to be made.

4.5 Thrombosis of Cerebral Venous Sinuses

Although the clinical course of a cerebral venous sinus thrombosis exhibits some differences from arterial ischemic infarction, there may be considerable difficulties in the differential diagnosis in individual cases. Fundamentally, sinus thromboses are divided into simple and septic forms, which differ clinically and require different types of treatment. In the majority of cases of cerebral venous sinus thrombosis the development of symptoms is fluctuating and subacute. The first warning symptoms may precede the manifestation of neurologic focal symptoms by weeks. Headache, epileptic attacks, and papilledema are some of the most common early signs before the appearance of central pareses, psychotic disturbances, or disorders of vigilance (Einhäupl 1988).

In the further course there may also be marked cerebral swelling and the CT demonstration of intracerebral hemorrhages and dilated hyperdense cortical venous markings. However, in many cases the diagnosis cannot be confirmed by CT and even the so-called delta sign is nonspecific; after injection of contrast medium there is absence of contrast accumulation at the site of thrombotic material at the junction of the straight and sigmoid sinuses. MRI is often better than CT in depicting thrombosis in the superior sagittal sinus. The diagnosis is confirmed by angiography; as well as failure to depict the sinuses and main veins there are indirect signs with delayed venous emptying and bypass circulation (corkscrew phenomenon). Obviously, in contrast to cerebral artery ischemias, a greater temporal window is available for treatment in sinus thromboses. This is due to the different mechanisms involved: occlusion of the afferent vessels in arterial ischemia and of the efferent vascular system in venous ischemias. This may largely explain why the administration of anticoagulants is not associated with secondary hemorrhages if reperfusion trauma fails to develop with reopening of the efferent vessel. Even with spontaneous hemorrhages (stasis bleeding) full heparinization is indicated, contrary to the long-held fears of some authors (Dörstelmann et al. 1981; Einhäupl 1988).

Therapeutically therefore the early administration of anticoagulants is advised, depending on the clinical severity and the neuroradiologic findings once the diagnosis has been made (Dörstelmann et al. 1981; Bousser et al. 1985; Einhäupl 1988). Fibrinolytic treatment has already been used in occasional cases (Bogdahn et al. 1980; Di Rocco et al. 1981; Zeumer and Hacke 1988).

In septic sinus thromboses, which rarely present difficulties in differential diagnosis from ischemic infarcts, antibiotics and the early surgical evacuation of inflammatory foci are the mainstays of treatment.

The search for causes should include, besides diseases with a raised risk of thrombosis (e.g., deficiency of antithrombin III or protein C), oral contraceptive intake, pregnancy or the puerperium, and often occult tumors.

References

Adams R (1943) Occlusion of the anterior inferior cerebellar artery. Arch Neurol Psychiatry 49:765

Adams RD, Eecken HM van der (1953) Vascular disease of the brain. Annu Rev Med 4:213

Babikian V, Ropper AH (1987) Binswanger's disease: a review. Stroke 18:2

Baquis GD, Pessin MS, Scott M (1985) Limb shaking. A carotid TIA. Stroke 16:444

Barnett HJM, Boughner DR, Taylor DW, Couper PE, Kostuk WJ, Nichol PM (1980) Further evidence relating mitral-valve prolapse to cerebral ischemic event. N Engl J Med 302:139

Berlit P, Kessler C, Storch B, Krause KH (1983) Immunvaskulitis und Nervensystem. Nervenarzt 54:497

Biller J, Hingtgen WL, Adams HP, Smoker WRK, Godersky JC, Toffol GJ (1986) Cervico-cephalic arterial dissections. Arch Neurol 43:1234

Blackwood W, Hallpike JF, Kocen RS, Mair WGP (1969) Atheromatous disease of the carotid arterial system and embolism from the heart in cerebral infarction: a morbid anatomical study. Brain 92:897

Bogdahn U, Dommasch D, Wodarz R (1980) Thrombolytische Therapie der Sinusthrombose. In: Mertens HG, Przuntek H (eds) Pathologische Erregbarkeit des Nervensystemes und ihre Behandlung. Springer, Berlin Heidelberg New York, p 675

Bogousslavsky J, Hachinski VC, Barnett HJM (1985) Causes cardiaques et artérielles de cécité monoculaire transitoire. Rev Neurol (Paris) 141:774

Bogousslavsky J, Vinuela F, Barnett HJM, Drake CG (1985) Amaurosis fugax as the presenting manifestation of dural arteriovenous malformation. Stroke 16:891

Bogousslavsky J, Regli F, Uske A (1988) Thalamic infarcts: clinical syndromes, etiology, and prognosis. Neurology 38:837

Bornstein NM, Krajewski A, Lewis AJ, Norris JW (1990) Clinical significance of carotid plague hemorrhage. Arch Neurol 47:958

Bousser MG, Chiras J, Bories JB, Castaigne P (1985) Cerebral venous thrombosis – a review of 38 cases. Stroke 16:199

Brown MS, Kovanen PT, Goldstein JL (1981) Regulation of plasma cholesterol by lipoprotein receptors. Science 212:628

Burton JL (1983) Livedo reticularis, porcelain-white scars, and cerebral thrombosis. Lancet I:1263

Cameron MM (1978) Chronic subdural hematoma: a review of 114 cases. J Neurol Neurosurg Psychiatry 41:834

Caplan LR (1988) Clinical course and lesion distribution in carotid and middle cerebral artery occlusive disease. In: Hennerici M, Sitzer G, Weger HD (eds) Carotid artery plaques. Karger, Basel, p 186

Caplan LR, Gorelick PB, Hier DB (1986) Race, sex and occlusive cerebrovascular disease: a review. Stroke 17:648

Cerebral Embolism Study Group (1983) Immediate coagulation of embolic stroke: a randomized trial. Stroke 14:668

Cerebral Embolism Task Force (1986) Cardiogenic brain embolism. Arch Neurol 43:71

Cerebral Embolism Task Force (1989) Cardiogenic brain embolism. The Second Report of the Cerebral Embolism Task Force. Arch Neurol 46:727

Chambers BR, Norris JW (1986) Outcome in patients with asymptomatic neck bruits. N Engl J Med 315:860

Chun CH, Johnason JD, Hofstetter M, Raff MJ (1986) Brain abscess. A study of 45 consecutive cases. Medicine (Baltimore) 65:415

Connett MC, Lanche JM (1965) Fibromuscular hyperplasia of the internal carotid artery: report of a case. Ann Surg 162:59

Corston RN, Kendall BE, Marshall J (1984) Prognosis in middle cerebral artery stenosis. Stroke 15:237

Countee RW, Vijayanathan (1979) Reconstruction of the "totally" occluded internal carotid arteries. Angiographic and technical considerations. J Neurosurg 50:747

Craig DR, Meguro K, Watridge C, Robertson JT, Barnett HJM, Fox AJ (1982) Intracranial internal carotid artery stenosis. Stroke 13:825

Critchley M (1930) The anterior cerebral artery and its syndromes. Brain 53:120

Currier R, Giles C, DeJong R (1961) Some comments on Wallenberg's lateral medullary syndrome. Neurology 11:778

Del Zoppo GJ, Hacke W (1987) Fibrinolytische Therapie bei ischämischen Hirninfarkten. Dtsch Med Wochenschr 112:603

Del Zoppo GJ, Harker LA (1984) Blood-vessel interaction in coronary disease. Hosp Pract [Off] 19:163

Del Zoppo GJ, Zeumer H, Harker LA (1986) Thrombolytic therapy in acute stroke: possibilities and hazards. Stroke 17:595

DePalma RG, Hubay CA, Insull W, Robinson AV, Hartman PH (1970) Progression and regression of experimental atherosclerosis. Surg Gynecol Obstet 131:633

Di Rocco C, Iannelli A, Leone G, Moschini M, Valori VM (1981) Heparin-urokinase treatment in aseptic dural sinus thrombosis. Arch Neurol 38:431

Dörstelmann D, Dobiasch H, Mattes W, Reuther R (1981) Hirnvenen und Sinusthrombose. Ein Beitrag zur Antikoagulantienbehandlung. Nervenarzt 52:243

Ehringer H, Bockelmann L, Konecny U, Koppensteiner R, Marosi L, Minar E, Schöfl R (1987) Verschlußkrankheit der extrakraniellen A. carotis: Spontanverlauf und frühe Phase nach Thromb-endarteriektomie im bildgebenden Ultraschall. Vasa [Suppl] 20:71

Einhäupl K (1988) Sinus- und Hirnvenenthrombosen. In: Brandt T, Dichgans J, Diener HC (eds) Therapie und Verlauf neurologischer Krankheiten. Kohlhammer, Stuttgart, p 275

Feinberg WM, Bruck DC, Ring ME, Corrigan JJ (1989) Hemostatic markers in acute stroke. Stroke 20:592

Feuer D, Weinberger J (1987) Extracranial carotid artery in patients with transient global amnesia. Stroke 18:951

Fisher CM (1980) Transient focal cerebral ischemia as a presenting manifestation of unruptured cerebral aneurysm. Ann Neurol 8:367

Fisher CM, Goore I, Okabe N, White PD (1965a) Atherosclerosis of the carotid and vertebral arteries – extracranial and intracranial. J Neuropathol Exp Neurol 24:455

Fisher CM, Goore I, Okabe N, White PD (1965b) Calcification of the carotid siphon. Circulation 32:538

Foster JW, Hart RG (1987) Hypoglycemic hemiplegia: two cases and a clinical review. Stroke 18:944

Freund HJ (1987) Abnormalities of motor behavior after cortical lesions in humans. In: The nervous system. (Handbook of physiology, vol 5) p 763

Freund HJ, Hummelsheim H (1985) Lesions of premotor cortex in man. Brain 108:697

Gaul JJ, Marks SJ, Weinberger J (1986) Visual disturbance and carotid artery disease. 500 symptomatic patients studied by non-invasive carotid artery testing including B-mode ultrasonography. Stroke 17:393

Glenner GG, Murphy MA (1989) Amyloidosis of the nervous system. J Neurol Sci 94:1

Goodwin JA, Gorelick PB, Helgason CM (1987) Symptoms of amaurosis fugax in atherosclerotic carotid artery disease. Neurology 37:829

Gorelick PB (1987) Alcohol and stroke. Stroke 18:268

Gorelick PB, Caplan LR, Hier DB, Parker SL, Patel D (1984) Racial differences in the distribution of anterior circulation occlusive disease. Neurology 34:54

Gotoh F (ed) (1983) Annual Report (1982) of the Research Committee on Spontaneous Occlusion of the Circle of Willis (Moyamoya disease). Ministry of Health and Welfare, Japan

Hacke W (1986) Clinical relevance of multimodal assessment of brainstem functions in severe vascular brainstem lesions. In: Kunze K, Zangemeister WH, Arlt A (eds) Clinical problems of brainstem disorders. Thieme, Stuttgart, p 101

Hacke W, Zeumer H (1986) Herpes simplex Enaphalitis. Dtsch Med Wochenschr 111:23

Hacke W, Del Zoppo GJ, Harker LA (1987) Thrombosis and cerebrovascular disease: In: Poeck K, Ringelstein EB, Hacke W (eds) New trends in the diagnosis and management of stroke. Springer, Berlin Heidelberg New York, p 59

Hacke W, Zeumer H, Ferbert A, Brückmann H, Del Zoppo GJ (1988) Intraarterial fibrinolytic therapy improves outcome in patients with acute vertebrobasilar occlusive disease. Stroke 19:1216

Hankey (1991) Isolated angiitis: angiopathy of the central nervous system. Cerebrovasc Dis 1:2

Hart RG (1988) Vertebral artery dissection. Neurology 38:987

Hart RG, Easton JD (1986) Hemorrhagic infarcts. Stroke 17:586

Hart R, Easton DF (1986) Dissections and trauma of cervico-cerebral arteries. In: Barnett HJM, Mohr JP, Yatsu FM, Stein BM (eds) Stroke. Churchill Livingstone, Edinburgh, p 293

Hass WK, Fields WS, North RR, Kricheff JI, Chase NE, Bauer RB (1968) Joint study of extracranial arterial occlusions: II. Arteriography, techniques, sites, and complications. JAMA 203:961

Healton EB (1986) Fibromuscular dysplasia. In: Barnett HJM, Mohr JP, Stein DM, Yatsu FM (eds) Stroke. Churchill Livingstone, Edinburgh, p 831

Healton EB, Brust JC, Feinfield DA, Thomson GE (1982) Hypertensive encephalopathy and the neurologic manifestations of malignant hypertension. Neurology 32:127

Helgason C, Caplan LR, Goodwin J, Hedges T (1986) Anterior choroidal artery-territory infarction. Arch Neurol 43:681

Hennerici M (1987) Hochauflösende Ultraschall-Duplexsystemanalyse der extrakraniellen Karotis-strombahn. In: Hartmann A, Wassmann H (eds) Hirninfarkt. Urban and Schwarzenberg, Munich, p 228

Hennerici M (1990) Regression of atherosclerosis. In: Norris JW, Hachinski VC (eds) Prevention of stroke. Springer, Berlin Heidelberg New York

Hennerici M, Aulich A, Sandmann W, Freund HJ (1981) Incidence of asymptomatic extracranial arterial disease. Stroke 12:750

Hennerici M, Rautenberg W, Mohr S (1982) Stroke risk from symptomless extracranial disease. Lancet II:1180

Hennerici M, Rautenberg W, Trockel U, Kladetzky RG (1985) Spontaneous progression and regression of small carotid atheroma. Lancet I:1415

Hennerici M, Hülsbömer HB, Hefter H, Rautenberg W (1986) Spontaneous history of asymptomatic internal carotid occlusion. Stroke 17:718

Hennerici M, Hülsbömer HB, Hefter H, Lammerts D, Rautenberg W (1987) Natural history of asymptomatic extracranial arterial disease – results of a long-term prospective study. Brain 110:777

Hennerici M, Klemm C, Rautenberg W (1988a) The subclavian steal phenomenon: a common vascular disorder with rare neurologic deficits. Neurology 38:669

Hennerici M, Sitzer G, Weger HD (1988b) Carotid artery plaques. Karger, Basel

Hennerici M, Steinke W, Rautenberg W (1989) High resistance Doppler flow pattern in extracranial carotid dissection. Arch Neurol 46:670

Hornig CR, Dorndorf W, Agnoli AL (1987) Hemorrhagic cerebral infarction – a prospective study. Stroke 17:179

Hutchinson EC, Yates PO (1957) Carotico-vertebral stenosis. Lancet I:2

Imparato AM, Riles TS, Gorstein F (1979) The carotid bifurcation plaque: pathologic findings associated with cerebral ischemia. Stroke 10:238

Jacobs L, Kinkel WR, Poladini I, Kinkel R (1986) Correlations of nuclear MRI, CT and clinical profiles in multiple sclerosis. Neurology 36:27

Jentzer A (1954) Dissecting aneurysm of the left internal carotid artery. Angiology 5:232

Kennard C, Swash M (1981) Acute viral encephalitis. Its diagnosis and outcome. Brain 104:129–148

Koskiniemi M (1981) Acute encephalitis. Acta Med Scand 209:115

Kunitz SC, Gross CR, Heyman A, Kase CS, Mohr JP, Price TR, Wolf PA (1984) The pilot stroke data bank: definition, design and data. Stroke 15:740

Leadbetter WF, Burkland CE (1938) Hypertension in unilateral renal disease. J Urol 39:611

Levine SR, Welch KMA (1987) The spectrum of neurologic disease associated with antiphospholipid antibodies. Lupus anticoagulants and anticardiolipin antibodies. Arch Neurol 44:876

Levine SR, Welch KMA (1989) Antiphospholipid Antibodies. Ann Neurol 26:386

Levine SR, Washington JM, Jefferson MF, Kieran SN, Moen M et al. (1987) "Crack" cocaine-associated stroke. Neurology 37:1849–1853

Levy RM, Bredesen DR, Rosenblum ML (1985) Neurological manifestations of the acquired immunodeficiency syndrome (AIDS): experience at UCSF and review of the literature. J Neurosurg 62:475

Little JR, Sawany B, Weinstein M (1980) Pseudotandemstenosis of the internal carotid artery. Neurosurgery 7:574

Luhan J, Pollock S (1953) Occlusion of the superior cerebellar artery. Neurology 3:77

Luken MG, Whelan MA (1980) Recent diagnostic experience with subdural empyema. J Neurosurg 52:764

Luxon LM, Harrison MJG (1979) Chronic subdural hematoma. Q J Med 48:43–53

Malcolm Stewart R, Samson D, Diehl J, Hinton R, Ditmore QM (1980) Unruptured cerebral aneurysms presenting as recurrent transient neurological deficits. Neurology 30:47

Malinow MR (1984) Atherosclerosis: progression, regression and resolution. Am Heart J 108:1523

Marx A, Messing B, Storch B, Busse B (1987) Spontane Dissektionen hirnversorgender Arterien. Nervenarzt 58:8

Marzewski DJ, Furlan AJ, Louis PS, Little JR, Modic MT, Williams G (1982) Intracranial internal carotid artery stenosis: long-term prognosis. Stroke 13:821

Matthews WB, Wattam JRB, Poutney E (1982) Evoked potentials in the diagnosis of multiple sclerosis. A follow up study. J Neurol Neurosurg Psychiatry 45:303

McGill H, Arias-Stella J, Carbonell L (1968) General findings of the internal atherosclerosis project. Lab Invest 18:498

Miller VT, Hart RG (1988) Heparin anticoagulation in acute brain ischemia. Stroke 19:403

Miller VT, Hart RG (1989) Heparin in acute stroke. Stroke 20:1284

Mitsuyama Y, Thompson LR, Hayashi T, Lee KK, Keehn RJ, Resch JA, Steer A (1979) Autopsy study of cerebrovascular disease in Japanese men who lived in Hiroshima, Japan and Honolulu, Hawai. Stroke 10:389

Mohr JP, Caplan LR, Melski JW et al. (1978) The Harvard Cooperative Stroke Registry: a prospective registry. Neurology 28:754

Mokri B, Sundt TM, Houser OW, Piepgras DG (1986) Spontaneous dissection of the cervical internal carotid artery. Ann Neurol 19:126

Morris GC, Lechter A, DeBakey ME (1968) Surgical treatment of fibromuscular disease of the carotid arteries. Arch Surg 96:636

Moster ML, Johnston DE, Reinmuth OM (1983) Chronic subdural hematoma with transient neurological deficits: a review of 15 cases. Ann Neurol 14:539

Müller HR (1989) Transient global amnesia. Schweiz Rundsch Med 36:970

Müller HR, Mase R (1981) Pathogenesis and prognosis of transient global amnesia. Gerontology 27:110

Nielsen H, Gyldensted C, Harmsen A (1982) Cerebral abscess. Etiology and pathogenesis, symptoms, diagnosis and treatment. A review of 200 cases from 1935–1976. Acta Neurol Scand 65:609

Norris JW, Bornstein NM (1986) Progression and regression of carotid stenosis. Stroke 17:755

Okada Y, Yamaguchi T, Minematsu K, Miyashita T, Sawada T et al. (1989) Hemorrhagic transformation in cerebral embolism. Stroke 20:598

Ott BR, Zamani A, Kleefield J, Funkenstein HH (1986) The clinical spectrum of hemorrhagic infarction. Stroke 17:630

Palubinskas AJ, Ripley HR (1964) Fibromuscular hyperplasia in extrarenal arteries. Radiology 82:451

Paullus WS, Pate TG, Rhoton AL (1977) Microsurgical exposure of the petrous portion of the carotid artery. J Neurosurg 47:713

Pessin MS, Kwan E, De Witt LD, Hedges TR, Gale D, Caplan LR (1987) Posterior cerebellar artery stenosis. Ann Neurol 21:85

Phillips SJ (1989) An alternative view of heparin anticoagulation in acute focal brain ischemia. Stroke 20:295

Powers WJ, Press GA, Grubb RL, Gado M, Raichle ME (1987) The effect of hemodynamically significant carotid artery disease in the hemodynamic states of the cerebral circulation. Ann Intern Med 106:27

Rautenberg W, Hennerici M (1988) Pulsed Doppler assessment of innominate artery obstructive disease. Stroke (in press)

Reivich M, Holling HE, Robberts B, Toole JF (1961) Reversal of blood flow through the vertebral artery and its effect on cerebral circulation. N Engl J Med 265:878

Ringelstein EB, Zeumer H, Angelou D (1983) The pathogenesis of strokes from internal carotid artery occlusion. Diagnostic and therapeutical implications. Stroke 14:867

Roederer GO, Langlois YE, Jager KA, Primozich JF, Beach KW, Phillips DJ, Strandness DWE (1984) The natural history of carotid arterial disease in asymptomatic patients with cervical bruits. Stroke 15:605

Ross R, Glomset J (1976) The pathogenesis of atherosclerosis. N Engl J Med 295:369, 1332

Rostrom B, Link H (1981) Oligoclonal immunoglobulins in cerebrospinal fluid in acute cerebrovascular disease. Neurology 31:590

Scharff RE, Hennerici M, Bluschke V, Lück J, Kladetzky RG (1982) Cerebral ischemia in young patients: is it associated with mitral valve prolapse and abnormal platelet activity in vivo? Stroke 13:454

Scheinberg P (1989) Heparin anticoagulation. Stroke 20:173

Schlesinger B (1976) The upper brainstem in the human. Springer, Berlin Heidelberg New York

Shinar D, Gross CR, Mohr JP et al. (1985) Interobserver variability in the assessment of neurologic history and examination in the Stroke Data Bank. Arch Neurol 42:557

Soria ED, Fine EJ, Paroski NW (1987) Lacunes: the pervasive strokes. NY State J Med 6:650

Spitzer K, Thie A, Becker V, Kunze K (1988) Klinische Verläufe bei ausgedehnten supratentoriellen Hirninfarkten mit Hirnödem. Intensivmedizin 25:192

Steinke W, Aulich A, Hennerici M (1989) Diagnose und Verlauf von Carotisdissektionen. Dtsch Med Wochenschr 114:1869

Steinke W, Klötzsch C, Hennerici M (1990a) Carotid artery disease assessed by colour Doppler flow imaging. AJNR 11:259

Steinke W, Klötzsch C, Hennerici M (1990b) Variability of flow patterns in the normal carotid bifurcation. Atherosclerosis (in print)

Takeuchi K, Shimitzu K (1955) Hypoplasia of the bilateral internal carotid arteries. Brain Verve (Tokyo) 9:37

Toole JF, Janeway R, Choi K, Cordell R, Davis C, Johnston F, Miller HS (1975) Transient ischemic attacks due to atherosclerosis. Arch Neurol 32:5

Toole JL (1984) Cerebrovascular disorders, 3rd edn. Raven, New York

Torvik H, Jörgenson L (1964) Thrombotic and embolic occlusions of the carotid arteries in an autopsy material, part I: prevalence, location and associated diseases. J Neurol Sci 1:24

Tour RL, Hoyt WF (1959) The syndrome of the aortic arch. Am J Ophthalmol 47:35

Unsöld R, Seeger W (1989) Compressive optic nerve lesions at the optic canal. Springer, Berlin Heidelberg New York

Wallis WE, Donaldson I, Scott RS, Wilson J (1985) Hypoglycemia masquerading as cerebrovascular disease (hypoglycemic hemiplegia). Ann Neurol 18:510

Waterston JA, Brown MN, Butler P, Swash M (1990) Small deep cerebral infarcts associated with occlusive internal carotid artery disease: a hemodynamic phenomenon? Arch Neurol 47:953

Wechsler LR, Kistler JP, Davies KR, Kampinski MJ (1986) The prognosis of carotid siphon stenosis. Stroke 17:714

Whisnant JP, Martin MJ, Sayre GP (1961) Atherosclerotic stenosis of cervical arteries. Arch Neurol 5:429

Yatsu FM (1986) Atherogenesis and stroke. In: Barnett HJM, Mohr JP, Stein BM, Yatsu FM (eds) Stroke. Churchill Livingstone, Edinburgh, p 45

Yatsu FM, Loeb J (1981) Atherosclerosis: The role of lipids. Clin Neurosurg 29:437

Zenker G, Erbel R, Krämer G, Mohr-Kahaly S, Drexler M, Harnoncourt K, Meyer J (1988) Transesophageal two-dimensional echocardiography in young patients with cerebral ischemic events. Stroke 19:345

Zeumer H (1985) Survey of progress: vascular recanalizing techniques in interventional neuroradiology. J Neurol 231:287

Zeumer H, Hacke W (1988) Ischämische Insulte. In: Hacke W (ed) Neurologische Intensivmedizin, 2nd edn. Perimed, Erlangen, p 86

Zeumer H, Hacke W, Kolmann HL, Poeck K (1982) Lokale Fibrinolysetherapie bei Basilaris-Thrombose. Dtsch Med Wochenschr 107:728

5 Diagnosis

The diagnosis of cerebral ischemia is based on the course, extent, and clinical features of neurologic deficit. The choice and timing of diagnostic methods are largely influenced by the general condition, age, and previous medical history of the patient. Particularly with the most common cause of cerebral ischemias, arteriosclerotically induced vascular disease, resulting disorders and the individual prognosis must be seen in terms of the neurologic features. All these factors, with their therapeutic implications, determine the course of diagnostic procedure in the acute phase as well as any monitoring that may be needed in the chronic stage. Noninvasive methods of examination have been applied to monitor the clinical course, both in patients who have already experienced cerebral ischemia and in those in whom various clinical findings indicate an increased risk. Such examination assumes particular significance in the context of today's increasingly critical discussion regarding principles of treatment. Moreover, the diagnosis and importance of a TIA – in its purely clinical definition as a completely reversible and therefore relatively harmless episode of disturbed cerebral circulation – must now be reconsidered since CT and MRI techniques have often demonstrated (in 20%–50% of cases) parenchymatous defects even at this stage (Waxman and Toole 1983).

5.1 History and Clinical Findings

5.1.1 General Impressions and General Findings

Even the general examination of the patient provides important information. This begins, for example, with biologic age, physical and nutritional status, nicotine abuse with corresponding skin changes in the fingers, and disorders of fat metabolism with xanthelasma. Further data provided by the general examination include signs of heart failure and arrhythmias, alterations in the pulse as evidence of arteriosclerosis of the large arteries, limitation of pulmonary function or skin lesions in the collagenoses, vasculitis (temporal arteritis), or other vasculopathies (e. g., Sneddon's syndrome; Fig. 4.13). Neuropsychological and psychopathologic factors are also often evident, such as changes in spontaneous speech, motor speech performance, or states of consciousness, and these will have an important influence on the further diagnostic procedures.

5.1.2 Neurologic History and Examination Findings

In all types of transient cerebral ischemia the data obtained from the history are of great importance, for the phenomenology of the neurologic features permits identification of the affected cerebral arteries, and the course of the disorder over time must be accorded special attention. The history presents problems when the patient is incapable of providing reliable information; for example, transient aphasic disturbances may not be discovered if the patient did not speak at the time of a cerebral ischemia (e. g., with a hemiparesis). The most varied types of speech and language disorders, appearing simultaneously with a hemiparesis and important for topical diagnosis (hemispheric versus infratentorial lesion), often remain indistinguishable. Motor and sensory disturbances may also not be differentiated by the patients, and different types of visual disorder may not be differentiated, for example, whether one eye or both eyes in homonymous visual field defects were affected.

Understanding the course of a cerebral ischemia is of importance in differential diagnosis for analyzing the underlying disturbance of cerebral function, especially in assigning the relevant pathomechanisms and etiology to these events. For instance, in cortical lesions TIAs may present throughout as focal convulsive attacks, or their course may show migratory signs of deficit imitative of a jacksonian attack. On the other hand, monosymptomatic cerebrovascular episodes may also be the expression of recurrent cardiac emboli, which usually come into consideration only with the appearance of symptoms affecting both hemispheres or different vascular territories (Fig. 5.1).

In cerebral insult, besides the features of focal neurologic deficit, the psychopathologic changes even in the early phase are of crucial prognostic importance. In hemispheric ischemias disturbances of consciousness are unfavorable signs as evidence of an influence on the opposite cerebral hemisphere even if no lesions are found on CT or MRI examination. In brainstem ischemias, which often develop progressively over several days, characteristic prodromes with disorders of waking and sleeping rhythm, attention, and concentration often develop long before the focal symptoms.

5.1.3 Neuropsychological Symptoms

While most physicians are familiar with the basic elements of neurologic and physical examination, there is still great uncertainty in the methods of investigation, description, and classification of neuropsychological symptoms. Therefore, the neuropsychological examination is described in detail here (see Poeck 1985).

5.1.3.1 Aphasias

Aphasias are central language disorders which affect speech, comprehension, reading, and writing. The speech-dominant hemisphere is the left half of the cerebrum in right-handed persons and the right half in most left-handed persons, although in some of the latter the speech centers are situated bilaterally or in the left hemisphere. Aphasias are to be distinguished from dysarthrias, which can also be caused by lesions

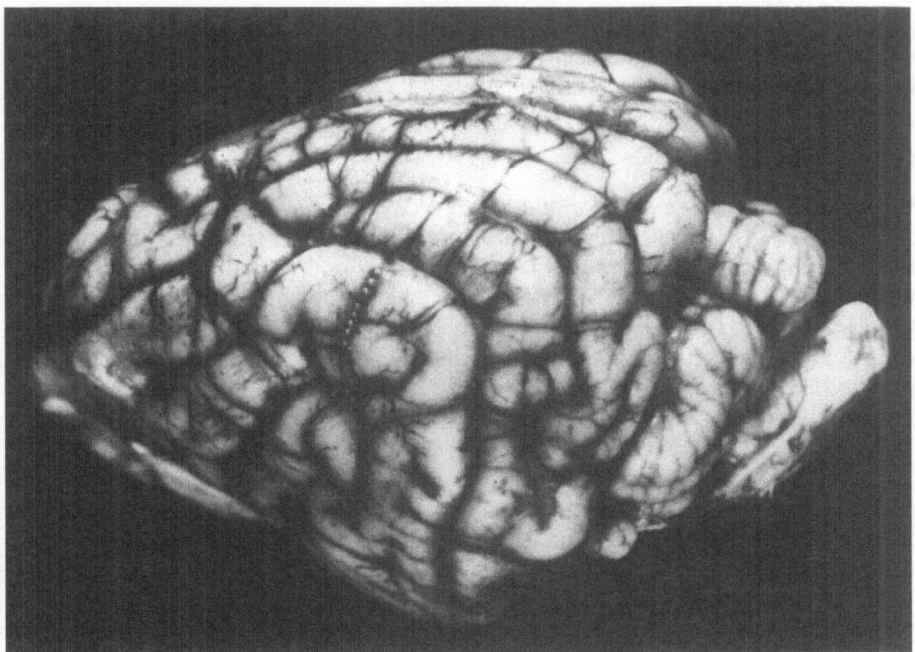

Fig. 5.1. Demonstration of several steel spherules (0.8 mm diameter) which have all embolized into the same branch of the middle cerebral artery after introduction into the left internal carotid artery. (From Whisnan: 1955, 1982)

in the non-speech-dominant hemisphere, basal ganglia, brainstem, or peripheral speech apparatus.

About one-half of patients with a left cerebral infarction experience aphasia. In the acute stage it is often difficult to determine the type of aphasia as the initial symptoms either fluctuate greatly, or no speech is produced. Identification with reasonable certainty is possible only after several weeks. Most important is assessment of the patient's spontaneous speech, in which answers are supplied to contrived questions in an open, structured conversation. Mimicry and gesture are assessed in connection with speech-relevant performance, and attention is also paid to articulation and prosody, which are characterized by rhythm and melody in speech. The rate of speech and the syntactic structure of connected sentences or phrases must also be described (are paraphrases used; does the patient closely miss the intended phrase?).

Phonematic paraphasias, i. e., alteration of the sound of a word (e. g., "bird" in place of "beard") are to be distinguished from semantic paraphasias. They may stem from the same semantic area ("pencil" or "writing" for ball-point pen), but nonexistent, quite aberrant words may also emerge which still retain some similarity with actual speech elements. Finally, there may occur perseverations, automatisms, and stereo-typed verbalizations ("yes, yes, yes").

Short supplementary tests should also be administered for reading and writing and for speech comprehension and nomenclature (parts of the body, objects of daily life). With stable deficits standardized tests (e. g., the Aachen Aphasia Test) are capable of providing an exact account of findings. Aphasic syndromes are various subtypes of aphasia following ischemic insults which are also found in less typical form after hemorrhage and in tumors or encephalitis.

Global Aphasia

Global aphasia is often found in the first few days after a stroke. Speech production and comprehension are both greatly impaired. Paraphasias, disordered comprehension, increased efforts at speech, agrammatisms, and verbal automatisms occur. Often, communication is no longer possible. As time passes speech comprehension usually improves first. Objective tests may frequently demonstrate persistent severe disorders of speech comprehension even when good communication has been restored.

Broca's Aphasia

Patients with Broca's aphasia speak very slowly and haltingly and must exert themselves to speak. Articulation is poor, and a dysarthria is almost always present. Speech melody (prosody) is disturbed, and there are usually one- or two-word phrases and agrammatism. Phonematic paraphasias are striking (e.g., "hanner" instead of "hammer," "carrion" instead of "crayon"). Speech comprehension is only moderately impaired. The phonematic paraphasias are maintained even when speech is repeated. Broca's aphasia is related to fronto-precentral and lateral parts of the brain which correspond only partially to Broca's area as historically described. Differentiation from anarthria and dysarthria is often difficult and frequently impossible from the history.

Wernicke's Aphasia

Patients with Wernicke's aphasia show a well-preserved flow of speech, sometimes even an exaggerated speech production. Grammatical mistakes occur in the form of paragrammatism (faulty sentence construction), not as agrammatism. Speech comprehension is considerably disturbed and abundant phonematic and semantic paraphasias occur in spontaneous speech which often have no similarity to the word aimed at and are actually neologisms. The extreme case is an excessive flow of speech production with exclusively semantic paraphasias, known as phonematic jargon. Reading and writing are usually disturbed in the same way as speaking and speech comprehension. Perseverations occur. The lesion is usually situated in the posterior part of the temporal lobe and always involves the first temporal convolution, corresponding to the territory of the posterior temporal artery.

Amnestic Aphasia

The prominent feature in amnestic aphasia is difficulty in finding the right word although speech flow is well preserved and sentence construction largely intact. The ability of the patient to communicate is good, and speech comprehension is only transiently disturbed. Semantic paraphasias predominate, which often deviate only slightly from the words actually aimed at. Paraphrases are common ("what one writes with" instead of "ball-point pen"), as are empty, general phrases ("approximately something like that") and perseverations (repetition of previously used and verbally altered words). The lesion is often in the temporoparietal region, and the prognosis, even for spontaneous recovery, is relatively good.

Special Types

Less common special types of aphasias include conduction aphasia, in which the patient speaks fluently with many phonematic paraphasias but is unable to repeat, and transcortical aphasia with virtual absence of spontaneous speech but good preservation of the ability to repeat even long sentences.

5.1.3.2 Apraxias

Apraxias are disturbances in the overall structuring of individual movement components toward providing a purposeful sequence of movements, while the separate component motor functions including coordination are intact. Apraxias are often overlooked or misinterpreted as pareses, especially when disturbed complex movement sequences cannot be recalled, and the individual motor functions are not investigated. Ideomotor apraxia, with its subtype buccofacial apraxia, is to be distinguished from ideatory apraxia.

Ideomotor apraxia, also known as ideokinetic apraxia, is characterized by the inability to perform simple motor procedures such as waving, raising a coffee cup to the mouth, or brushing the teeth either on command or by imitation. However, the separate movement components, for example, the upward and downward movements of the arms or hands which make up waving, are undisturbed. The patient does not know *how* to carry out the motor sequence. Often during testing there is a marked perseveration of motor elements recalled from earlier tests when new requests are made.

Buccofacial apraxia is a special type of ideomotor apraxia, marked mainly by disorders of movement sequences in the region of the mouth and tongue. This causes many apraxia patients considerable difficulty in relearning how to speak because of impairment of the rapid movement sequences required in articulation.

In the uncommon and most complex ideatory type of apraxia the patient can no longer correctly perform specific sequential procedures; for example, he is unable to spread butter on a slice of bread with a knife or to stir sugar in coffee and then raise the cup to the mouth, although each separate movement is perfectly practicable. Therefore, the patient does not know *what* he must do in the movement sequence. Usually he is incapable of performing the procedure either on verbal request or imitatively.

Sometimes an apraxia of limb kinesis is distinguished, described as a slowing, increased formality, or stiffness of movements (e.g., breaking a boiled egg with a spoon or selecting a key from a key-ring with one hand). However, this type of apraxia is very difficult to distinguish from a paresis, and apraxic and paretic elements are often combined.

When testing for apraxia, the patient is asked verbally to perform simple and more complex movements (waving, menacing, touching the opposite earlobe or the tip of the nose with the nonparalyzed hand, removing and replacing spectacles) and to perform these movements imitatively. He is also asked to make certain noises (whistling, tongue clicking), to stick out the tongue, to open or close the mouth. Attention is paid to how the movements are performed, and whether stereotypes or perseverations occur.

Besides motor apraxia, which includes ideomotor and ideatory apraxia, there is also a constructional apraxia which is not discussed in detail here and is not uncommonly associated with spatial disorientation.

5.1.3.3 Anosognosia and Neglect

Anosognosia is failure to recognize the state of illness and occurs with lesions of both the speech-dominant and – especially in infarcts – of the non-speech-dominant hemisphere. This is striking, for example, when patients are unaware of paralysis on one side of the body. Anosognosia may exist even with unilateral visual field restriction or complete blindness.

Neglect refers to a unilateral disregard of perceptual or physical functions in the absence of a sensorimotor deficit of any severity. In most cases (80%–90%) neglect occurs in lesions of the non-speech-dominant hemisphere, less often also in left-hemispheric lesions. In motor neglect the initial impression on clinical examination is that there is a severe hemiparesis, especially when bilateral motor exertions are studied. When the patient's attention is directed to the paralyzed limb, the individual functions remain well preserved on both sides. The same applies to sensory and visual field disturbances. Also here, neglect is often only noticed in that, with closed eyes and simultaneous touching of both sides of the body, one-half of the body is ignored, or, in confrontational perimetric examination, bitemporally presented movement stimuli are localized only in one-half of the visual field.

5.1.4 Vascular Diagnosis

Traditionally, the cerebral arteries are palpated and auscultated in the neck to detect obstructive lesions of the carotids. While both techniques have an established place in general angiologic diagnosis, they are now obsolete for the cerebral arteries because of the high rate of error and the far more reliable noninvasive ultrasound techniques. High-grade stenoses of the internal carotid may be overlooked if there is no murmur on auscultation, and murmurs conducted asymmetrically from the heart or external carotids may be incorrectly identified. Merely the unilateral absence of a pulse in the cervical triangle may occasionally indicate occlusion of the common carotid.

On the other hand, measurement of the blood pressure in both arms is important to demonstrate the possible association of subclavian flow impairment with a vertebral steal phenomenon, provided always that the individual pressures are correctly measured. Not uncommonly treatment required for hypertension is not carried out for years because the blood pressure is always taken in the same arm without recognizing the existence of a communicating high-grade subclavian flow impairment. Differences of 30 mmHg in systolic pressure between the two arms should arouse suspicion of subclavian stenosis. Absence of temporal artery pulsations may be evidence of obstructions of the external carotids. If there are also tender thickenings, a history of headaches, and a raised ESR, the characteristic features of a temporal arteritis are present.

Fundoscopy directs attention to signs of diabetic and hypertension-induced vascular lesions, arterial and venous occlusions, emboli (e. g., cholesterol, platelet aggregates, calcified material), hemorrhages, microaneurysms, and signs of an ischemic optic nerve lesion or of raised intracranial pressure (papilledema; Fig. 5.2). However, even in recurrent attacks of typical amaurosis fugax emboli are seldom directly demonstrable in the arteries as it is rapidly subject to lysis.

In recent years, various indirect instrumental techniques for the demonstration of high-grade flow impairment in the internal carotid artery in the neck have been abandoned in favor of ultrasound methods; these include ophthalmodynamometry and thermography. Oculoplethysmography is still used mainly in English-speaking countries, partly because objective recording is better than with periorbital Doppler ultrasound. By applying a feather-weight measuring instrument to the cornea, the

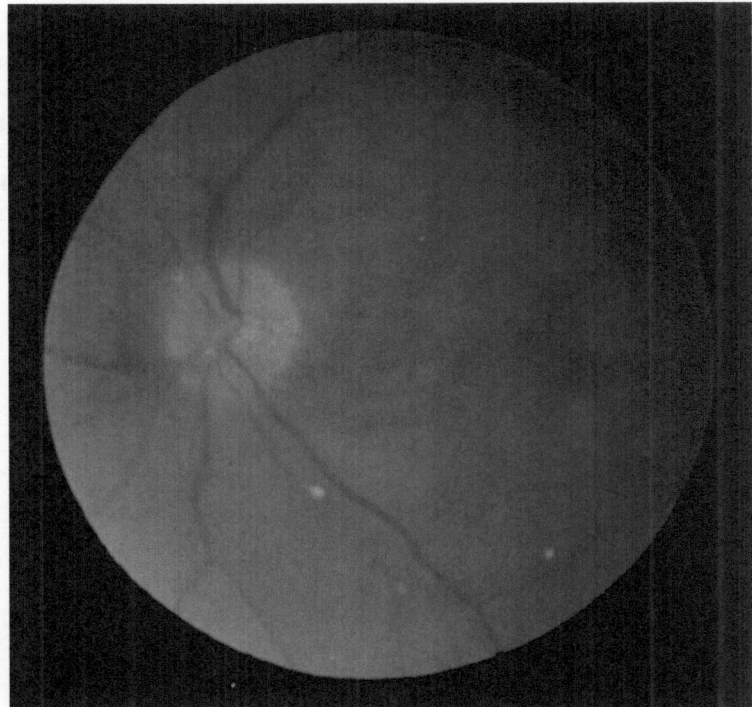

Fig. 5.2. Optic fundus of a patient with recurrent monocular visual disturbances of varying expression in embolizing carotid stenosis. The glittering golden cholesterol crystals seen in several arterial branches are characteristic

intraocular pressure is altered after the creation of a vacuum; if the intraocular pressure exceeds the systolic blood pressure, no pulsation in the ophthalmic artery can be recorded, and if it is less than the systolic pressure, the pulsations reappear. Gee's method determines the systolic pressure in the ophthalmic artery, which, according to Kartchner and McGray, assesses the relative arrival time of the ocular pulse wave.

5.1.5 Cardiologic Diagnosis

While cardiologic diagnosis is usually limited to the ECG and a chest X-ray in cases of acute cerebral insult, the search for a cardiac source of emboli should be accompanied by a wide-ranging electrocardiographic diagnostic procedure (e. g., stress ECG, long-term ECG; Table 5.1). Cardiac ultrasound occupies an intermediate position and is clearly indicated if there is any suspicion of a cardiac source of embolism. Unfortunately, the sensitivity of the traditional transthoracic technique in objectivizing such sources has proven unsatisfactory so far, so that they are much less often diagnosed than pathologic studies would suggest (Blackwood et al. 1969). Thrombi are the most often overlooked; only when they exceed 1 cm in size are they demonstrable by ultrasound with any degree of reliability. Most recently, transesophageal examination has brought an increase in sensitivity and specificity for the diagnosis of sources of embolism.

However, growing importance is being assigned to thrombi with the decline in heart valve defects following inflammatory diseases because of modern antibiotic treatment. Thus, intra-atrial and less often intraventricular thrombi in aneurysms after myocardial infarction may develop in the context of a cardiomyopathy (up to 50%), with and without arrhythmias and even with a diameter of several centimeters. We can presume that the importance of cardiac emboli in cerebral ischemia compared with stenosing vascular lesions of the extracranial cerebral arteries has been consider-

Table 5.1. Diagnostic criteria of cardiac cerebral embolism

Probable cardiac criteria
    Atrial fibrillation and flutter (paroxysmal or permanent)
    Mitral valve defects (with or without atrial fibrillation)
    Other valvular lesions (including postoperative states)
    Endomyocarditis
    Sick sinus syndrome
    Completed myocardial infarcts (3–6 months earlier)
    Aneurysms of the heart wall
    Cardiomyopathy (with or without demonstration of thrombus)
    Mitral valve prolapse
    Atrial myxoma
    Persistent foramen ovale

Suggestive neurologic criteria
    Demonstration of different affected vascular territories
    Epileptic attacks at the onset of cerebral ischemia
    Branch occlusion of intracranial arteries at angiography
    Multiple infarcts or hemorrhagic infarcts at CT
    Simultaneous peripheral emboli

ably underestimated. It remains to be seen to what extent a more accurate description can be obtained by the use of contrast agents in echocardiography, transesophageal ultrasound, or the new techniques of CT and MRI. According to new and encouraging findings, a patent foramen ovale as the cause of cerebral ischemias is more common in patients aged under 45 years (after excluding other possible causes) than has hitherto been supposed and can be demonstrated using contrast echocardiography (Lechat et al. 1988).

Evaluating of the pathogenetic relevance of abnormal echocardiographic findings is particularly problematic, for example, in the case of mitral valve prolapse (MVP; Barnett et al. 1980). This phenomenon is encountered in long-term studies in healthy individuals (up to 18%) without an increased rate of embolism. It may be that active complementary mechanisms have not so far been identified. Two patients with MVP in fact showed disturbances of thrombocyte function (Scharff et al. 1982), which might serve as mediators of thromboembolic lesions of the heart valves, but no significant incidence was found compared with asymptomatic sufferers from MVP. Paradoxic cerebral emboli associated with a persistent foramen ovale can now be shown to have a distinctly higher incidence (Lechat et al. 1988; Biller et al. 1986) by means of transesophageal echocardiography and the use of contrast media in ultrasound (bubble technique).

In a high proportion of cases (up to 40%) cardiac cerebral emboli tend to become secondarily hemorrhagic, possibly due to greater and faster autolysis. This situation, familiar from pathologic studies in fatal cases, has been verified by the CT findings in cases with a favorable clinical outcome (Hornig et al. 1986). It is not possible to decide what the therapeutic implications of these observations may be (e. g., as regards early anticoagulant treatment) without a prospective study. Also, the treatment of cardiac arrhythmias, especially of atrial fibrillation and arteriovenous block grade III, is still disputed and the object of two large prospective randomized studies. As in patients with aortic defects or after the implantation of synthetic valves, the risk of ischemia seems to be markedly raised.

A detailed account of the problem of cerebral infarcts of cardiac origin, with numerous references, is to be found in the publications of the Cerebral Embolism Task Force for the years 1986 and 1989.

5.1.6 Laboratory Diagnosis

Clinical laboratory diagnosis is important in the choice and monitoring of treatment for cerebral ischemias; it is also useful for establishing the diagnosis of obscure or rare causes. One distinguishes on practical grounds among a range of laboratory parameters, which include: (a) those essential in the early phase of cerebral ischemia, (b) those routinely employed with only minor deviations for the inpatients of most hospitals, and (c) those that can be selectively added in the further course of diagnostic deliberations (Table 5.2)

In view of the extremely large number of strokes of undetermined etiology even after the most exhaustive use of modern instrumental techniques (about one-third according to the results of the NINCDS Stroke Data Bank; Mohr 1986), particular significance attaches to the third set in the above list. These are to be employed after

Table 5.2. Clinical laboratory studies in patients with cerebral ischemias

Absolutely essential basic information (general practice, emergency unit)	Hospital admission routine[a]	Laboratory studies for special problems
ESR, red blood count (Hb, red cells, hematocrit), leukocytes, creatinine, glucose Also desirable: Sodium, potassium, Quick test, PTT	Differential blood count, platelets, ESR, urea, creatinine, sodium, potassium, SGOT, SGPT, AP, GLDH, γGT, CK, glucose, T_3, T_4, Quick, PTT Total protein, electrophoresis, cholesterol, triglycerides, uric acid	Additional clotting studies such as fibrinogen, protein C, protein S, antithrombin III, fibrinogen depletion products, factor VIII Platelet function test, lupus anticoagulant, anticardiolipin antibodies For diagnosis of vasculitis, see Table 4.5, including: immunoelectrophoresis, CSF immunology, rheumatoid status, blood cultures, specific inflammatory parameters such as serology for syphilis and HIV Lipid electrophoresis, HDL, LDL, VLDL, apolipoproteins

[a] Admission routine differs from hospital to hospital; this is a laboratory routine for ordinary wards. A series of studies (urea, creatinine, T_3, T_4) are used to safeguard the patient in the event of contrast studies.

completing the imaging techniques if the etiology of the disease is still undetermined. Especially in younger patients (under 45 years) the possibility of a nonarteriosclerotic vascular disease must be suspected and an extensive range of supplementary diagnostic procedures undertaken. In the context of arteriosclerosis, on the other hand, those factors should be specially analyzed which are accessible to therapeutic influence. Therefore the measurement of only triglycerides and total cholesterol is not sufficient and the subfractions of the serum lipids should be analyzed too. CSF examinations are seldom diagnostically decisive, so that as a rule lumbar puncture can be avoided in cerebral ischemias. Of course, it is important to know that pleocytosis and increased protein, including positive demonstration of cerebral immunoglobulin production, is possible, especially in cortically situated infarcts, and this should not be taken as evidence of focal encephalitis in differential diagnosis.

5.2 Ultrasound Diagnosis

Numerous ultrasound techniques have been developed for the demonstration of flow impediments in the neck arteries and the intracranial arteries at the skull base. Some are capable of analyzing the hemodynamic conditions in the carotid and vertebral arteries (continuous and pulsed Doppler ultrasound, various spectrum analysis techniques using Doppler and auscultation signals). Other methods image the morphology of the cervical arteries in ultrasound B-mode and yet others combine the B-mode and Doppler ultrasound in the so-called duplex system. The latest development provides color-coded Doppler echotomographs which superimpose the flow pattern in an artery upon the two-dimensional image.

Transcranial pulsed Doppler techniques have been introduced in recent years for the investigation of flow conditions in the cerebral arteries at the skull base (Aaslid 1986). Here, too, a two-dimensional reference technique to demonstrate the position of the measured volume in a coordinate system has recently been introduced to compensate for the disadvantages of the initial hand-held method. The low transmission frequencies of high energy used in the pulsed Doppler technique are indicated particularly for depicting lesions at the origins of the cerebral arteries from the aortic arch in the thorax and in the submandibular region (Rautenberg and Hennerici 1988).

The various techniques mentioned above supplement each other, and their appropriate use provides an accurate and complete analysis of flow changes in the entire intrathoracic, extracranial, and intracranial portions of the large arteries supplying the brain with their essential collateral circulations (Büdingen et al. 1982; Hennerici and Neuerburg-Heusler 1988; Widder 1985). They are suited preferentially for monitoring the course; the importance of this for the treatment of various types of cerebrovascular diseases is growing continually. The following can now be monitored: obstructive or dilative arteriopathies, inflammatory or degenerative vascular disorders, transient or permanent lesions of the cerebral circulation, possibly with vasospasms, abnormal collateral circulation, and arteriovenous malformations.

5.2.1 Continuous and Pulsed Doppler Techniques

5.2.1.1 Indirect Methods

Like ophthalmodynamometry, oculoplethysmography, and thermography, periorbital Doppler ultrasound is an indirect diagnostic technique introduced primarily for the demonstration of extracranial carotid lesions, mainly on the basis of altered flow direction in the fronto-orbital end-branches of the ophthalmic artery (Fig. 5.3). With the directional Doppler system it is possible to demonstrate flow reversal in the fronto-orbital branches of the ophthalmic artery (supratrochlear and supraorbital arteries); because of frequent coil formations at the recording sites, compression tests of the external carotid branches (e. g., superficial temporal and facial arteries) maintaining the retrograde flow are necessary. Of course, the reliability of periorbital Doppler ultrasound is limited to hemodynamically pronounced (over 80%) stenoses of the internal carotid artery, and even here it reaches an accuracy of only some 80%, since with intact collateralization via the opposite carotid system or the arterial circle of Willis from the vertebrobasilar pathway the ophthalmic collaterals are not opened. While this method has been largely abandoned for diagnostic purposes in recent years in favor of direct techniques for the demonstration of carotid stenoses, it may be of major clinical significance for demonstration of the ophthalmic collaterals. The latest studies comparing vascular and metabolic aspects using positron emission tomography (PET) have shown that the ophthalmic collaterals are more often patent in patients with symptomatically marked extracranial vascular obstructions than in patients with asymptomatic lesions (Powers et al. 1987; Kuwert et al. 1990). Retrograde perfusion of the ophthalmic artery is therefore regarded as a sign of

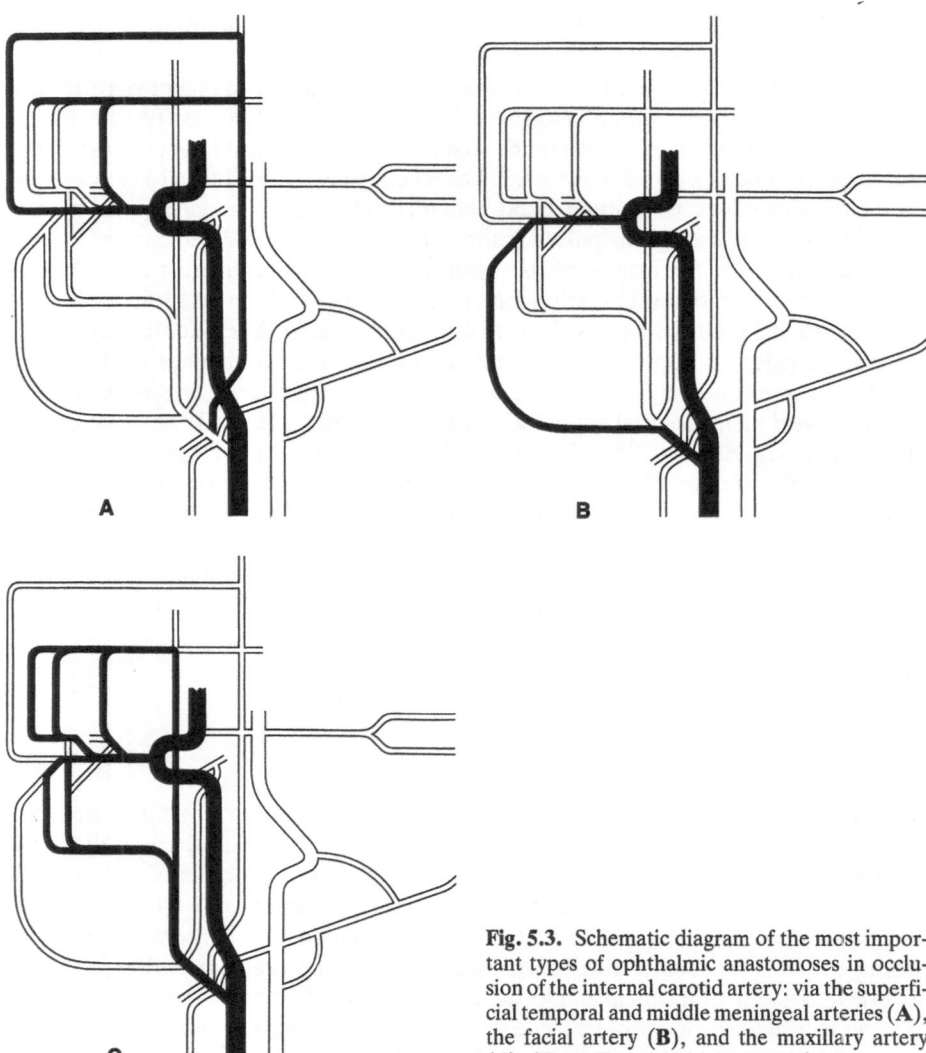

Fig. 5.3. Schematic diagram of the most important types of ophthalmic anastomoses in occlusion of the internal carotid artery: via the superficial temporal and middle meningeal arteries (**A**), the facial artery (**B**), and the maxillary artery (**C**). (From Krayenbühl et al. 1979)

insufficiency of the far more important collateral circulation via the circle of Willis and seems to be of negative prognostic value in the sense of exhausting the intracranial collateral capacity.

5.2.1.2 Direct Methods

Direct investigational techniques are important in demonstrating structural and hemodynamic lesions of the carotid system in the neck. The Doppler technique permits demonstration of the site and severity of stenoses due to plaque formations with greater reliability, provided the vessel lumen is narrowed by at least 40%. This applies to both the continuous-wave Doppler technique and the pulsed-wave system, in which waves of ultrasound are emitted in bursts and received again after a variably defined interval, permitting localization of the echo-reflecting structure in the tissue. In North America pulsed Doppler techniques are widely used in duplex systems, whereas in Europe continuous Doppler ultrasound with the hand-held probe is preferred. By sequential performance of a series of pulsed Doppler elements

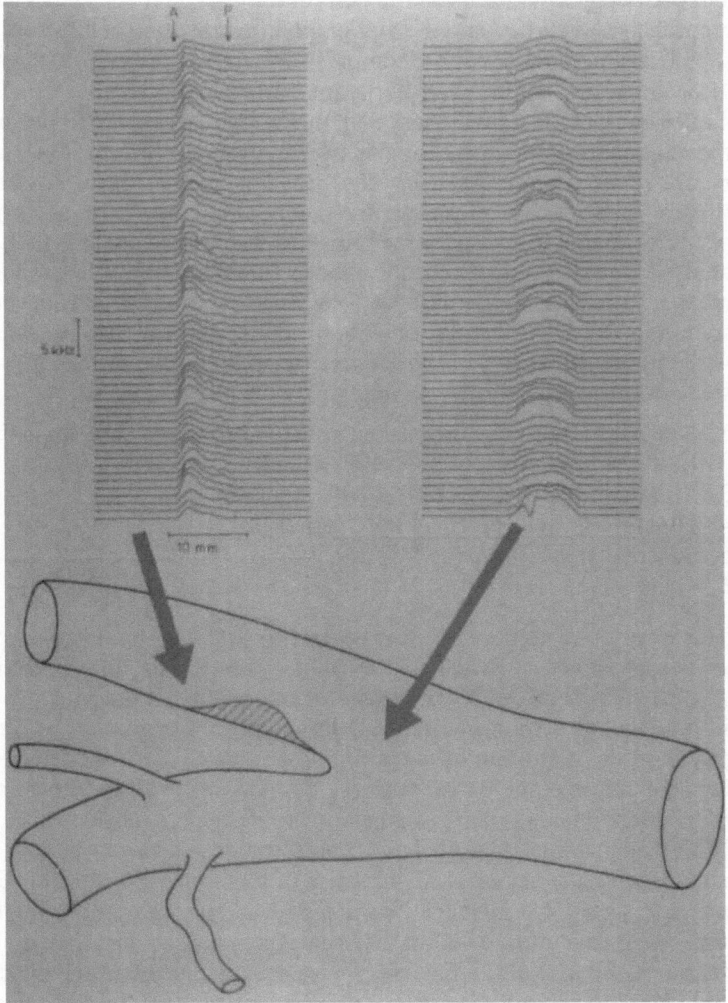

Fig. 5.4. Doppler ultrasound recording of a small plaque formation (< 40%) in the internal carotid artery with a multichannel pulsed Doppler. The flow profiles recorded over several cardiac cycles show a normal laminar distribution pattern proximal to the plaque; immediately distal to the plaque there is an evident asymmetry with flow acceleration opposite the mural lesion. *A*, Anterior wall; *P*, posterior wall of vessel

(Reneman et al. 1986) the intra-arterial flow profiles can be analyzed simultaneously, which is not possible with the continuous techniques. Asymmetries help to recognize even low-grade mural lesions which would otherwise be accessible only to an imaging B-mode technique (Fig. 5.4). Calculations to determine flow volumes can be added. With the direct method, all the extracranial vessels in the neck supplying the brain can be investigated: the common carotid, the bifurcation, the internal carotid up to the submandibular region, and individual branches of the external carotid (e.g., the superficial temporal, facial, occipital, and superior thyroid arteries). The large neck arteries can be differentiated and pathologic processes demonstrated under normal and pathologic conditions on the basis of the characteristic audiosignals, the shape of recorded pulse curves, and the topographic interrelation of different arteries, possibly supplemented by appropriate compression tests of the external carotid branches. The most important diagnostic criteria are summarized in Table 5.3. In addition to the audiosignal, the recorded changes in the Doppler signal are important in interpreting the examination findings. For this two methods are useful. One is the recording of mediated flow velocities using the principle of the "zero-crossers," a technically simple, economic technique but one that does not represent the Doppler spectrum in adequate detail. The other is the principle of spectrum analysis (e.g., sequential filter analysis or fast Fourier transformation, FFT), whereby flow velocities included in measured volumes are imaged differentially by their amplitude through the corresponding Doppler frequencies without topographic allocation (Figs. 5.5, 5.6). Even with the simple "zero-passage counter" technique, a crude classification of degrees of stenosis into six groups is possible:

1. Normal findings or nonstenosing plaque formation (less than 40% stenosis)
2. Low-grade stenoses (40%–60% stenosis)
3. Middle-grade stenoses (60%–80% stenosis)
4. High-grade stenoses (over 80% stenosis)
5. Subtotal stenoses (over 95% stenosis)
6. Complete occlusion

This hemodynamic classification correlates well with the angiographic evaluation of grades of stenoses, as verified by numerous studies. Interpretation of the angiographic images depends essentially on the quality of the imaging techniques (e.g., intravenous or intra-arterial digital subtraction angiography, conventional angiography) and the definition of the method of determining stenosis (measurement of the local or relative degree of stenosis). Difficulties arise in allocating the findings of individual hemodynamic investigations to particular classes.

While this simple method is adequate for acute diagnosis and has proven itself abundantly, a series of problems arise in long-term monitoring. Complex hemodynamic changes, for instance, are not adequately represented by the mediated flow velocity alone; moreover, an adequate comparison of a previous with a present finding after an observation interval is not possible. Also, the division into grades of stenosis is too rough for reliably determining the progression, persistence, or even regression of the vascular lesion in the individual case. This is more easily achieved if several parameters of the Doppler spectrum are recorded and analyzed (Table 5.4). It was long unclear which of these parameters are useful in semiquantitative analysis, and what points in the cardiac cycle are suitable for their documentation; however,

Table 5.3. Ultrasound diagnosis in the differentiation of stenoses in the carotid flow territory. (From Hennerici and Neuerburg-Heusler 1988)

	Nonstenosing plaque	Low-grade stenosis	Middle-grade stenosis	High-grade stenosis	Subtotal stenosis
Local stenosis grading	< 40%	40%–60%	60%–70%	ca. 80%	> 90%
Stenosis grading relative to distal lumen	0	< 30%	≈ 50%	≈ 70%	> 90%
Indirect criteria	No evidence of flow impairment			Ophthalmic artery: no or retrograde flow Common carotid artery: reduced flow	
Direct criteria analog curve	Unremarkable	Altered audiosignal, local flow increase	Marked flow increase, loss of pulsatility, systolic deceleration	Strong local flow increase, systolic deceleration	Variable stenosis signal with reduced intensity
Spectrum analysis		Spectrum widened	Spectrum widened, increased, increased intensity of low-frequency component	Inverse frequency components with reduced frequency spectrum	
Poststenotic	Unremarkable			Reduced systolic flow velocity	Difficult to detect, markedly reduced signal
Systolic peak frequency in stenosis region related to 4 MHz transmission frequency	< 3 KHz		4–8 KHz	> 8 KHz	Variable
Quality of B image demonstration	+++	+++	++	+	+

the latest statistical-analytic studies show that the individual parameters contribute differently to the determination of the grade of stenosis (Fig. 5.6). Daffertshofer (1988) has shown in multivariate analysis that the reliability of these parameters can be assessed individually, and that in descending order the systolic peak frequency, the mean frequency, and the systolic spectrum width provide an optimal combination of parameters for discrimination of the degree of stenosis. Arbeille et al. (1985) have

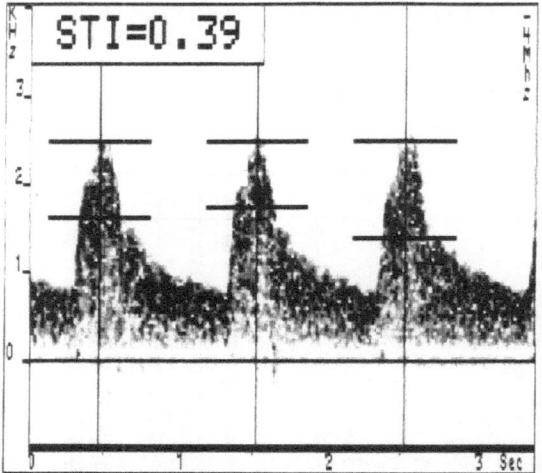

Fig. 5.5. FFT spectrum of internal carotid artery using the principle of Arbeille et al. (1985). *Upper horizontal lines,* FM (2520 Hz); *lower horizontal lines,* FO (1400 Hz)

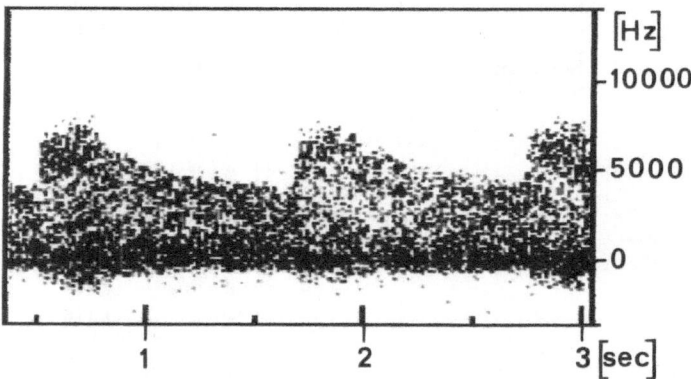

Fig. 5.6. FFT spectrum of an approximately 70% ICA stenosis after discriminant analysis. *1,* Maximal frequency 7420 Hz; *2,* mean frequency 2240 Hz, peak frequency 840 Hz; *3,* window breadth 16%. Function (1) contributes 94.9% to assessment of degree of stenosis, function (2) 4.9%, and function (3) only 0.2%. (From Daffertshofer 1988)

suggested an index for determination of the degree of stenosis (STI), calculated from the maximal flow velocity (FM) and the mean band width of the spectrum (FO; Fig. 5.5):

$$STI = 0.9 \ (1\text{-}FO/FM)$$

An empirical comparison of the Doppler signal analysis with the angiographically obtained grades of stenosis yields an equally good correlation (Fig. 5.7) as that reported for the STI values from postoperatively measured carotid endarterectomy specimens. The lower limits of resolution that can be attained with the two techniques, however, are not yet entirely clear. Changes of around 10% can be distinguished with certainty by discriminant analysis, i. e., progression from 70% to

Table 5.4. Criteria for spectral analysis of the Doppler signal

– Systolic and diastolic peak frequency
– Mean frequency
– Frequency band with highest signal amplitude (mode frequency)
– Systolic frequency window, spectral broadening
– Negative retrograde flow component

80% or regression from 70% to 60% can be diagnosed. Alterations in flow profile occur even under physiologic conditions (juxtamural reflux phenomena or vortex formation), which are not distinguishable from similar phenomena in an initial arteriosclerosis, and such early structural mural lesions are therefore often difficult to diagnose using hemodynamic techniques. Their analysis is the field of ultrasound, which is superior in sensitivity even to selective angiography. Moreover, it affords the possibility (within certain limitations) of a differential analysis of the mural structure and especially of the surface properties of some of the plaque formations, which may allow evaluation of the prognosis for the associated risk of embolism.

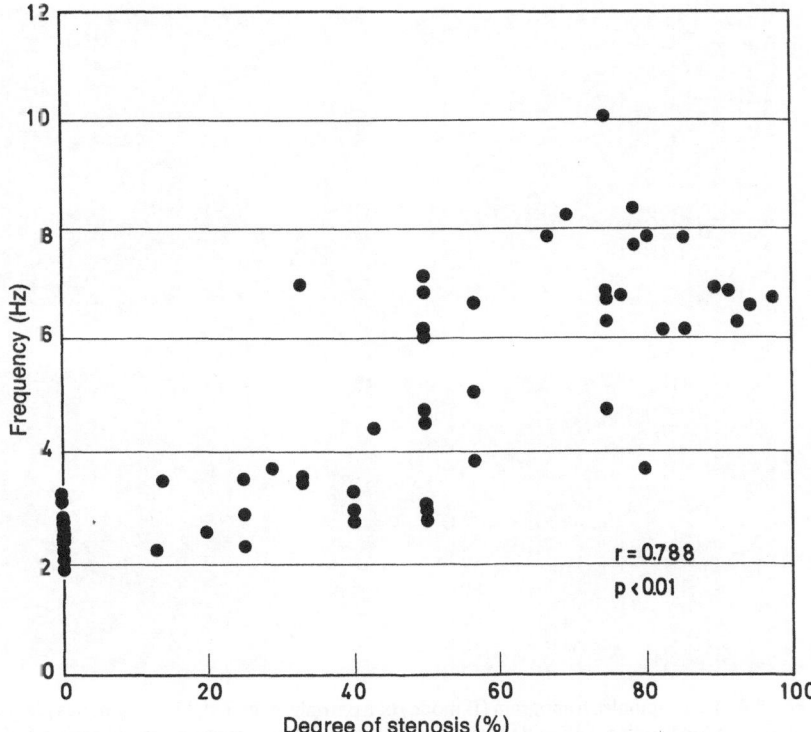

Fig. 5.7. Relationship of degree of stenosis as assessed angiographically (in lateral view) and maximal frequency of the FFT spectrum in the Doppler sonogram. (From Daffertshofer 1988)

5.2.2 B-Mode Ultrasound, Duplex System Analysis, and Color-Coded Doppler Flow Imaging

The high-resolution, two-dimensional ultrasound techniques allow imaging and differentiation of early forms of arteriosclerotic mural lesions in the directly accessible region of the carotids in the neck. In the case of a normal vessel wall a hypoechoic region appears bordered by two bright reflections. Externally, against the echo line facing the vessel lumen (intima-media reflection) is a further border surface reflection, corresponding to the adventitia (Fig. 5.8C).

Different types of plaque formation consistent with the pathologic findings can be distinguished using simple criteria (Table 5.5):

1. Flat plaques constitute the earliest detectable form of arteriosclerotic lesion in the B image and are characterized by an increasing broadening and destructuring of the normally hypoechoic intermediate layer and a thickening of the internal reflection line, the morphologic substrate of which is usually an accumulation of subintimal fibers, intimal thickenings, and proliferated smooth muscle cells (Fig. 5.8D).

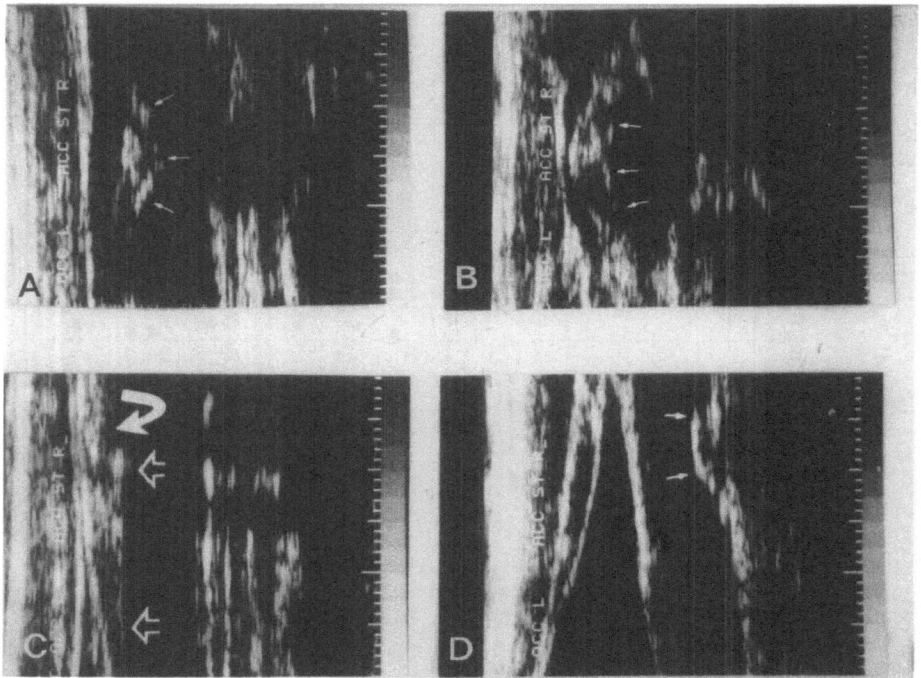

Fig. 5.8. Echo-impulse tomogram (B mode) of a partially calcified, heterogeneous plaque with sound shadow in longitudinal (**A**) and transverse (**B**) section of the common carotid artery. **C** An extensive, flat, soft plaque on the anterior wall of the common carotid which is partly ulcerated (*curved arrow*). **D** A flat plaque with smooth surface

Table 5.5. Ultrasound parameters for assessment of the extracranial carotid system

Vessel size
Length, diameter

Vessel movement
Transverse, axial
Systolic, diastolic

Course
Relative position of external and internal carotid arteries
High bifurcation, low bifurcation
Extent and conformation of carotid bulb
Kinking and coiling

Pathologic lesions
Plaque site and size
Plaque surface (regular, irregular, ulcerated, cavitated)
Echogenicity (homogeneous, heterogeneous, with and without signal-shadow)
Plaque shape (eccentric, concentric, irregular)

2. With increasing size, the so-called soft plaque extends into the vessel lumen. Its initially usually homogeneous structure becomes heterogeneous; hypo- and hyperechoic components alternate and may impede assessment (Fig. 5.8 B). Such advancing mural lesions are characterized pathologically by an atheromatous core which is usually packed with a mixture of cholesterol, cholesterol ester, neutral fats, and proteins and covered with a fibrous sheath on the luminal aspect. This consists predominantly of smooth muscle, collagen, elastin, and proteoglycans and usually contains considerable amounts of intra- and extracellular lipids.

3. With further development, complications of plaque formation are compounded. In addition to acute hemorrhages (hemorrhagic plaques), a layered reconstruction with calcified deposits may occur (hard plaques; Fig. 5.8), while rupture of the plaque sheath and ulceration is possible at the surface. It is often difficult to distinguish normal states of the vessel wall from uncomplicated (flat and soft plaques) and complicated (hard and hemorrhagic) plaque formations; extensive superficial lesions can generally be defined by their smooth contours. However, sensitivity in demonstrating ulceration by B-mode imaging (40%–70%) is poorer than specificity (approximately 90%); therefore ulcers may often be missed, while false-positive findings are rather rare. With the in vitro and in vivo examinations so far available and even with high-resolution ultrasound systems (10 MHz transmission frequency), an ulcer must have an extent of at least 2–3 mm to be demonstrable. It is also not clear whether hemorrhages can be reliably distinguished from soft plaques with central detritus, despite the increased reliability of the method due to improved quality of B imaging and scrupulous exclusion of the more important sources of error (Fig. 5.9).

If exclusively two-dimensional techniques are employed, the quantitative evaluation of luminal narrowing and the assessment of lesions during serial observations are problematic. This also applies to comparison with angiographic techniques, where superimposition effects must be taken into account, and to the interpretation of

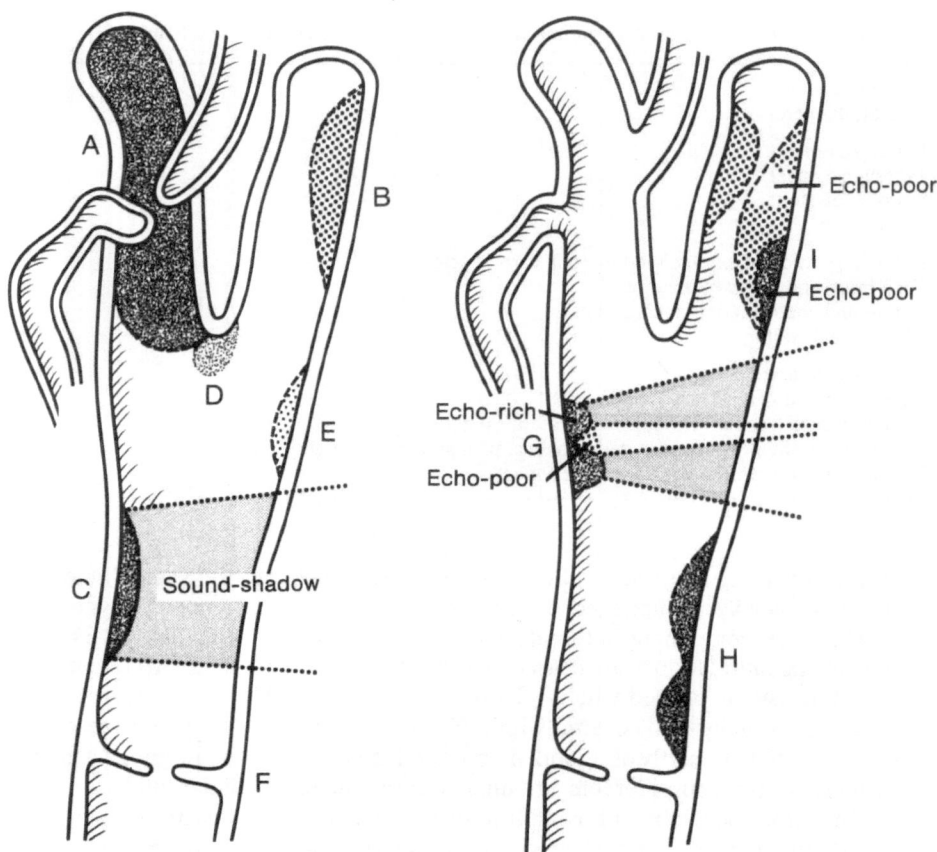

Fig. 5.9. Diagrams of problem situations in B-mode imaging. *A*, Occlusion of external carotid; *B*, high-level stenosis; *C*, calcified plaque on anterior wall with extensive signal-shadow; *D*, stenosis at bifurcation at division of flow; *E*, sound-transparent (nonechogenic) plaque; *F*, buttonhole stenosis; *G*, nonuniform calcified deposit at proximal and distal plaque margin (no ulcer!); *H*, oblique surfaces at plaque margins (no ulcer!); *I*, possible hemorrhage, central plaque necrosis

operative and even of pathologic specimens. Three-dimensional reconstruction is indispensable for this purpose and is possible by means of relatively simple computer-based graphic techniques. By means of additional analysis of vessel wall pulsation and the flow profile at the site of plaque formation it is possible to describe the interaction of hemodynamic and morphologic parameters in more detail (Fig. 5.10); from this one may deduce important prognostic parameters, such as the embolism risk of a vascular lesion. Predictive indices for these frequent causes of cerebral ischemia have not as yet been identified. Thrombotic deposits of arteriosclerotic vascular lesions probably play an important role. Depending on their structural composition, they frequently undergo spontaneous lysis, but as yet direct demonstration of such intravascular phenomena has not been possible with imaging ultrasound techniques. Only now, by the simultaneous analysis of the B-mode image and flow profile using special methods, can they be demonstrated. In this context the color-coded Doppler

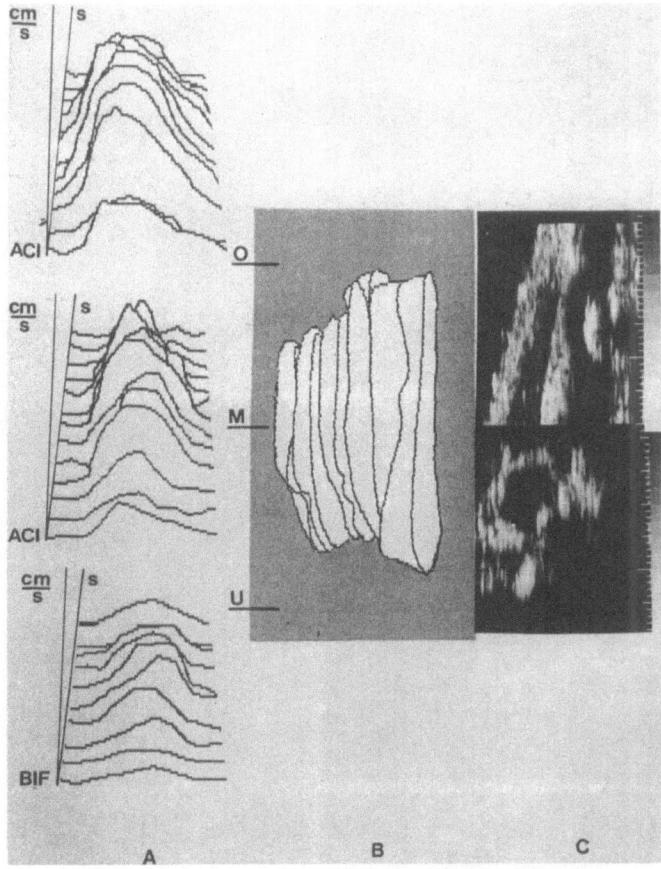

Fig. 5.10. Three-dimensional reconstruction of contour (**B**) and flow profile from a multichannel pulsed Doppler (**A**) below (*U*), in the middle (*M*), and above (*O*) a shallow plaque, which is also shown in two-dimensional high-resolution sonograms (**C**) in longitudinal section (*above*) and transverse section (*below*). The interaction of flow signal and plaque morphology shown by three-dimensional reconstruction can provide important guidelines in monitoring the course and prognosis of plaque formation

flow imaging recently introduced into diagnosis (Fig. 5.11) is important, although the equipment is still very expensive. It allows the portrayal of complex mural and flow changes; as the Doppler signals can be observed simultaneously over the entire vascular cross-section, the B-mode image can be optimized at regions with altered flow and thus the underlying mural lesion more easily identified. Conversely, a search can be made for low-grade flow changes in the vicinity of a structural lesion in the B-mode image. This is particularly valuable in the analysis of postoperative changes. Even with simple ultrasound techniques low-grade lesions of the mural structure are regularly found which usually undergo regression. Among 1720 cases analyzed in the literature with a mean observation period of 2.5 years, there was a restenosis rate of 8.6% annually (Table 5.6). Asymptomatic restenoses are much more common than symptomatic ones.

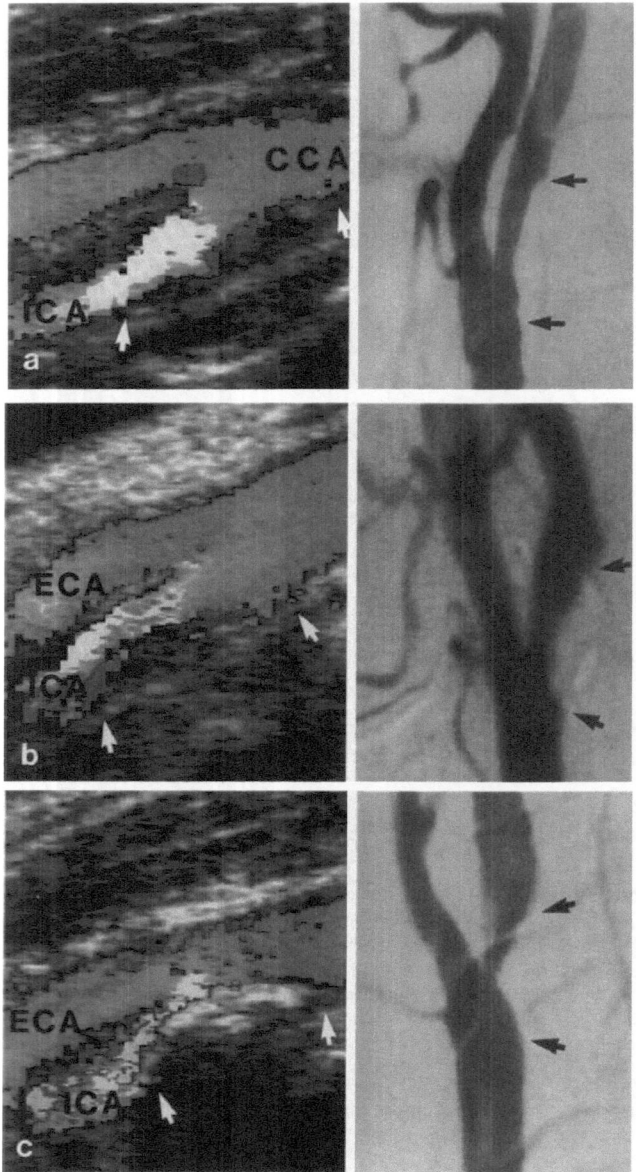

Fig. 5.11a–c. Color-coded Doppler sonograms and angiograms of stenoses of the internal carotid artery (*ICA*) of varying severity. **a** Longitudinal plaque formation at the posterior wall of the bifurcation, leading to approximately 40% luminal narrowing in the ICA and causing marked increase in flow velocity with color loss. **b** Heterogeneous plaque on posterior wall of carotid, leading to a middle-grade stenosis of the ICA of around 60% with moderate poststenotic turbulence (*blue*). **c** Longitudinal calcified plaque producing high-grade stenosis with about 80% luminal constriction. Characteristic color loss over a short segment with marked distal turbulence and retrograde flow build-up. *ECA*, external carotid artery. (From Steinke et al. 1990)

Table 5.6. Restenosis rates after carotid disobliteration as shown by noninvasive observations

Source	Year	Method	No. of operations	Mean observation period (months)	Restenosis rate (%) Symptomatic	Asymptomatic	Total
Aukland	1982	Doppler	84	1–60 (21)	10.7	6.0	16.7
Zierler	1982	Duplex	89	1–46 (16)	5.6	30.4	36.0
Norrving	1982	Doppler	64	12–156 (72)	15.0	22.5	37.5
Baker	1983	OPG/CPA/Doppler	133	1–60 (20)	1.5	12.0	13.5
Padayachee	1983	Doppler	54	< 72 (34)	9.3	3.7	13.0
Thomas	1984	Doppler	257	1–54 (20)	1.6	4.2	5.8
O'Donnell	1985	Doppler/B-mode	276	6–180 (29)	1.4	10.9	12.9
Nicholls	1985	Duplex	145	3–48 (18)	2.8	19.3	22.1
Keagy	1985	Duplex	122	1–142 (26)	—	—	22.1
van Berge	1985	Doppler	87	(13.4)	1.1	12.6	13.7
Colgan	1985	Doppler/IV-DSA	80	(22)	1.3	12.5	13.8
Barnes	1986	Doppler	47	3–77 (32)	0	6.4	6.4
Russell	1986	Doppler/IV-DSA	60	3	—	1.6	1.6
Zbornikova	1986	Duplex/IV-DSA	113	1–112 (62)	6.2	17.7	23.8
Sanders	1987	Duplex/IV-DSA	109	12			7.3
			1720		8.6% ± 5.9% year		

OPG, Oculoplethysmography; CPA, carotid phonoangiography; IV-DSA, intravenous digital subtraction angiography.

The advantage of color-coded Doppler flow imaging, even compared with angiography, lies in the better classification that it provides of carotid stenoses. This is because the examination is possible in several planes in addition to the analysis of longitudinal and transverse sections, the texture of the mural lesion can be portrayed, and even so-called hypoechoic regions can be reliably detected by absence of the Doppler signal. This demonstration is particularly important for the problem of the embologenic capacity of a vascular lesion, and hence for the overwhelming number of cerebral ischemias caused by an embolic source. Comparative studies between angiography and Doppler ultrasound have also shown significant advantages in the differentiation of total and subtotal carotid occlusions, assuming that slow-flow analysis is available (Steinke et al. 1990). Moreover, training in this technique requires less time than that with all traditional angiographic ultrasound techniques and documentation of the findings is more objective. Thus, an ideal method is now available for prospective, course-monitoring studies.

5.2.3 Transcranial Doppler Ultrasound

Low-frequency pulsed Doppler techniques are used both for the investigation of flow conditions at the juxtabasal intracraninal arteries and for the analysis by continuous Doppler or duplex techniques of inaccessible parts of the vessels (proximal carotid and truncal lesions, submandibular portion of the carotids, distal part of the vertebral artery). For this, ultrasound frequencies of 1.5–2 MHz are used with 10–20 times the ultrasound energy compared with simple continuous Doppler ultrasound in the neck (10–100 mW/cm²). This is necessary to overcome the signal absorption at the calvarium. Intracranially, for the *anterior circulation,* it is generally possible quite reliably to identify the siphon of the internal carotid transorbitally and the various parts of the arterial circle of Willis transtemporally by audiosignal, Doppler spectrum, flow direction, and reaction to compression tests of the ipsi- or contralateral common carotid in the neck. Criteria for the demonstration of stenoses and occlusions analogous with extracranial examination findings have been established (Lindegaard et al. 1986; Hennerici et al. 1987; Mattle et al. 1988). A prerequisite is finding an appropriate "echo window" at the skull, which is occasionally difficult. It should be noted that there are considerable positional variants of the circle of Willis (Fig. 5.12) so that every second case does not correspond to the textbook pattern. The stepwise identification of the vessel segments is essential to reliable diagnosis. Accuracy in identifying vessels on the basis of their flow signals is further enhanced by recording the position of the Doppler measured volume in fine-caliber vessel segments compared with adjacent wider segments of the circle of Willis. In pathologic processes, sometimes with severe hemodynamic changes and impaired spatial orientation, this is the essential advantage of a new two-dimensional scanning system over the originally blindly performed, hand-held, transcranial examination technique (Fig. 5.13).

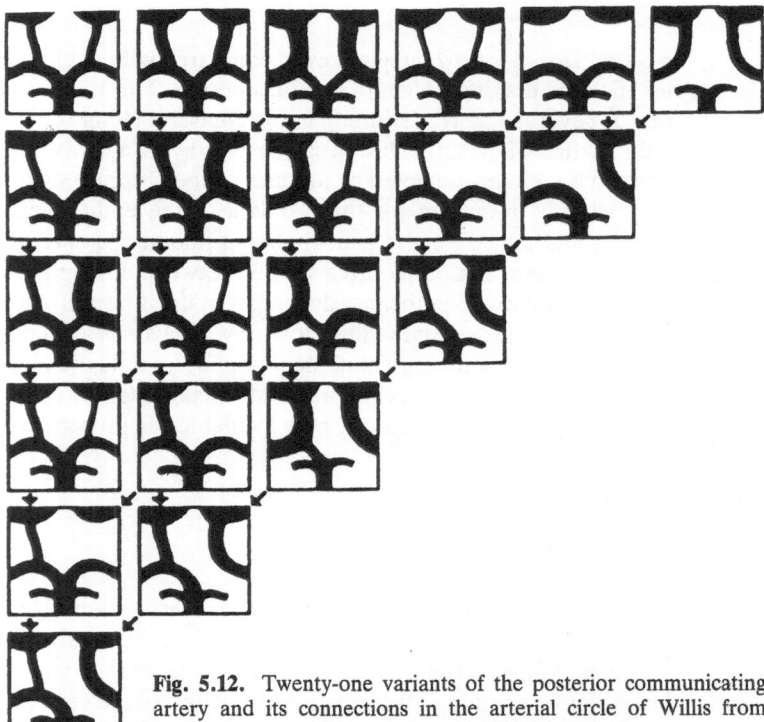

Fig. 5.12. Twenty-one variants of the posterior communicating artery and its connections in the arterial circle of Willis from examination of 2727 autopsies. (From Padget 1944)

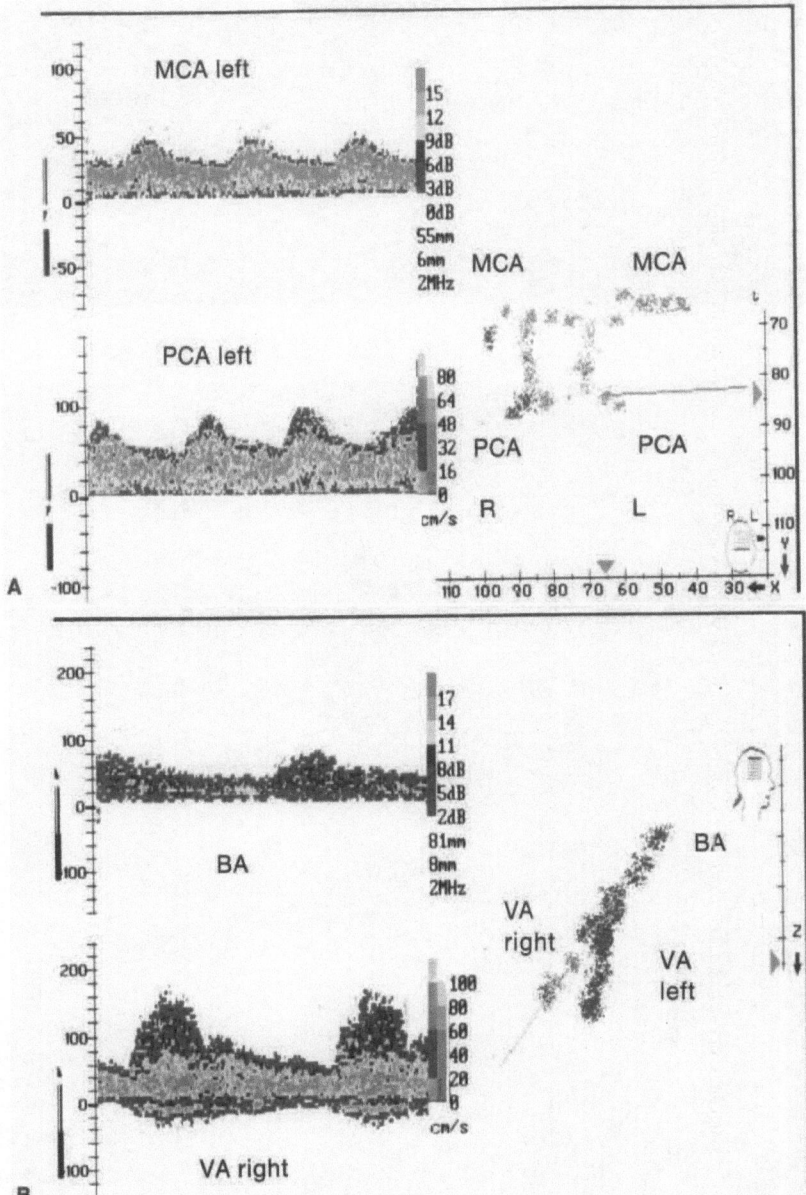

Fig. 5.13. Image obtained from a two-dimensional, transcranial scanning system showing the arterial Willis' circle from a transtemporal (**A**) and a transnuchal (**B**) approach. On the *right side* of each part, the position of the Doppler probe is shown on a head model given in the coordinate system of the measurement points of the information volume. The flow direction is color coded (*red* and *yellow* towards the probe, *blue* and *green* away from the probe). **A** *Left part* shows the FFT spectra of the middle cerebral artery (M1 segment; *above*) and the posterior cerebral artery (P1 segment; *below*) in a control individual. **B** *Left part* shows the FFT spectra of the basilar artery (*above*) and a stenosis of the vertebral artery (*below*)

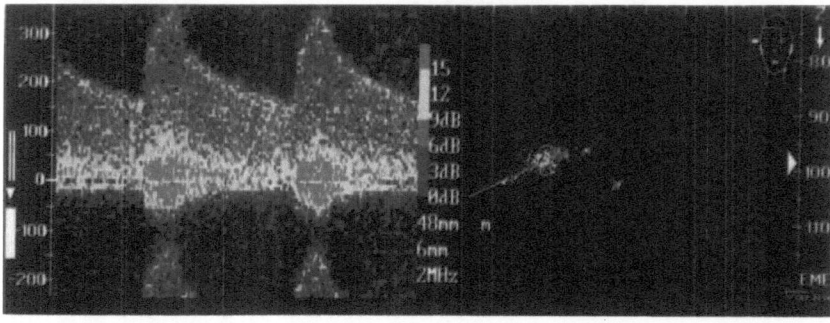

Fig. 5.14. Images obtained from a two-dimensional transcranial scanning system (**A**) and an angiogram (**B**) in a woman with moderate stenosis of the middle cerebral artery (M1 segment) on the right. **A** Frontal section shows the M1 segment of the MCA (for details see Fig. 5.13). In variable lengths of the labeled zone of the measurement volume characteristic changes of stenosis with flow acceleration, increased intensity at lower flow rates, and backflow phenomena are shown around the base line as an expression of the angiographically confirmed middle-grade stenosis (*arrow* in **B**)

This applies particularly to the *posterior circulation* and the vertebrobasilar system in the posterior cranial fossa with its extremely variable anatomy, where misinterpretations frequently occur with the hand-held method without radiotopographic findings (Mull et al. 1990). The variable choice of measurement volume as against an initially standardized excessive volume ($4 \times 10 \times 10$ mm) is a further advantage of the new system in view of the dimensions of the middle and anterior cerebral arteries (Fig. 5.14): in the M1 segment (pars sphenoidalis) the lumen of the middle cerebral artery is 3–5 mm, the internal diameter of the anterior cerebral (A1 segment) 1–3 mm, while, according to Wollschlaeger and Wollschlaeger (1974), hypoplasias (< 1 mm diameter) occur on the right in 8.6%, the left in 4.1%, and bilaterally in 3.2% of cases.

The importance of transcranial Doppler ultrasound consists in the noninvasive demonstration of intracranial stenoses and occlusions, and especially in monitoring the course of patients with a known vascular process. Examples include patients with vasospasm after subarachnoid hemorrhage, those with spontaneously evolving arteriovenous malformations, and those after neuroradiologic, neurosurgical, or radiotherapeutic measures. Further uses are in monitoring the course of extracranial vascular lesions, recording of changing collateral circulations, supervising of patients under intensive medical care, and after fibrinolysis connected with a cerebral ischemia.

5.3 Computer-Assisted Imaging Techniques

The major radiologic techniques for examining stroke patients are cranial CT and cerebral (arterial) angiography. We no longer employ cerebral scintigraphy in the diagnosis of strokes. With only a few exceptions, conventional plain X-ray of the skull and spine is of no value in patients with acute stroke.

PET is of scientific interest and widens the understanding of metabolic processes in stroke, but its application is restricted to a few research centers because of the costs in terms of personnel and equipment. Here, too, the acute stages of the disease can be studied so far only in exceptional cases. Single photon emission computed tomography (SPECT) is more widely available and technically easier to perform, also in connection with the isotopes used, but has the major disadvantage of poor image resolution. It is currently not very valuable in patient care. MRI is being employed with increasing frequency for the detection of small lesions, chiefly in the posterior cranial fossa. Hemispheric lacunes are also better demonstrated using this method. However, unconscious and intubated patients cannot yet be examined by this method with sufficient reliability because of problems with the equipment.

5.3.1 Cranial Computed Tomography

5.3.1.1 Temporal Development of CT Findings

The nature and extent of the changes on CT depend on the time after the stroke at which the examination is performed. In the early phase of stroke CT permits the exclusion of a cerebral hemorrhage. Within the first 8–12 h the majority of ischemic infarcts still escape CT demonstration; with large infarcts early signs of brain swelling can be detected early.

Demarcation of the infarct region begins only between 8 and 24 h. A relatively reliable definition of the size of infarct and its localization to particular vascular territories is possible after 2–3 days. In this phase the use of contrast does not improve on the information from the examination. After 3–5 days at the earliest the administration of contrast produces enhancement at the margin of the infarct zone, which becomes increasingly marked during the next 1–2 weeks (Fig. 5.15).

This phenomenon is particularly important between the 10th and 20th days after an infarct, especially if the first CT examination is made at this time; around the 14th day after a stroke the infarct zone may not be detectable in the unenhanced CT image. Because of reparative processes, edema, and increased perfusion in the infarcted region, density values are measured which correspond to those of the healthy brain

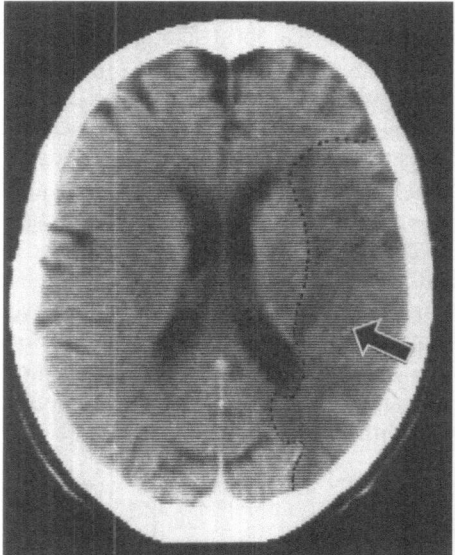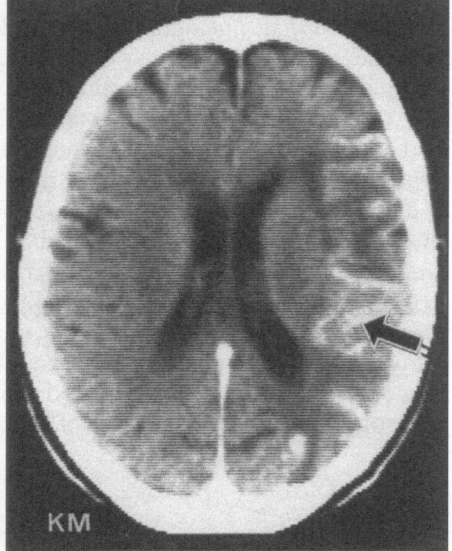

Fig. 5.15. Fogging effect and contrast enhancement. CT of a relatively extensive left middle cerebral infarct some 12 days old (extent indicated by *dotted line*). In the unenhanced scan (*left*) the infarct zone is quite recognizable; however, chiefly in the middle group of middle cerebral branches there is a virtually normal density (fogging effect). After administration of contrast (*right*) there is more marked depiction of the infarct zone due to hyperemia in the cortical region, especially in the region not clearly demarcated in the untreated CT due to the fogging effect (*arrow*)

tissue (fogging effect). A minor edematous swelling of the infarct zone may certainly remain detectable, but small lesions may escape CT demonstration in this phase. Significant contrast accumulation in the infarct zone may then permit positive demonstration of that zone despite the fogging effect (Fig. 5.15).

Most infarcts show an increase in size after 4–7 days due to edema formation. With very small infarcts this does not appear as a space-occupying lesion, but with large infarcts it may lead to a harmful space-occupying swelling of the brain with transtentorial herniation. In complete, noncollateralized occlusions of the middle cerebral or internal carotid arteries the swelling may affect the entire hemisphere, a state in which survival is rare. In infarcts of the cerebellar hemisphere the edema may cause impaired CSF drainage by compression of the aqueduct. The resulting obstructive hydrocephalus must then be treated by ventricular drainage and decompressive craniotomy to prevent superior or inferior infratentorial herniation. Ventricular drainage alone is probably inadequate as the considerable pressure gradient in the posterior fossa still persists. The volume increase with small and medium-sized infarct zones may be manifested by obliteration of the cortical sulci or compression of a lateral ventricle or even by a midline shift (Figs. 5.16, 5.17).

After transient ischemic attacks or other completely reversible ischemic disorders the CT remains normal in about 75% of cases. In many patients with a high-grade but still asymptomatic extracranial vascular stenosis, corresponding lesions may already be found at CT examination (see p. 109). However, other patients show lesions indicative of a microangiopathy and therefore probably of another pathogenesis.

In the following series of infarct patterns (see also Fig. 1.10) with illustrative images (Ringelstein et al. 1985; Zeumer and Ringelstein 1988; Zülch 1985) we classify the infarcts into macroangiopathies (hemodynamically induced infarcts and territorial infarcts) and microangiopathies (Fig. 1.14). For reasons of clarity, and unless otherwise stated in the legends, definitive lesions are shown, i. e., lesions at about 3–4 weeks after the stroke. Lateralization is determined by radiologic criteria, i. e., unless otherwise indicated, the left side of the head is at the *right* of the image.

5.3.1.2 Macroangiopathies

Macroangiopathies are caused by arteriosclerotic, inflammatory, traumatic, or thromboembolic diseases of the extracranial arteries supplying the brain and of the large cerebral (pial) vessels.

Hemodynamically ·Induced Infarcts

Hemodynamically caused infarcts are produced by significant restriction of perfusion pressure with loss of the pressure gradient in the vascular periphery or at the center of a collateralized vascular zone. The degree of stenosis of extracranial vessels which may lead to hemodynamically induced infarcts cannot be specified with certainty. Under normal blood pressure conditions (which frequently correspond to hypertensive values in these patients), with normal collateralization and functioning autoregulation, internal carotid stenoses of less than 80% may still be hemodynamically asymptomatic.

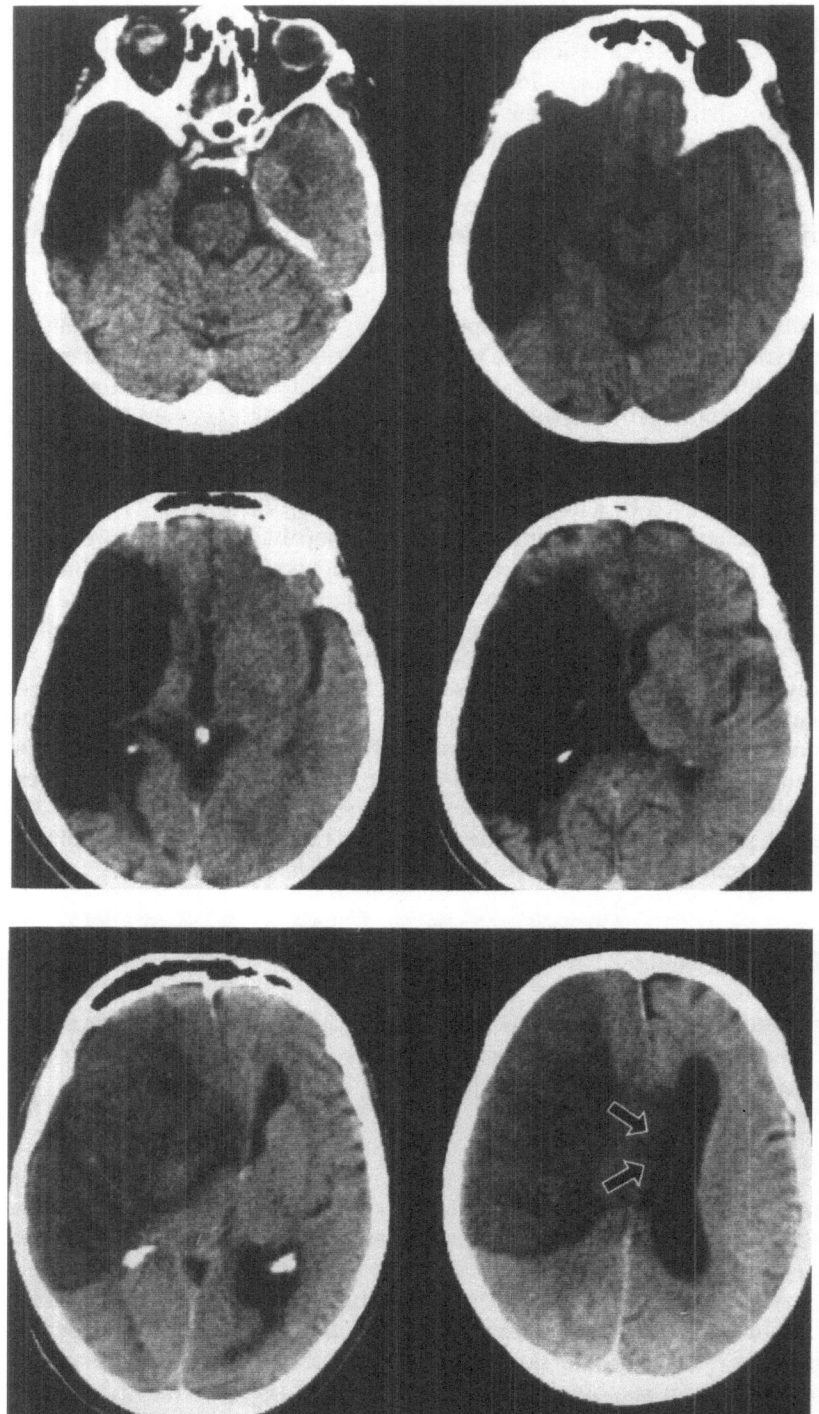

Fig. 5.16

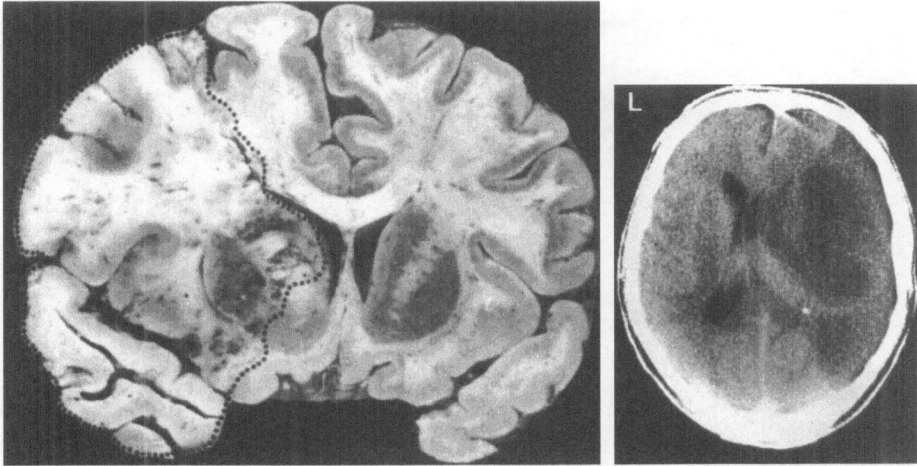

Fig. 5.17. Pathologic specimen of an extensive, space-occupying middle cerebral infarction including part of the lenticulostriate arteries. (From Zülch 1985)

The situation is different if several afferent vessels have stenoses and the collateral capacity is thereby impaired. Also, severe anemia, systemic hypotension, shock, delayed resuscitation, and altered rheologic parameters of the blood may produce hemodynamic effects even in low-grade stenoses. In hemodynamically induced strokes, end-flow and borderzone infarcts can be distinguished.

Low-flow infarcts occur in the distribution territory of the long, noncollateralized perforating arteries. The pressure drop beyond extracranially situated stenoses is often first noticed in these vessels. The zones of softening in low-flow infarcts appear on CT as hypodense lesions in the paraventricular, subcortical white matter. It is sometimes very difficult to distinguish these lesions from lacunar insults (see below). Figures 1.10c and 5.18 show such low-flow infarcts in the left and right paraventricular white matter. Clinically, there is commonly a fluctuating hemiparesis, often more marked in the lower limbs.

Borderzone infarcts occur in the border region between the supply zones of two or more cerebral arteries. They are also known as extraterritorial infarcts, and border area or watershed infarcts. In addition to often multiple extracranial and intracranial vascular stenoses or occlusions, other factors such as systemic hypotension and altered rheologic parameters may be involved in the etiology of these infarcts.

The decisive restrictive effect is due to multiple stenoses or to structural anomalies. Here the loss of the pressure gradient in the connecting collaterals between the

Fig. 5.16. Extensive right middle cerebral infarct. *Upper four images* show the findings 3 months after the event. *Lower two images* are from another patient and show the marked space-occupying effect of an extensive middle cerebral insult in the early phase: 4 days after the insult the infarct zone is demarcated; a marked midline shift with compression (*arrow*) of the left lateral ventricle is demonstrated

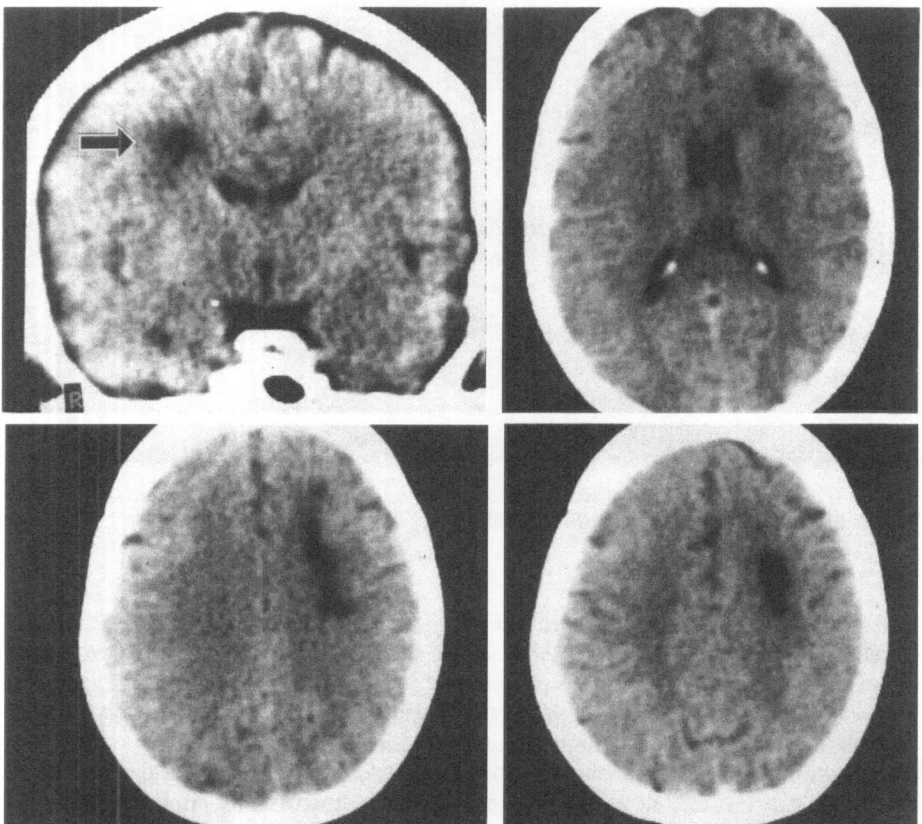

Fig. 5.18. Extensive, strictly subcortical, low-flow infarct in para- and supraventricular position. The subcortical position is particularly well shown in coronary section (*arrow*)

vascular territories (Figs. 1.10d, 1.11d) leads to typical necroses in the fronto-parasagittal borderzone (between the anterior and middle cerebral arteries) and the parieto-occipital borderzone (between the anterior, middle, and posterior cerebral arteries, the so-called triangle area). Figure 5.19 shows the pathologic findings in an anterior borderzone infarct which manifests unmistakably as an additional vertical parallel to the longitudinal cerebral fissure. Examples of posterior borderzone infarcts are given in Fig. 5.20.

Territorial Infarcts

Territorial infarcts are usually caused by embolic or local thrombotic occlusion of end-branches of the large supra- or infratentorial superficial arteries. Larger subcortical infarcts in the lentiform nucleus and thalamus may also be territorial infarcts, in which case differentiation from lacunar infarcts is difficult. Emboli leading to occlusions

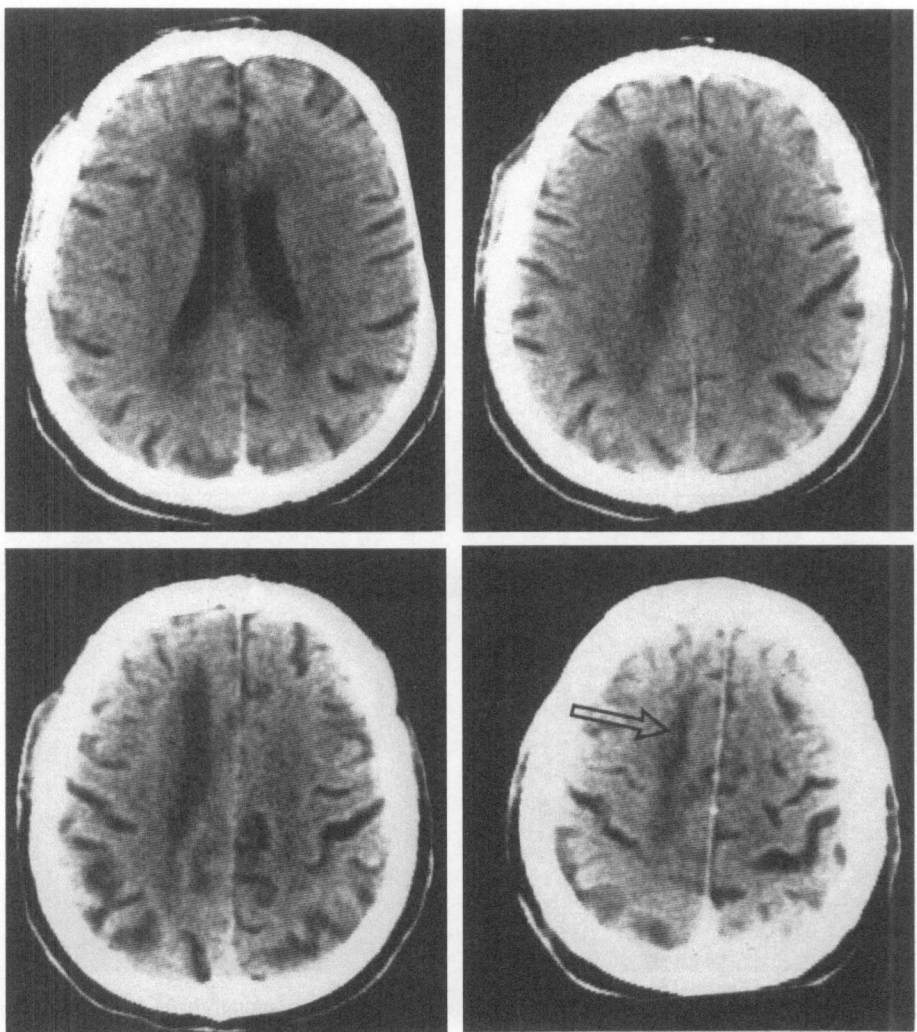

Fig. 5.19. Extensive borderzone infarct in the anterior cerebral/middle cerebral borderzone area, *right.* The lesion reaches the cortex (*arrow*)

with resulting cerebral infarcts originate largely from arteriosclerotic, even low-grade, stenoses of the carotid bifurcation. Cardiac emboli in arrhythmias, valvular defects, or occasionally mitral valve prolapse constitute the second important cause of territorial infarcts. In many cases a direct source of the embolism cannot be demonstrated despite close investigation, in which case a hypercoagulopathy may exist (see also Sect. 4.2.6, diagnosis in juvenile insults, p. 89).

The vascular occlusion described above leads to rhombus- or wedge-shaped necrotic areas affecting the cortex and white matter, corresponding to the anatomic supply

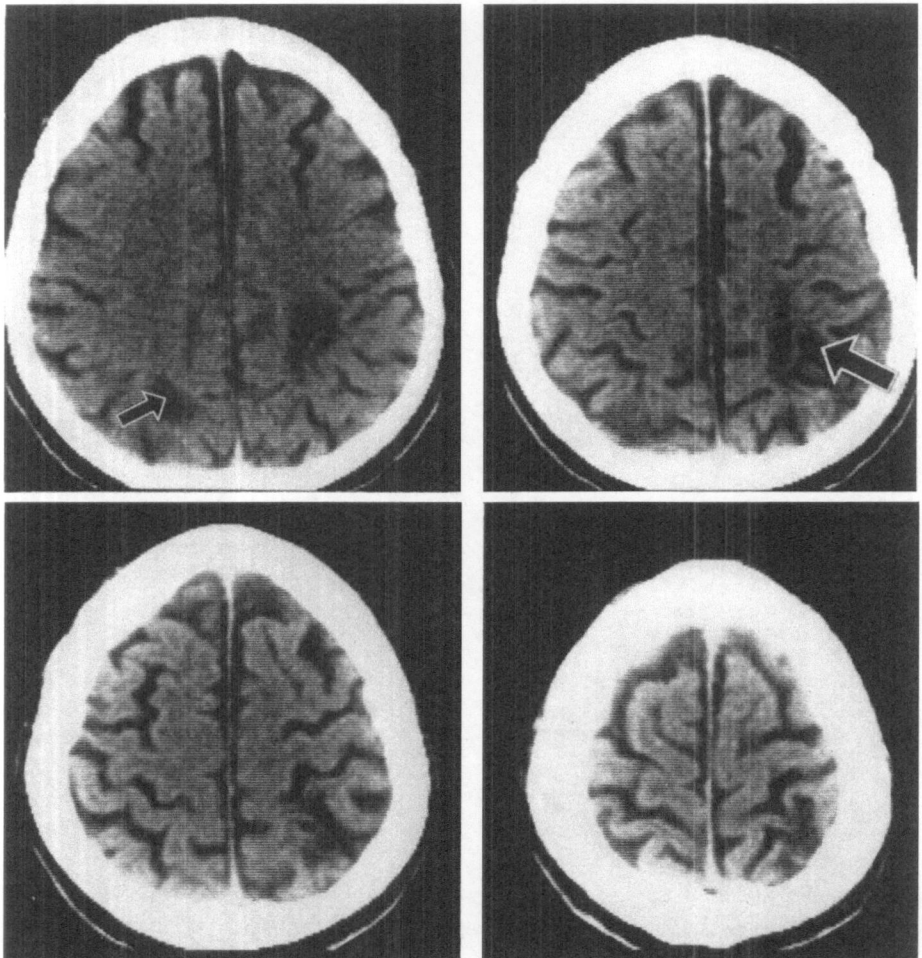

Fig. 5.20. Bilateral posterior borderzone infarcts, extending further parietally in the left hemisphere

territory of the artery. Deviations from these territories occur with good collateralization. Territorial infarcts in the distribution of the middle cerebral artery are particularly common. Here there may develop either a total softening of the entire middle cerebral territory (Fig. 5.16) as a space-occupying, life-threatening infarct, or infarcts of the anterior, middle, and posterior groups of middle cerebral branches (Figs. 5.21 and 5.22). With emboli in the proximal middle cerebral artery, the thrombus in the M1 segment of the artery can often be detected as a primary hyperdense region in CT. This finding is termed the hyperdense middle cerebral sign (Tomsick et al. 1989) or the malignant middle cerebral artery sign. It is found in the presence of an extensive middle cerebral territorial infarct. The MRI equivalent to this CT finding consists of suppression of the flow signal over the middle cerebral

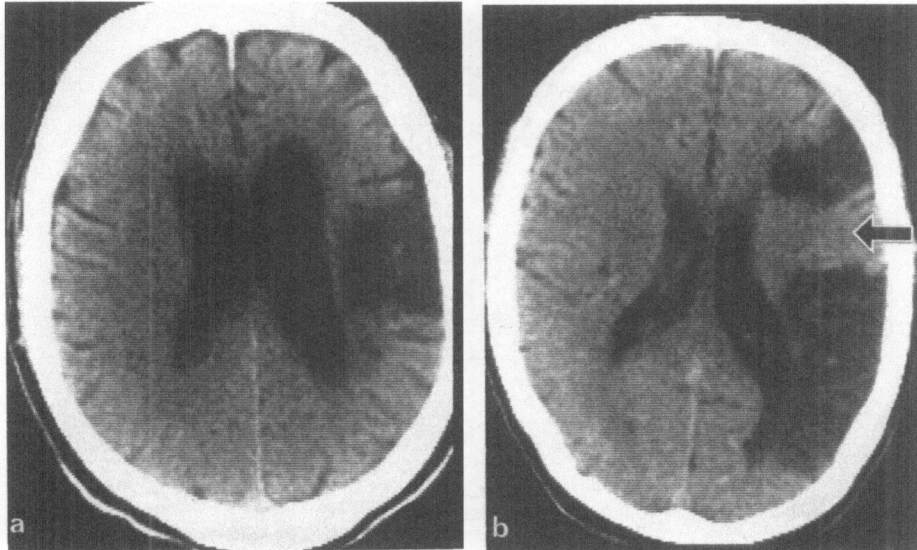

Fig. 5.21. a Territorial infarct in the supply zone of the middle group of branches of the left middle cerebral artery. **b** Territorial infarcts in the distribution area of the anterior and larger part of the middle and posterior group of branches of the middle cerebral artery. Only one part of the territory supplied by the middle branches of the left middle cerebral artery is not infarcted (*arrow*)

artery. The same applies to loss of the flow signal in occlusions of the carotid siphon and of the distal basilar artery. Sometimes, as already mentioned, the infarct is related only to the strictly subcortically located and inadequately collateralized territory of the lenticulostriate arteries (extensive or partial lentiform nucleus infarct; Figs. 1.11f, 5.23), while good collateralization exists at the periphery, and extension of the insult to the cortex is prevented. In a similar way there arise the so-called central middle cerebral infarcts, in which, for instance, only the insular groups of branches of the middle cerebral are affected – often difficult to distinguish from a focally emphasized atrophy. The lesional pattern of an extensive infarct of the lentiform nucleus is explained by the simultaneous blockage of the origins of the lenticulostriate arteries from the M1 segment of the middle cerebral artery. This occlusion can also be demonstrated angiographically if this examination is made early. However, the M1 segment of the middle cerebral artery may be patent again at the time of angiography due to autolysis of the embolus. Territorial infarcts in the anterior cerebral artery territory are less common. Figure 5.24 shows such an extensive infarct in the territory of the right anterior cerebral artery. Examples of infarcts in the posterior cerebral artery territory and the cerebellum are shown in Fig. 5.27.

The subject of internal carotid occlusion does not easily fit into this description. Quite a number of patients tolerate unilateral internal carotid occlusion with good collateralization without clinical features or lesions demonstrable by CT. There are even patients who remain asymptomatic with bilateral internal carotid occlusion. Carotid occlusions become symptomatic either hemodynamically with inadequate collaterali-

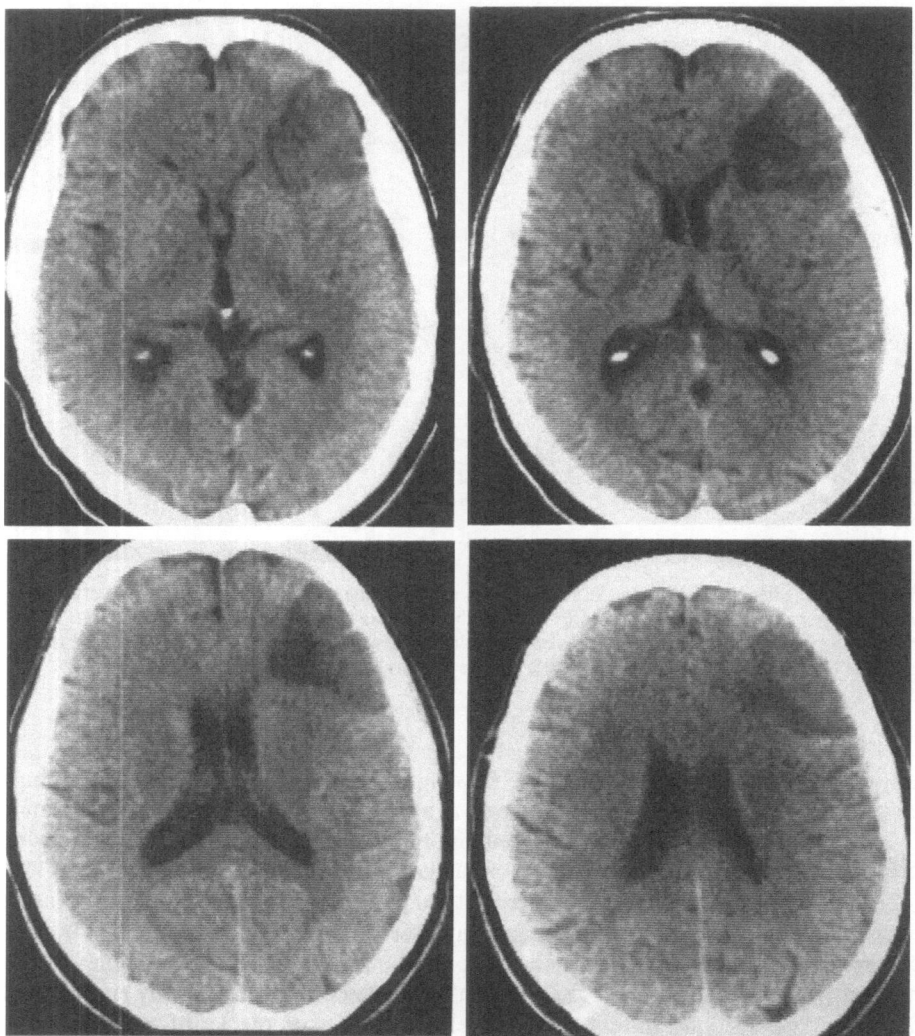

Fig. 5.22. A 24-hour-old infarct in distribution zone of the anterior group of branches of the left middle cerebral artery. Its extent is shown in different CT sections

zation, or through secondary embolism into the intracranial vessels, usually of the middle cerebral artery (arterioarterial embolism, periocclusional embolism). Since the therapeutic implications differ in hemodynamic and embolic complications of internal carotid occlusion, one should investigate angiographically also the opposite carotid to show the extent of cross-filling and to exclude or confirm the presence of secondary embolism.

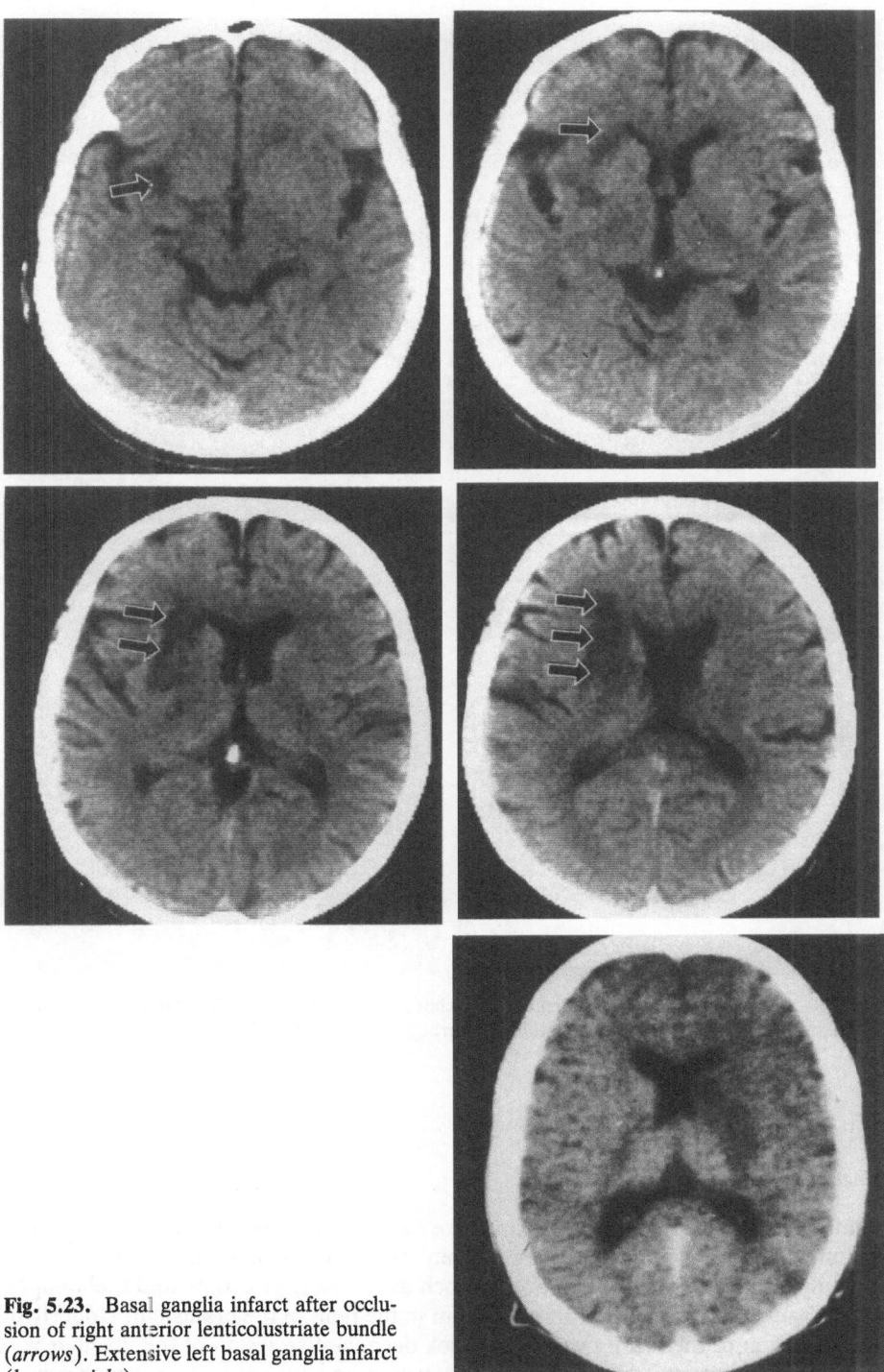

Fig. 5.23. Basal ganglia infarct after occlusion of right anterior lenticulustriate bundle (*arrows*). Extensive left basal ganglia infarct (*bottom right*)

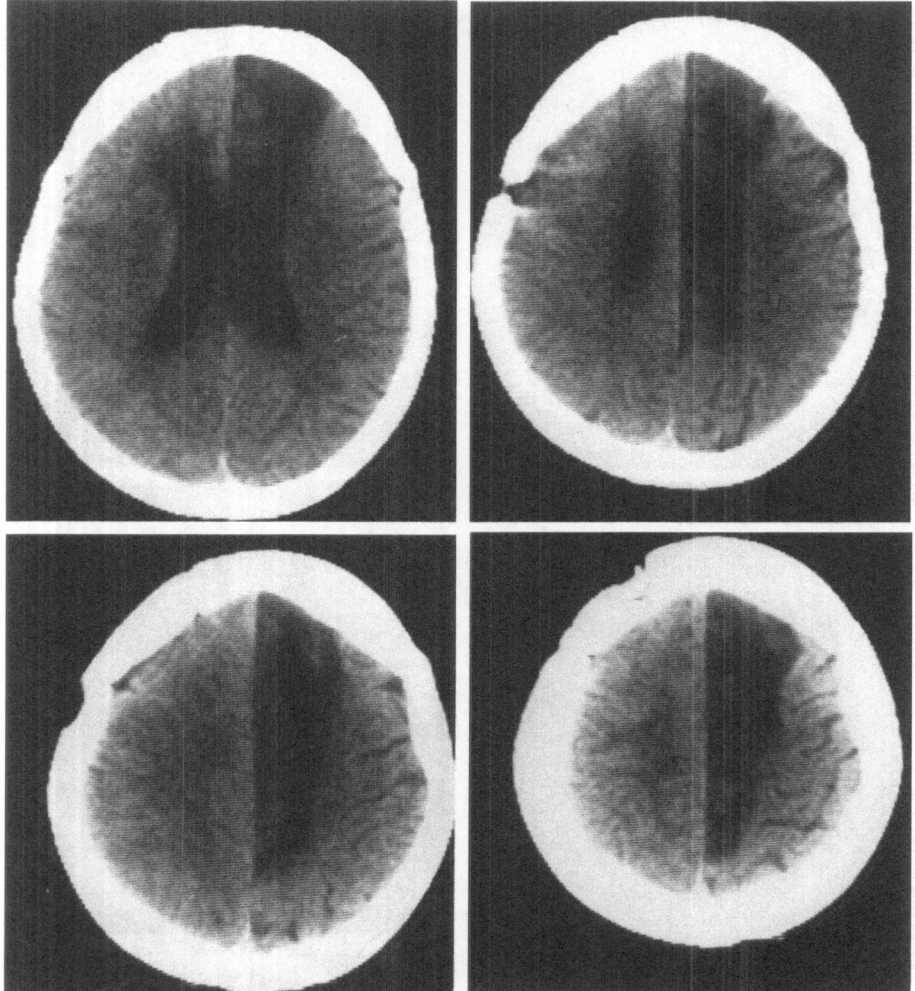

Fig. 5.24. Extensive infarct in the territory of the left anterior cerebral artery. This infarct was due to extensive vasospasm after a subarachnoid hemorrhage (see operative defect)

5.3.1.3 Microangiopathies

Lacunar Infarcts

Pathologically defined, lacunar infarcts are small, central, pseudocystic defects of 2–10 mm, rarely 15 mm in diameter. They arise from occlusion of intracerebral, noncollateralized, penetrating arteries such as the lenticulostriate and thalamoperforating arteries and the (perforating) rami to the pons in the brainstem. Underlying the occlusion of these arteries is a complex degenerative lesion of the vascular wall (hyalinosis), the cause of which must be taken to be a long-term hypertension.

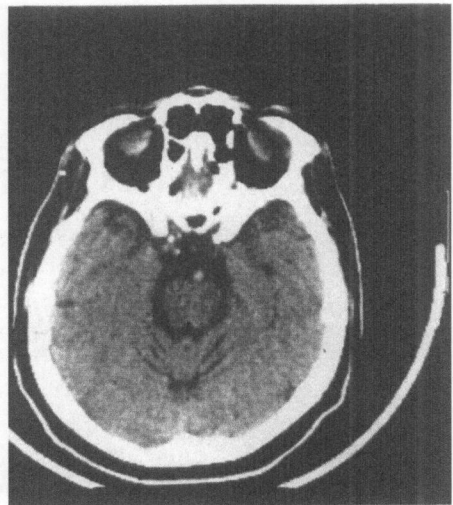

Fig. 5.25. Lacunar brainstem infarct in right cerebral peduncle

The usually multifocal necroses are found especially often in the basal ganglia and internal capsule, the juxtaventricular portions of the medulla, and the pons. Lacunar infarcts of the basal ganglia and medullary lacunes are usually easily recognized on CT (Fig. 1.10a), but those of the brainstem often evade demonstration (Fig. 5.25). Sometimes it is possible to demonstrate involvement of the brainstem by supplementary electrophysiologic studies. The lacunes shown on CT may be situated in clinically silent regions of the brain and need not necessarily correspond with the actual clinical features. However, the demonstration of infarct areas of lacunar size at typical sites leads to the conclusion that other lacunes exist which evade demonstration for technical reasons and may form the basis of the clinical presentation ("the tip of the iceberg"). Only rarely can lesions of lacunar size be confused with residues of hemorrhages. Recent lacunes in the edematous phase are sometimes more extensive than the definitive lesion proves to be.

Subcortical Arteriosclerotic Encephalopathy

Subcortical arteriosclerotic encephalopathy (SAE), or Binswanger's disease, is characterized by lacunar infarcts associated with a vacuolated demyelination of the white matter layer (Olszewski 1962; Zeumer et al. 1980). It is evidenced on CT by hypodensity of the white matter. In addition, many of these patients also have a dilative arteriosclerosis of the great vessels. These patients repeatedly develop neurologic features corresponding to different parts of the brain; often these are brainstem symptoms, which are capable of limited regression. Often also, but by no means necessarily, the patient shows an increasing intellectual and affective flattening; in such cases the SAE may be the basis and expression of a multi-infarct dementia. Figures 1.10g and 5.26 show the typical CT findings in SAE. The relationship between status lacunaris and Binswanger's disease is also supported by the pathologic findings. In microangiopathy there is a subendothelial hyalinosis or possibly atheromatosis. Occlusion of individual small vessels then leads to lacunes. As the disease progresses,

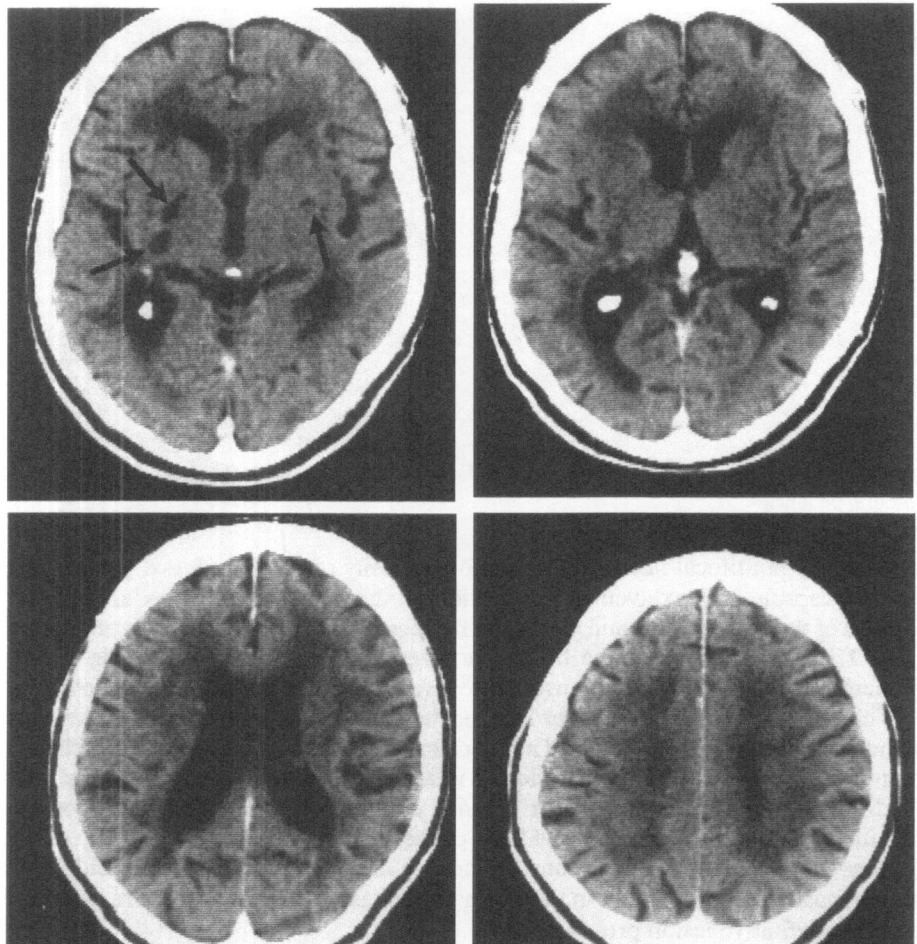

Fig. 5.26. Subcortical arteriosclerotic encephalopathy with lacunar infarcts (*arrows*), particularly in the region of the right basal ganglia, and diffuse hypodensity of the paraventricular and supraventricular white matter

there may be extravasations rich in protein from the as yet not finally occluded vessels, which are responsible for the demyelination of the white matter.

Knowledge of the microangiopathic causes of infarction is important for several reasons. In patients in whom CT shows lesions definitely indicative of a microangiopathy, it cannot be concluded that operation on a coexistent carotid stenosis constitutes a causal therapy. The angiography which is a necessary precursor to such an operation and the operation itself further endanger patients with microangiopathies. Many patients with microangiopathies have initially poor rheologic values which may be still further impaired by the use of contrast media, although this risk is considered to be reduced since the introduction of digital subtraction angiography into the intra-arterial technique.

5.3.1.4 CT Findings in the Vertebrobasilar Territory

Macro- and microangiopathic infarct patterns may also be found in the posterior circulation. An example of a borderzone lesion between the territories of two cerebral arteries with the corresponding pathologic findings is shown in Fig. 5.27. Hemodynamically induced symptoms usually occur only if there are added systemic factors, such as hypotension or an impairment of the rheologic parameters.

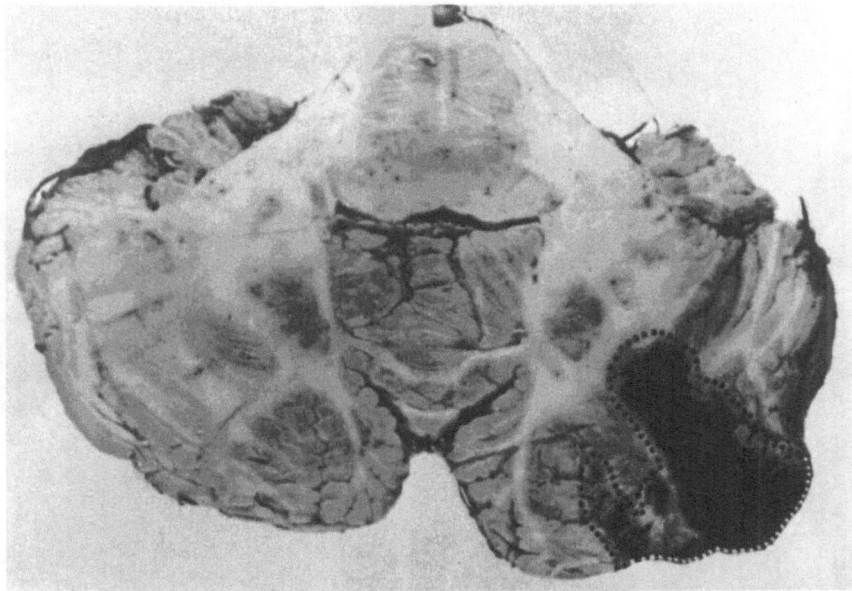

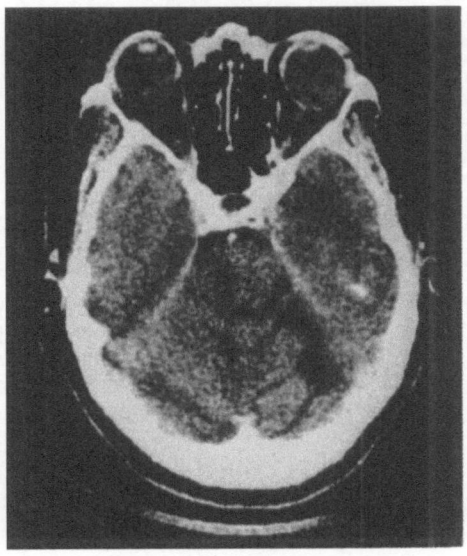

Fig. 5.27. Pathologic specimen of a hemorrhagic borderzone infarct in the posterior cranial fossa. *Lower part* shows the CT finding of a comparable (but as yet not hemorrhagic) lesion. (From Zülch 1985, by kind permission)

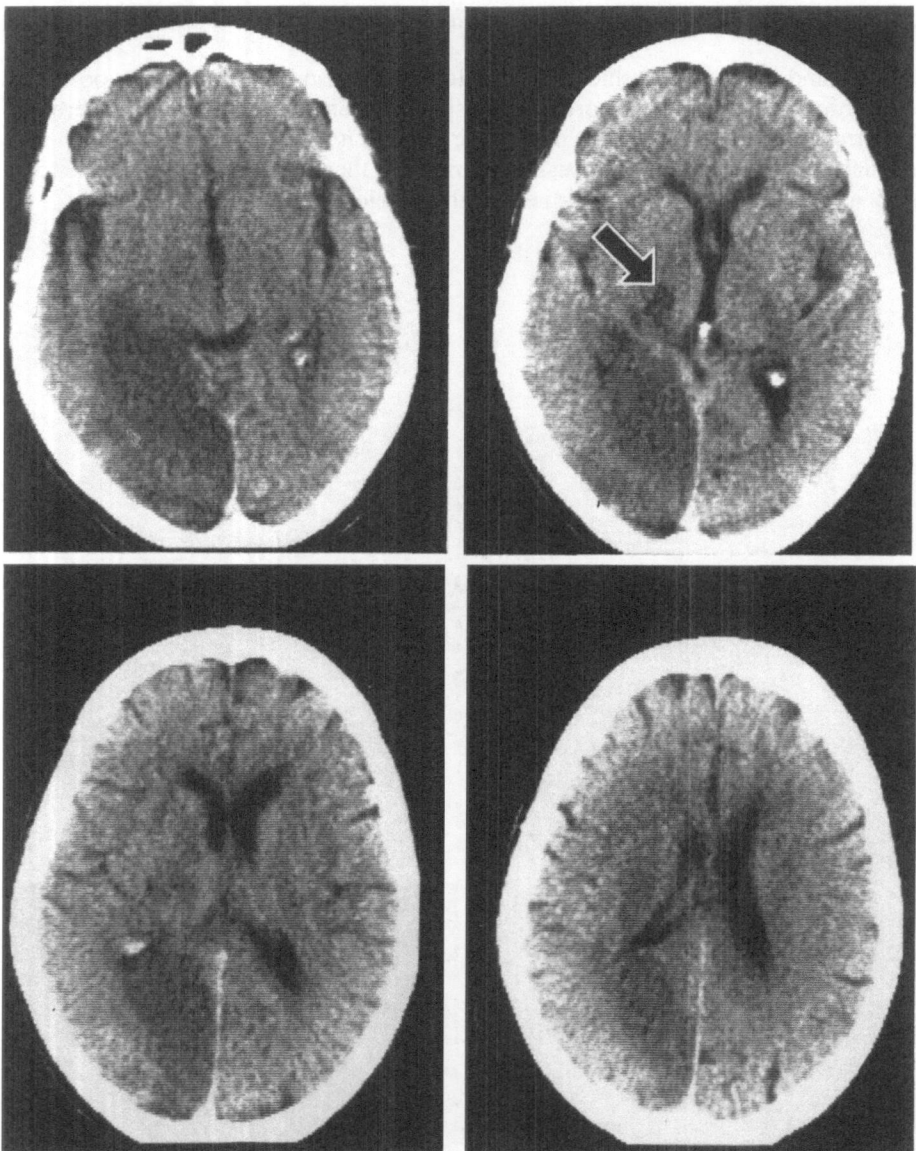

Fig. 5.28. a Extensive recent territorial infarct in the distribution of the right posterior cerebral artery, with demonstration of a hypodense lesion in the left thalamic region, presumably the expression of involvement of the posterior thalamoperforating arteries (*arrow*). **b** Territorial infarction in the distribution of both posterior cerebral arteries

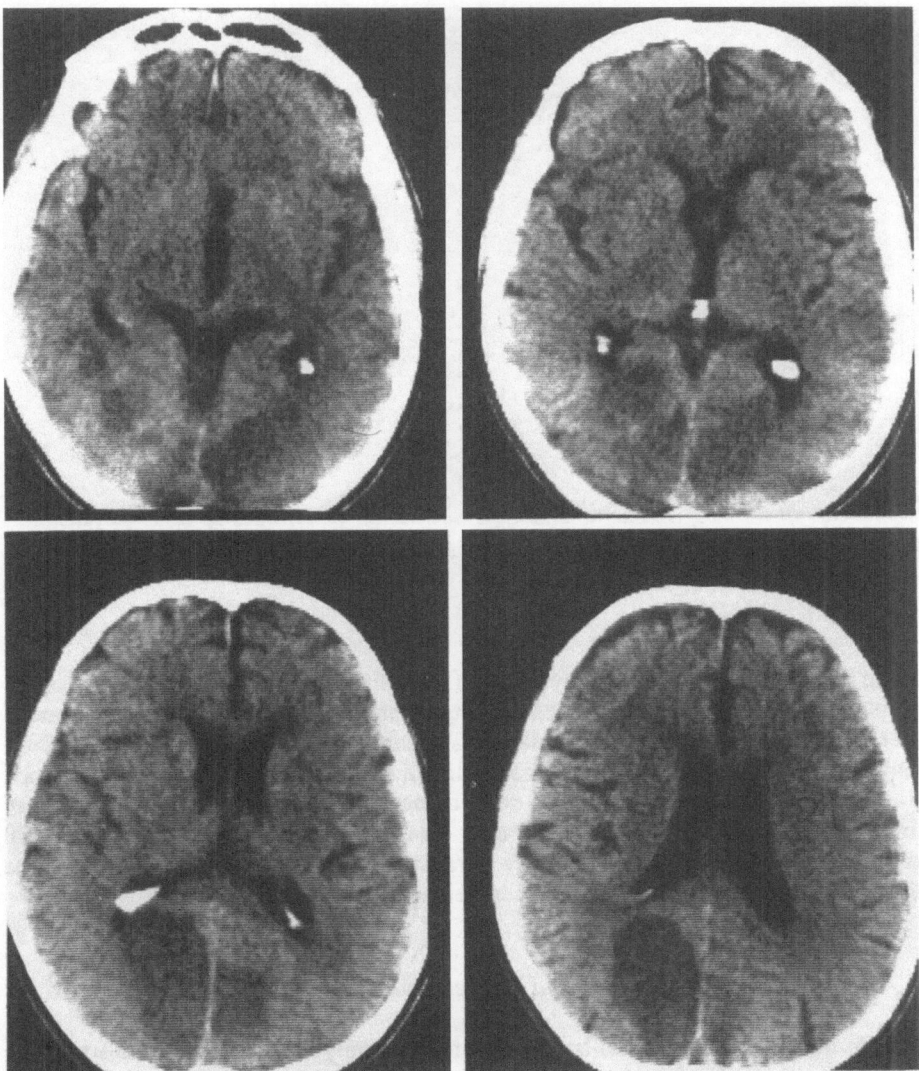

Fig. 5.28b

Occlusions of the main trunk or individual branches of the posterior cerebral artery, even bilateral, lead to territorial infarcts in the region of the posterior cerebral distribution as shown in Fig. 5.28.

Territorial infarcts in the posterior cranial fossa are easy to detect on CT only when they are infarcts of the cerebellar hemispheres. Figure 5.29 shows such an infarct of the superior cerebellar artery. With larger cerebellar softenings an obstructive hydrocephalus may develop as a consequence of the space-occupying effect of the infarct, and ventricular drainage may be required. Figure 5.30 shows a lacunar infarct

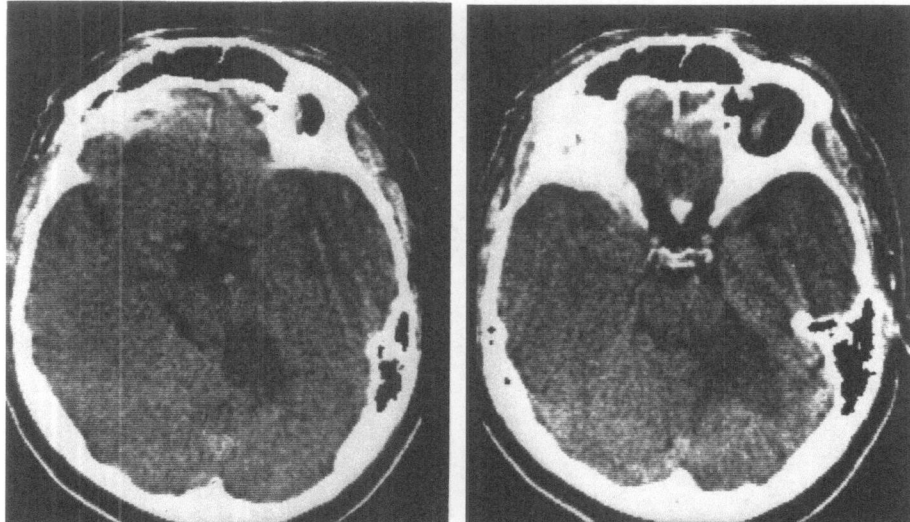

Fig. 5.29. Territorial infarct in distribution of left superior cerebellar artery

of the (left) brainstem and possibly a further territorial infarct in the distribution of the right paramedian brainstem branches. After embolism in the basilar artery, and if there is good collateralization via the long circumferential arteries, isolated lesions may occur in the brainstem and in the paramedian noncollateralized branches which supply the bulk of the thalamus and other diencephalic components. An example of this is given in Fig. 5.31. In the extreme case a softening of all the infratentorial structures results, but sometimes only a transverse type of hypodense lesion of the pons; the functional outcome, however, remains equally catastrophic.

5.3.1.5 Technical Limitations and Fogged Images

The demonstration of lesions by CT depends not only on their size but also on the interval between insult and examination. Between the 10th and 15th and sometimes even the 20th days after an insult, the extent of the insult zone may be difficult to assess correctly because of the fogging effect. Similar densities are measured in the necrotic area as in the surrounding undiseased cerebral tissue. It is important to distinguish between a large medullary lacune and a small borderzone infarct as each has a different underlying mechanism. It is usually necessary to look for a hemodynamic cause by (initially) noninvasive methods, although the question of angiography may arise. Finally, many patients are found to have combinations of macro- und microangiopathic lesions (Fig. 5.32), which may make it difficult to plan treatment.

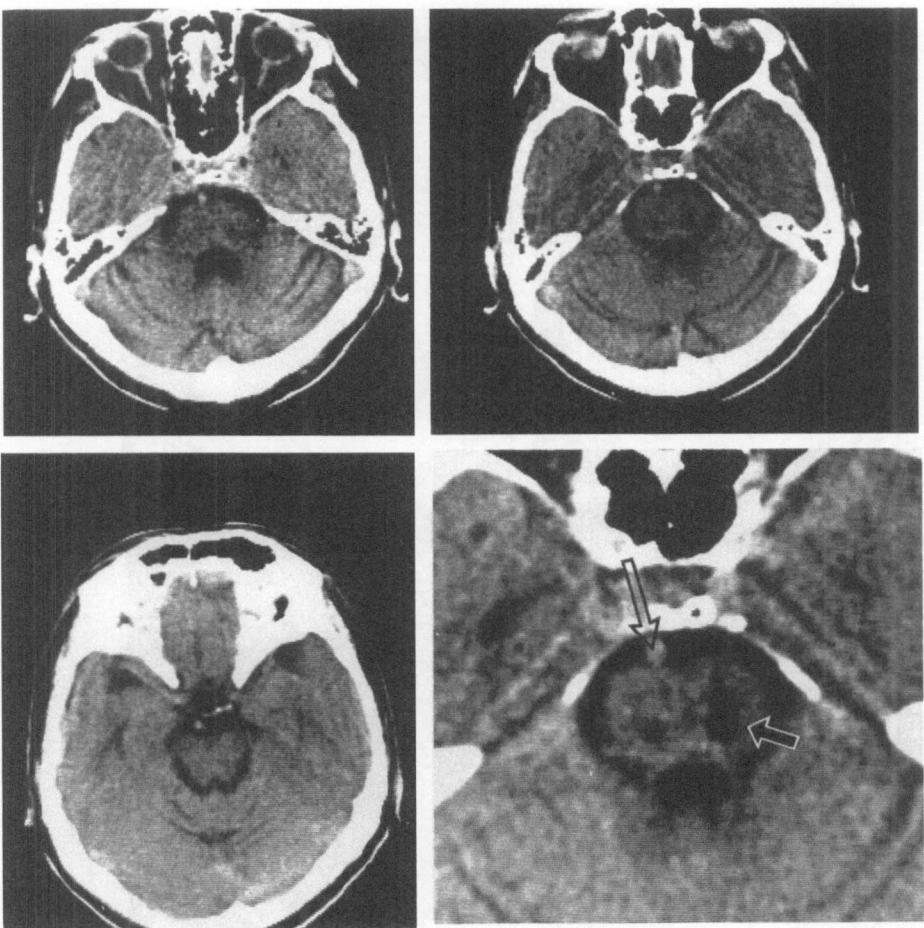

Fig. 5.30. Multiple vascular lesions of the brainstem. Lesion on the *right* corresponds to a lacune; lesion on the *left* (*black arrow*) is more extensive and could be attributable to a partial or complete blockage of the paramedian branches of the basilar artery. The examination was made without contrast; note the high density of the basilar artery (*open arrow*)

5.3.1.6 Secondary Hemorrhagic Infarcts

If early pathologic examination is made, many recent ischemic insults show some slight extravasation of blood which is sometimes detectable in vivo at CT. Rarely, this amounts to confluent hemorrhages with a space-occupying effect (see Fig. 5.33). Secondary hemorrhagic infarction occurs mainly in the marginal zones of the insult (Hart and Tegeler 1986).

Such secondary hemorrhages often develop after infarctions due to emboli, when this has led to autolysis of the embolic occlusion. After restoration of patency of the vessel lumen, the resumption of full-pressure perfusion of the ischemically damaged vessels

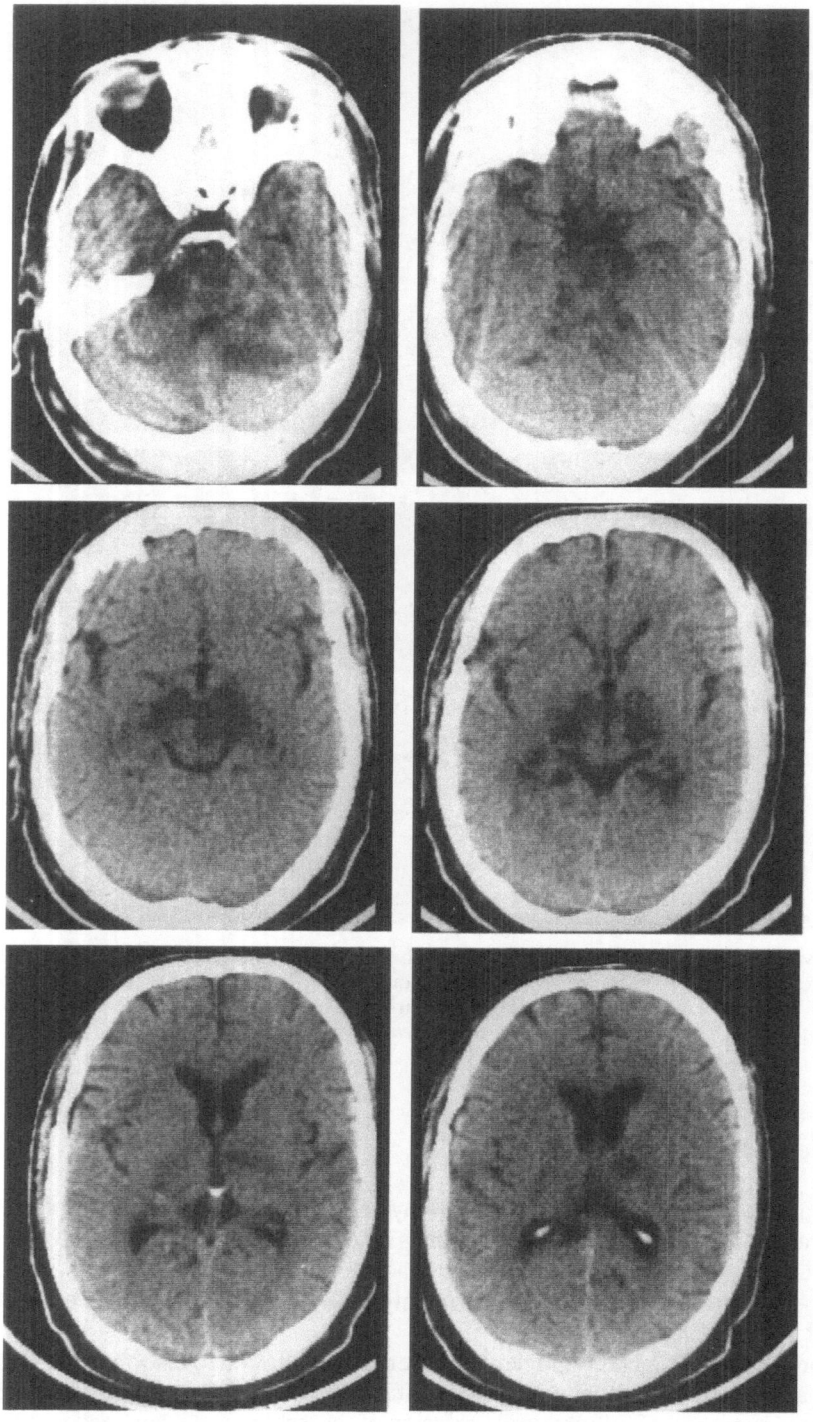

Fig. 5.31

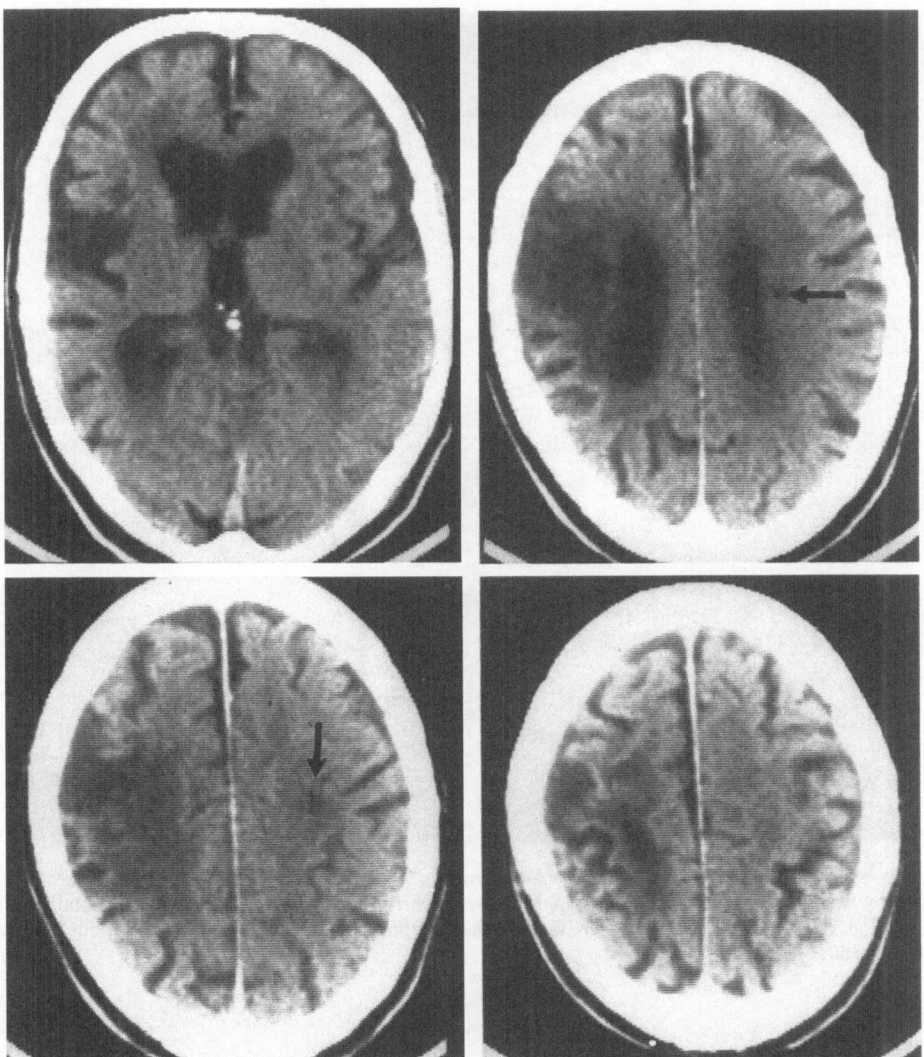

Fig. 5.32. More extensive, recent territorial infarct of the middle group of right middle cerebral branches with marked subcortical parietooccipital extension (borderzone). Doppler ultrasound showed a subtotal stenosis of the right ICA. Simultaneous lacunar insults of the left hemisphere (*arrows*)

Fig. 5.31. Extensive, confluent, hypodense lesions in the brainstem, thalamic region, and suggested also in the left posterior cerebral artery distribution. Isolated hypodense areas can also be detected in the left cerebellar hemisphere. Basilar thrombosis was not demonstrable in these patients despite angiography 5 h after the onset of clinical symptoms

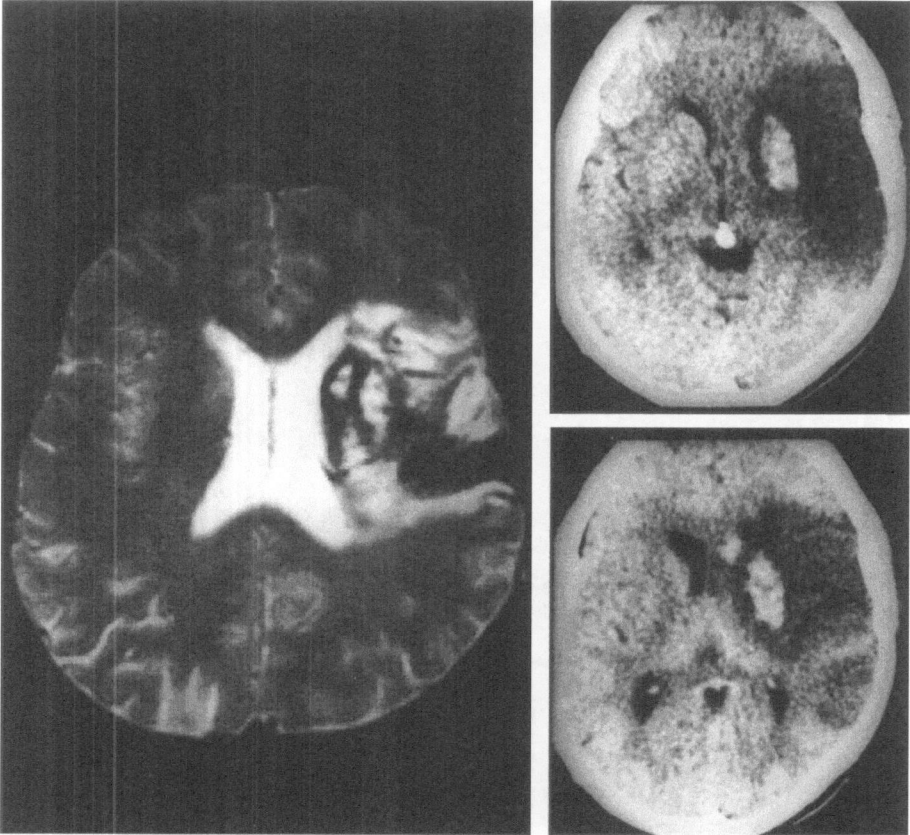

Fig. 5.33. MRI and CT of a secondary hemorrhagic, left middle cerebral infarct. MRI image in T2 shows the hemorrhage as a partly signal-intensive, partly signal-poor zone. The corresponding CT sections are some days older and were made with a very fast scan time in a very restless patient, and the image quality is therefore poorer

leads to extravasation of blood (reperfusion trauma). Animal experimental data indicate that these vascular lesions occur when noncollateralized vessels have been occluded for about 5–6 h. No precise data exist as to how often this secondary hemorrhagic extravasation actually occurs in the natural course after ischemic insults. The incidence reported in the literature ranges from 0% to over 40%. Hence it is impossible to say with certainty whether there is an increased risk of hemorrhage with the employment of aggressive methods of treatment, such as routine anticoagulation or even fibrinolytic therapy. In two prospective studies of patient groups with acute stroke and heparinization, hemorrhagic transformation of the infarct zone was found in 15% and over 40% of patients. However, there was associated clinical deterioration in no case or only four cases, respectively. The demonstration of small, hemorrhagic transformations is very reliably made using MRI (Fig. 5.33).

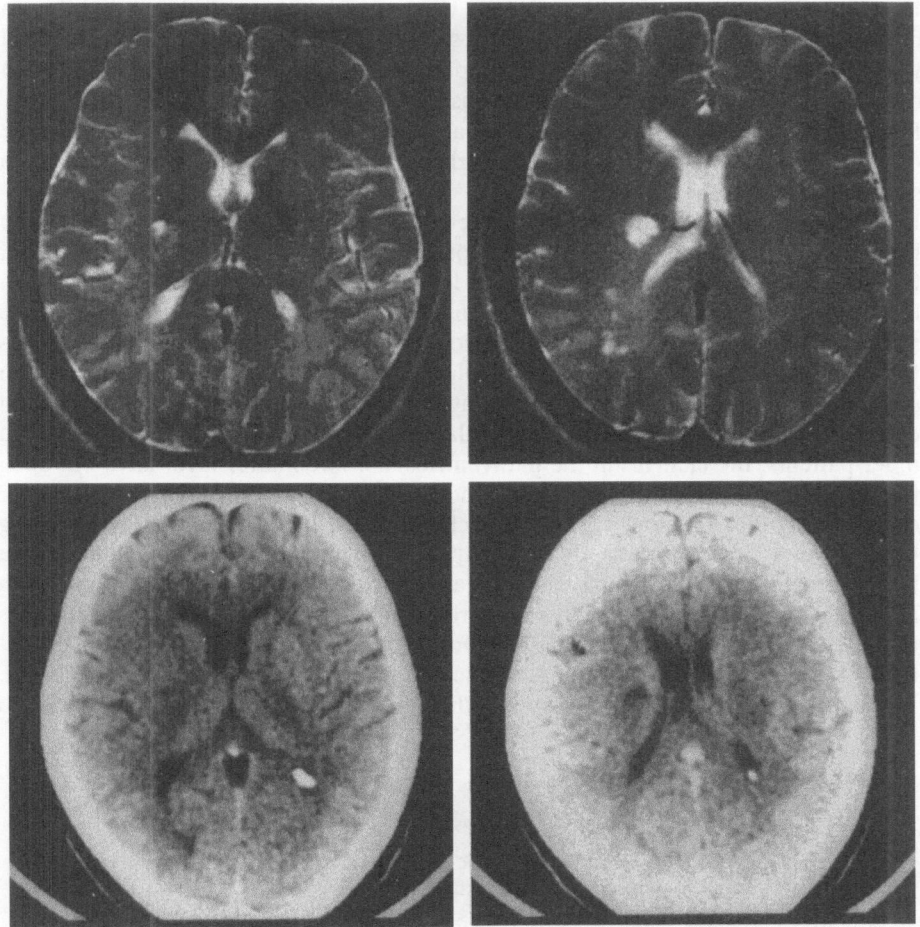

Fig. 5.34. MRI and CT imaging of a recent lacunar infarct. Especially in the *left half* of the figure the lower limit of the lacune is better demonstrated in the MRI image

5.3.2 *Magnetic Resonance Imaging*
(see Brant-Zawadzki and Norman 1987; Elster 1988)

MRI has already proven to be of great practical value in the diagnosis of inflammatory or tumorous disorders of the spinal cord and brainstem, epilepsy with complex-partial seizures, and multiple sclerosis. The diagnostic value of routine MRI in ischemic insults is becoming more and more important. Ischemic insults are visualized by MRI somewhat earlier than by cranial CT, and lacunar lesions are better demonstrated by MRI (Rothrock et al. 1987; Brant-Zawadzki et al. 1985; Ramadan et al. 1989). Better identification of the sites of territorial infarcts of the posterior cranial fossa, especially of the brainstem, has been demonstrated with MRI (Bogousslawský et al. 1986;

Ross et al. 1986; Ramadan et al. 1989). However, patients with limited ability to cooperate or with decreased consciousness cannot be investigated by this method without risk at the present time. MRI in patients with severe brainstem insults with disorders of consciousness or respiration is therefore still restricted.

Figure 5.33 shows an extensive territorial infarct in the middle group of middle cerebral branches with secondary hemorrhage. Here, the use of MRI provides no significant further evidence.

In older hemorrhages, the characteristic signal behavior of the iron ions in the hemosiderin deposits leads to the diagnosis. Figure 5.34 shows the CT and MRI findings in a patient with a recent lacunar lesion. Here, MRI helps to demonstrate a lacune which is at the limit of resolution in CT. This may be an important diagnostic aid in the occasional case with uni- or bilocular lacunes if the differential diagnosis from low-flow infarcts or an older small hemorrhage is to be made. Further, in subcortical arteriosclerotic encephalopathy there is a marked confluent modification of the relaxation times in the periventricular white matter (Fig. 5.35). Particularly in older patients, the changes in the paraventricular white matter layer have not been finally clarified as far as their actual diagnostic value is concerned. It is certainly the case that, in older patients, MRI can detect changes in the white matter layer ("aging brain") which do not necessarily have any pathologic significance, the clinical state being unremarkable. Particularly in the evaluation of such zones in older patients with abnormal signal intensity should strict priority be accorded to the clinical findings (Bradley et al. 1984; Awad et al. 1986; Dougherty et al. 1986; Kertesz et al. 1987). Figure 5.36 shows the MRI findings in a search for vascular lesions in the brainstem. While the CT was normal in a patient with clinical features unequivocally related to

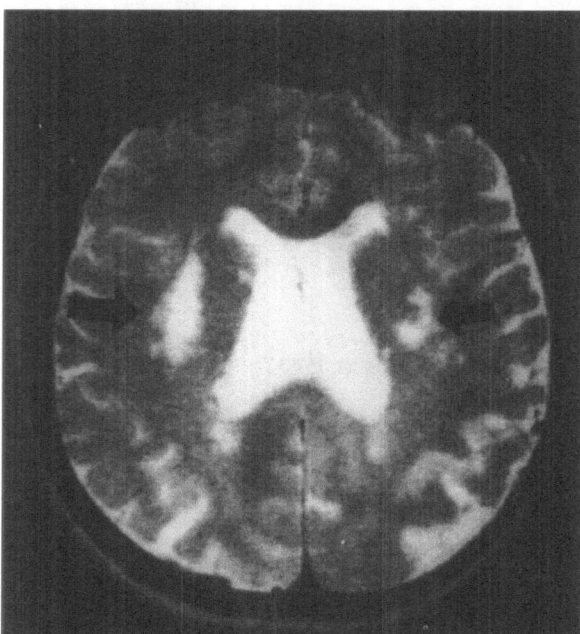

Fig. 5.35. Extensive subcortical, confluent, signal-intensive zones in the T2-weighted image correlated with a subacute arteriosclerotic encephalopathy. In addition, marked expansion of the subarachnoid space as in hydrocephalus ex vacuo. A communicating hydrocephalus is excluded by absence of signal-intensive areas covering the anterior portions of the ventricles

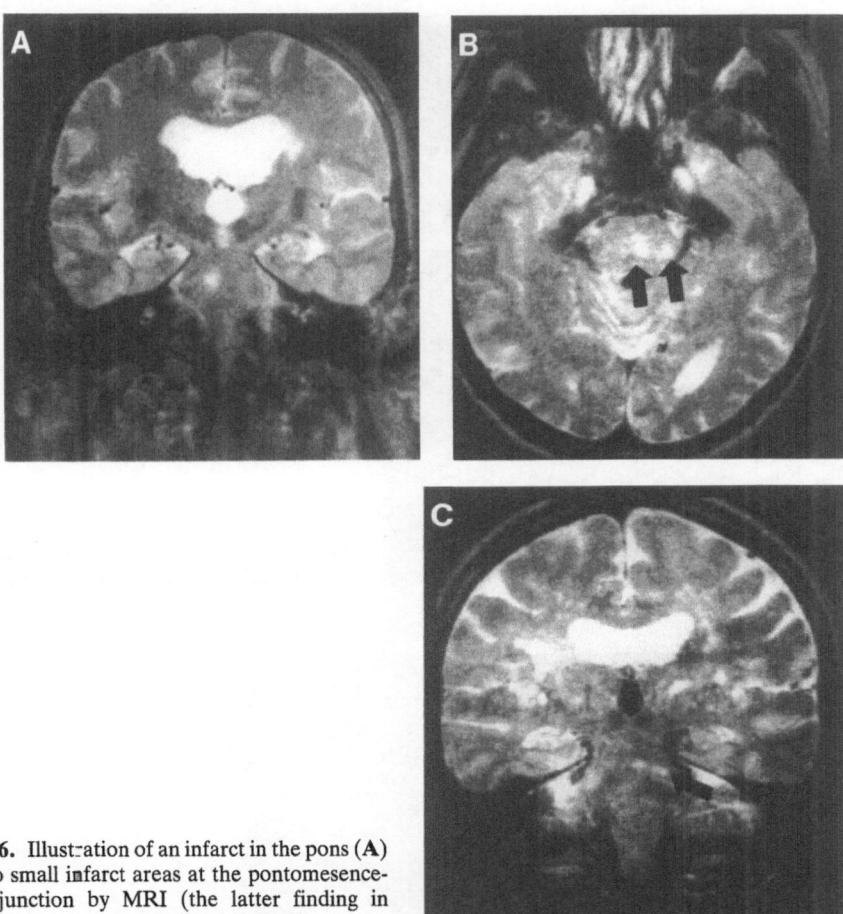

Fig. 5.36. Illustration of an infarct in the pons (**A**) and two small infarct areas at the pontomesence-phalic junction by MRI (the latter finding in coronal and conventional sections, **B, C**)

the brainstem, MRI in a T2-weighted image showed a clearly demarcated lesion (left) while in the middle and right images two small brainstem lesions in two different planes can be identified. This leads to the conclusion that the changes in signal behavior of particular structures after ischemia do not necessarily indicate the actual size of the final defect. The differentiation of territorial infarcts of the cerebellum and brainstem by MRI is particularly impressive. Examples are given in Figs. 5.37–5.39. By using paramagnetic contrast media, ischemically induced disturbances of the blood-brain barrier can be just as clearly demonstrated in the T1-weighted image as in the corresponding CT image (Fig. 5.40). In suitable cases, the falling-off in flow signal in one of the basal cerebral vessels can be assessed as the expression of a local vascular occlusion (Fig. 5.41).

MRI should not be employed as a screening investigation after TIAs or in cerebrovascular insufficiency. It takes some time to assess the clinical significance of many MRI findings, such as the abnormal relaxation time in the white matter mentioned above,

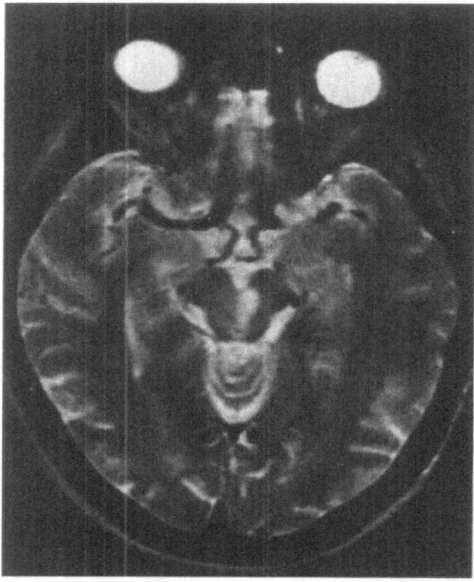

Fig. 5.37. Territorial infarct in tectum of left midbrain sparing the crus cerebri

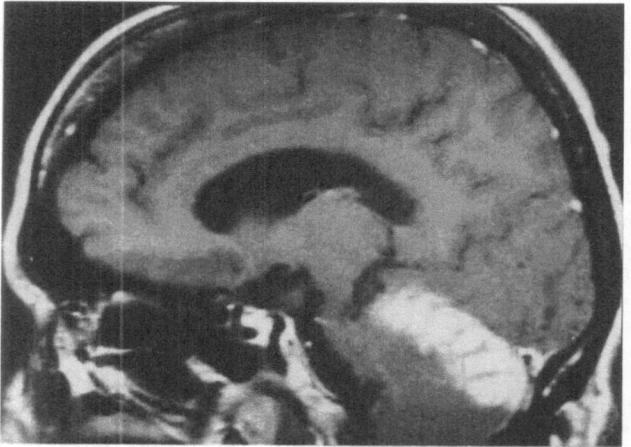

Fig. 5.38. Extensive superior cerebellar artery infarct in sagittal depiction

in migraine, or after TIAs. Until then we must interpret these findings with caution. Currently, MRI is proving the method of choice in cerebral ischemias, especially in the posterior circulation and in microangiopathies. In sinus thromboses MRI is far superior to CT and falls little short of cerebral angiography in diagnostic reliability (Macchi et al. 1988; Ramadan et al. 1989). Magnetic resonance spectroscopy could be used in future for the demonstration of biochemical markers in the early stages of stroke to provide guidance in prognosis and treatment planning (Levine et al. 1987; Brant-Zawadzki et al. 1987). Adaptations to measure CBF, oxygen utilization, and

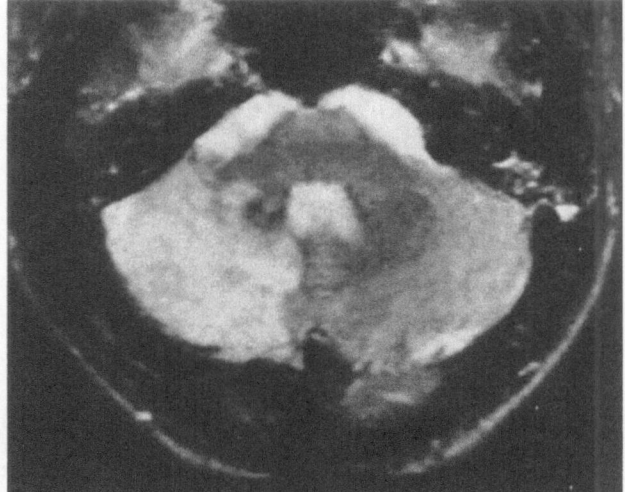

Fig. 5.39. Extensive right-sided posterior inferior cerebellar infarct with right vertebral occlusion

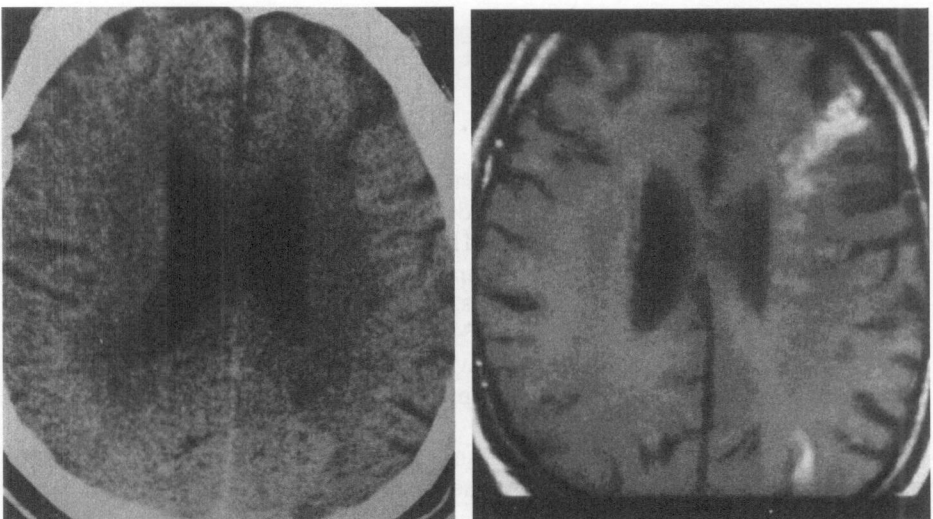

Fig. 5.40. Ischemic lesions after spontaneous lysis of MCA embolism in CT (*left*) and gadolinium contrast MRI (*right*). Note the obvious disturbances of the blood-brain barrier in the wedge-shaped subcortical left fronto-precentral infarct zone, a minor streaky paraventricular, and an additional, comma-shaped area of abnormal signal intensity occipitally in the borderzone to the posterior cerebral territory

glucose metabolism by means of magnetic resonance technology are being developed (Ewing et al. 1989; Eidelberg et al. 1988; Nakada et al. 1988). Development in this field is so rapid that assessments valid a year ago are already out of date (Ramadan et al. 1989; Gelmers et al. 1989).

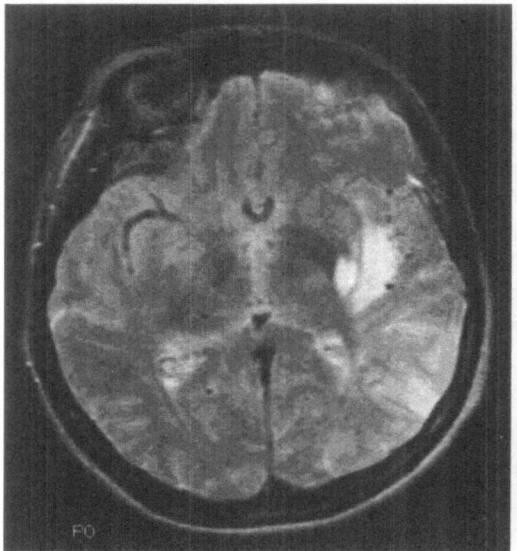

Fig. 5.41. Defect in flow signal in the left middle MCA in angiographically demonstrated MCA occlusion. A signal increase in the basal ganglia is already detectable. Manifest dilation of insular MCA branches, which have retrograde perfusion

5.3.3 Other Imaging Techniques (PET, SPECT)

In 1948, Kety and Schmidt described a quantitative method for the measurement of cerebral circulation which permits the determination of CBF volume from the difference between gas quantities obtained from the brain under constant distribution coefficients and the arteriovenous concentration. Before the development of SPECT and PET the xenon clearance method was the technique most widely used scientifically, with limitations, clinically (Heiss 1984). Numerous modifications and improvements in data analysis and illustration have contributed to the documentation of a regional impairment of blood flow in patients with ischemic infarcts, to observation of the mode of action and indications for various principles of treatment, and to quantitative analysis of the cerebral perfusion in different types of central nervous system diseases as well as analysis from the functional aspect.

PET allows measurement of the local concentration of positron emitters in sectional images similar to those of CT or MRI and permits, by means of marked improvements in the temporal and spatial resolution capacities of the camera system, an insight into the metabolism of the brain. For this, positron-emitting isotopes are used that emit gamma quanta in the opposite direction for the localization of metabolic processes, employing synthetic agents administered to the organism as tracers. In the early years, ^{15}O and other gaseous compounds were used for the measurement of oxygen consumption, circulation, and blood volume in the brain; sugar metabolism was also measured using ^{18}F-labeled deoxyglucose. Numerous studies with various labeled tracers made it possible to obtain new and far-reaching knowledge about the pathophysiologic mechanisms of the brain. It has been known for years from animal experimental studies that a reduction in circulation below 20% of the normal value leads to reversible functional deficits, whereas irreversible morphologic lesions appear only when the residual circulation of the cerebral tissue falls below 10%–12% of the normal value.

This concept opened a whole range of new therapeutic approaches aimed at the therapeutic windows, in which improvement of perfusion above the critical threshold could save brain tissue. More complicated still, although probably decisive for the success of treatment, are the mechanisms involved during the reperfusion phase, in which, through ATP deficiency and membrane depolarization, intracellular sodium and calcium influx with anaerobic glycolysis increased liberation of transmitters (e.g., glutamate) develops plus arachidonic acid metabolites (e.g., leukotrienes, thromboxane, prostacyclin) as well as free oxygen radicals. Individual pathobiochemical mechanisms can be studied using PET even in patients; the typical pattern of the infarct course has been described in the literature (Baron et al. 1981; Gibbs et al. 1984). In acute ischemia there is a reduced perfusion which is initially compensated by an increase in cerebral blood volume, but which cannot be completely adjusted. Increased oxygen extraction acts as a further and partly overlapping compensatory mechanism. With reduced perfusion, reduced oxygen consumption, and increased glucose turnover in a context of anaerobic glycolysis, ischemia and ultimately infarction develop if the compensatory mechanisms fail over a critical period (Table 5.7). How long and to what extent this is the case, and what therapeutic measures are indicated at different stages to combat the development of ischemic cell damage can be excellently investigated by metabolic studies with the aid of PET and later transferred to clinical practice. New methods for the demonstration of dopamine receptors, the measurement of the pH of cerebral tissue, and the observation of protein synthesis have expanded this extremely productive research technology. Its application to the clinical care of patients has, however, not as yet acquired any importance; this is linked with the extremely high costs in terms of personnel and equipment which this method entails. Model studies are of practical importance for understanding the behavior of pathophysiologic processes and for the development of simpler, related investigational techniques that can be used clinically. Figure 5.42 shows an example of different tracer studies in a patient with bilateral occlusion of the internal carotid artery and an infarct in the territory of the angular gyrus of the nondominant hemisphere.

Also, SPECT provides insights into disturbed metabolic processes in stroke, including the demonstration of metabolic disturbances in areas of the brain not shown to be

Table 5.7. The sequence of hemodynamic failure from a mild fall in rCPP to infarction is shown diagrammatically with reference to rCMRO$_2$, rOER, rCBF, and CBF:CBV. (From Frackowiak 1985)

	CMRO$_2$	CBF/CBV	OER	CBF
↓ Hemodynamic reserve	↔	↓	↔	↔
↓ Oxygen carriage reserve	↔	↓	↑	↓
Ischemia	↓	↓	↑	↓
Infarction	↓	Variable	↓	Variable

CMRO$_2$, Cerebral O$_2$ metabolism rate; CBF, cerebral blood flow; CBV, cerebral blood volume; OER, oxygen extraction rate.

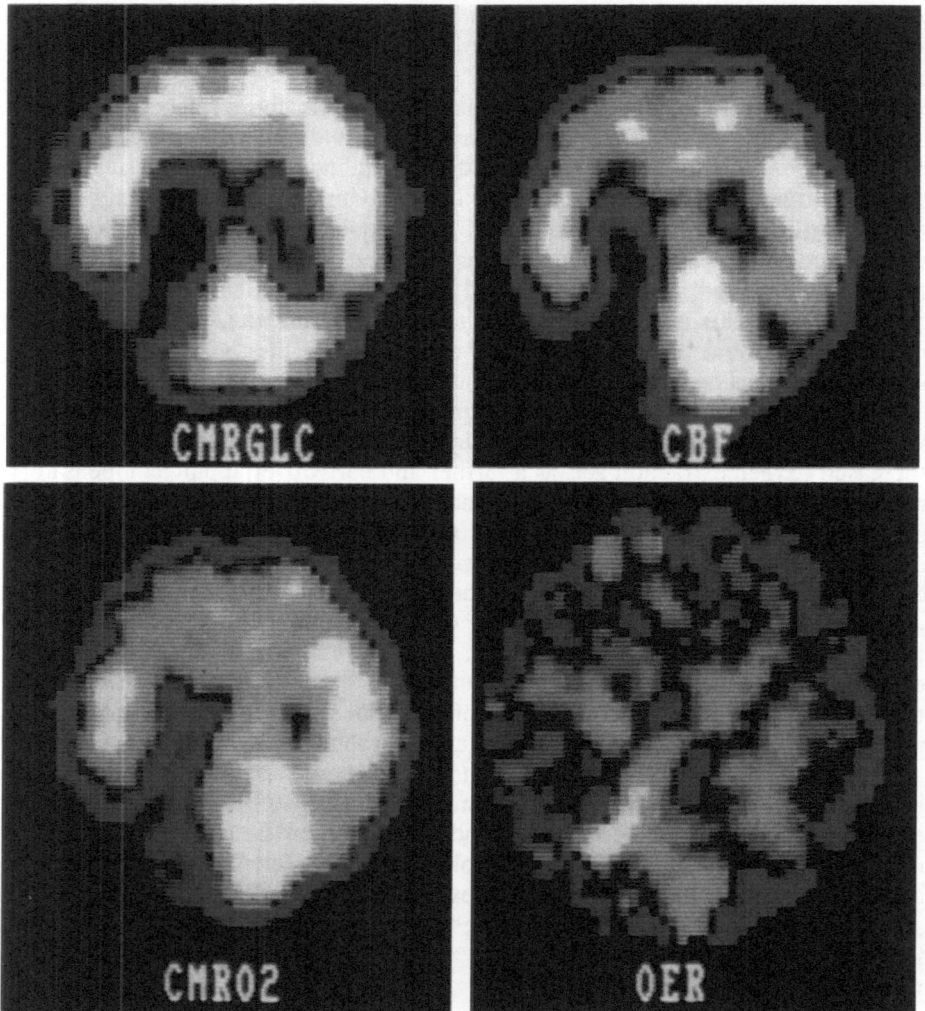

Fig. 5.42. PET in a patient with an infarct in the angular gyrus territory of the nondominant hemisphere with bilateral ICA occlusion. The regional blood flow (*CBF*) in this region is markedly reduced, but the increased oxygen extraction rate (*OER*) in one part of the ischemic region indicates metabolic compensation. Actually, in this subcortical region the zone of reduced oxygen metabolism (*CMRO2*) is also smaller than the CBF tomogram would suggest. This contrasts with the glucose metabolism (*CMRGLC*) and shows an uncoupling of the metabolism. (In cooperation with the Kernforschungsanlage Jülich, FRG, Prof. Feinendegen)

structurally damaged at CT examination. The major disadvantages of this method are the poor spatial resolution and the absence of absolute values. As yet, definitive statements can be made only in terms of lateral comparisons. Not uncommonly SPECT confirms the clinical (and electroencephalographic) suspicion of involvement of additional brain areas in patients with a circumscribed morphologic lesion on CT.

SPECT constitutes a functional method which can only be definitively evaluated when taken together with other functional and especially clinical findings.

5.4 Electrophysiologic Investigations

5.4.1 Electroencephalography

Electroencephalography (EEG) is not the diagnostic method of first choice in stroke. However, as the EEG is very widely used, we consider here the limitations of this method, its actual indications, and its value in stroke patients (see Aminoff 1982; Christian 1982).

In EEG potential variations which presumably correspond to the summation potentials of the excitatory and inhibitory synapses of the cerebral cortex are detected by electrodes applied to the scalp. The activities of specific parts of the cerebral hemispheres are examined in lateral comparison. Indirect conclusions as to subcortical functions and brainstem functions are possible. In the EEG typical waveforms can be distinguished which show a topographic distribution over the hemispheres in healthy subjects. Thus, in most adults occipital alpha waves dominate with a frequency of 8–13 Hz and an amplitude of 20–70 μV. They may be blocked by sensory impressions, for example, by opening the eyes. Slower components usually indicate local or global functional disturbances; faster elements (beta waves) occur as effects of medication or genetically determined normal variants. The frequency of the beta waves exceeds 13 Hz; the slower waves are termed theta waves (3.5–7.5 Hz) and delta waves (0.5–3 Hz).

Alterations in the shape of the curve may be marked by a general slowing (systemic change), by focal asymmetries (focal lesions), or by suddenly appearing focal or generalized potential variations (paroxysmal alterations). Features such as spikes, sharp waves, or spike wave complexes are indicative of predisposition to convulsions. These, too, may be focal or generalized.

The introduction of the new neuroradiologic techniques has led to a change in the importance of EEG in the diagnosis of neurologic emergencies. Instead of the description of focal lesions to be evaluated for topical diagnosis, the EEG has emerged as a measuring instrument for the general state of cerebral activity. Thus, typical changes are found in the different stages of loss of consciousness. With increasing unconsciousness after extensive infarcts, an EEG pattern can be found that is known as the burst suppression pattern. This is marked by single large outbreaks of high-voltage, slow EEG activity, followed by a phase of curve depression.

Only when functional disturbances markedly precede the demonstration of a morphologic lesion in an imaging technique does the EEG also possess topically diagnostic importance. In certain forms of encephalitis, for example, herpes simplex encephalitis, and if the CT findings are still normal, focal changes in the EEG are important diagnostic evidence.

It is often surprising that in many patients with severe unilateral symptoms no EEG findings are registered while in others they may be very marked. The most important reason for this evidently weak diagnostic value of the EEG in ischemic infarcts is obviously our altered understanding of the pathogenesis of ischemia. Before the introduction of CT there was virtually no possibility of establishing during life whether the cause of the stroke was a large territorial infarct, a middle cerebral occlusion, a lentiform nucleus infarct, or perhaps only a "strategically" located deep lacune.

When a completed stroke has occurred, the affected nerve cells are no longer electrically active and can no longer be "revived." These cells no longer participate in the group of synchronously active nerve cells. If the lesion is juxtacortical, a diffuse low-grade slowing and reduction in rhythmic basal activity results. A clinically suspicious and morphologically complete infarction of individual parts of the brain may correspond to this focal finding. Beyond this, focal EEG changes develop which also occur in the marginal zones of an ischemic region, leading to the relatively poor spatial resolution of the EEG in stroke.

EEG changes after a territorial infarct often appear in the form of theta foci or dysrhythmic groups even *before* demonstration of the ischemic lesion in CT. In larger infarct zones (and in intracranial hemorrhages), focal slow theta waves and slow theta dysrhythmias with sporadic delta waves predominate. After complete occlusion of the middle cerebral artery or its branches, a focal delta activity is found. However, this also occurs over juxtacortically situated intracerebral hemorrhages, in cerebral abscess, or in the vicinity of a tumor. In disorders near the midline rhythmic, bilaterally synchronous theta waves of around 5–6 Hz are sometimes found over the anterior and middle parts of the brain. Especially in borderzone infarcts, when unstable perfusion and oxygenation oscillate between functional and maintenance metabolism, high-amplitude steep potentials are found which are designated as periodic, lateralized, epileptiform discharges or "extraterritorial spike activity" (Chatrian et al. 1964; Karbowski 1974).

In rather rare cases, larger recent lacunar infarcts can lead to lateralized steep theta waves, but usually in the microangiopathies there is a diffuse, low-grade slowing and no focal changes. Small but clinically relevant branch occlusions can, like deep lacunar lesions, remain without EEG changes.

The EEG changes in young patients with *hemiplegic migraine accompagnée* are particularly impressive. Here there are quite extensive slow and high-amplitude delta foci, the demonstration of which in this case tends to be reassuring. An acute hemiplegia based on a middle cerebral embolism is usually associated with less marked EEG changes. The EEG changes in hemiplegic migraine may persist for days, rarely weeks, after the migraine attack even if there has been complete regression of the symptoms by then. These findings correspond to changes in cell metabolism, as demonstrated using PET. Vasospasm after a subarachnoid hemorrhage may likewise give rise to quite impressive focal changes in the EEG, which is therefore an appropriate examination for monitoring the course after subarachnoid hemorrhage.

5.4.2 Evoked Potentials

Potential changes in EEG associated with external stimuli are known as evoked potentials (EPs). They can be identified against the randomly distributed basal activity and are reproducible using electronic averaging (see Chiappa and Ropper 1982; Desmedt 1980; Lowitzsch et al. 1983; Stöhr et al. 1982).

EPs are of minor importance in the diagnosis of ischemic insults, but have proven useful in the monitoring of severe strokes in intensive care units. In brainstem infarcts and basilar thrombosis, multimodal EPs provide valuable information about the extent of the functional disturbances within the brainstem (Ferbert et al. 1988; Hacke 1986). Hence the use of EPs is confined to the monitoring of clinical course.

In the microangiopathies, pathologic EPs may support the suspicion of a multiplicity of lesions. The blink reflex, which is not discussed in detail here, may exhibit pathologic findings in both situations.

5.4.2.1 Visual Evoked Potentials

Visual evoked potentials (VEPs) may be elicited by checkerboard pattern stimuli with contrast reversal (or flash stimuli). The eyes can be stimulated separately in the entire visual field and for parts of the visual field. Normally there is a high-amplitude positive discharge (P100) 100 ms after a change of pattern. Depending on the stimulus pattern, VEPs are subject to major intra- and interindividual variations. VEPs are greatly influenced by disorders of vigilance and consciousness and by medication. VEPs need to be investigated only in those rare cases in which the differential diagnosis of intermittent ischemic insults from multiple sclerosis in younger patients needs clarification. They are pathologically altered in multiple sclerosis in many cases, but only very rarely in ischemic lesions. After posterior artery infarcts a hemianopia may be objectivized by potentials related to the visual field (Fig. 5.43), but this is possible even by clinical or perimetric examination. These effects are not necessarily always as marked as in the chosen example, although they can be demonstrated with adequate accuracy by multichannel recording. In SAE the VEPs are abnormal in a large number of patients; this is attributed to demyelinization of the white matter.

5.4.2.2 Brainstem Auditory Evoked Potentials

The brainstem auditory evoked potentials (BAEPs) are low-amplitude potentials which arise in the first 7 ms after a click stimulus due to stimulation of individual structures of acoustic conduction in the peripheral auditory nerve and in the brainstem, usually evoked by click stimuli. The potential components are labeled I–V (VI). Waves I and II probably arise in the acoustic nerve, waves III and IV in the medulla oblongata, and wave V at the pontomesencephalic junction. The BAEPs can be used for examination of the central auditory tract. The close topical relationship that was earlier presumed between particular BAEP components and specific locations on the auditory pathway is no longer supported. In brainstem diseases the latency between the usually well reproducible waves I and V (interpeak latency I–V) is particularly important.

In brainstem infarcts and basilar thromboses the changes in the BAEPs are impressive (Ferbert et al. 1988; Fig. 5.44). Patients in whom a rostrally placed basilar circulatory disorder exists often have normal BAEPs or perhaps a minor flattening of wave V. In patients with a lesion of the middle basilar, on the other hand, there occur marked changes in the middle and late potential components and a prolongation of the I–V

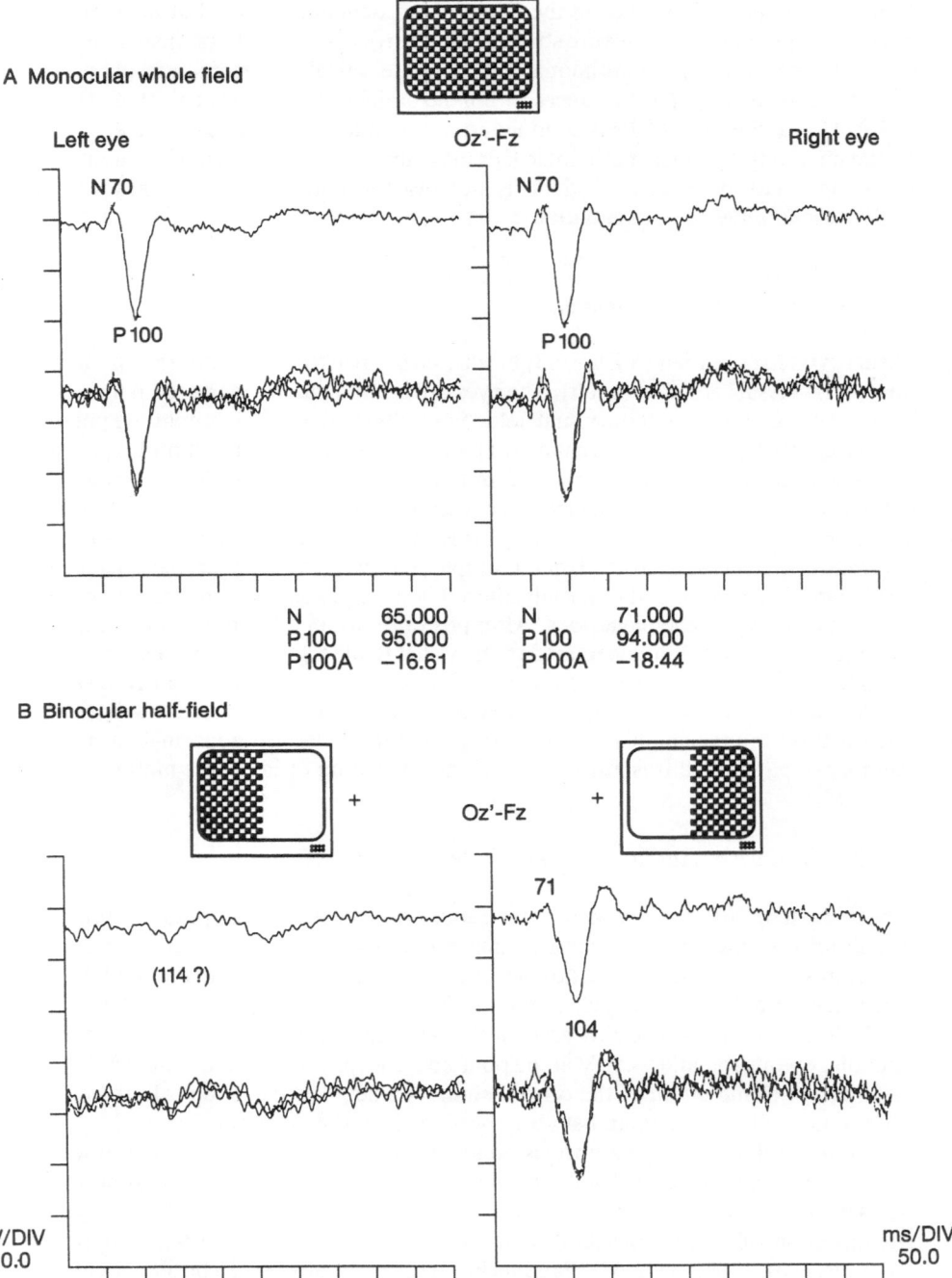

Fig. 5.43. Visual evoked potentials in whole-field (**A**) and half-field (**B**) stimulation. In the hemianopic visual field (*left*) there is no reliably reproducible potential on half-field stimulation

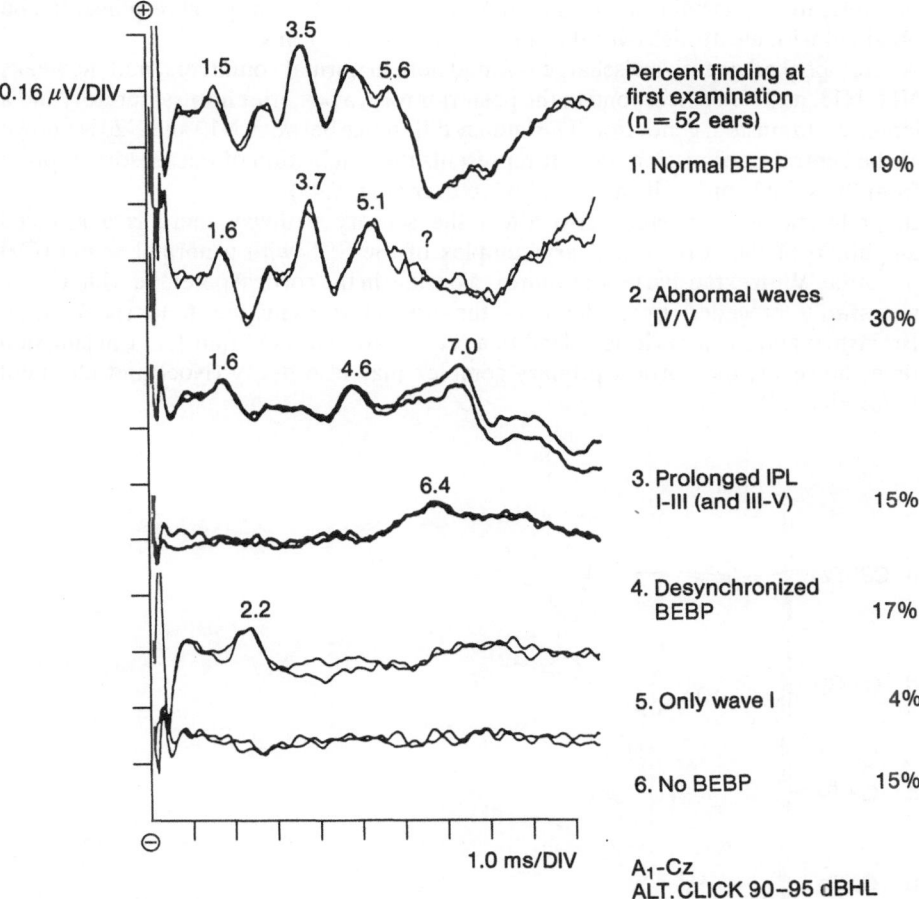

Fig. 5.44. BEBP pattern in basilar thrombosis

interpeak latency. If the labyrinthine artery is included in the circulatory disorder, the resulting pattern is one of cochlear hearing loss.

5.4.2.3 Somatosensory Evoked Potentials

Rectangular current impulses are applied to the peripheral mixed nerve trunks to evoke somatosensory evoked potentials (SEPs), which can be derived from both the cortex and the spinal cord. The cortical EPs are easier to reproduce. On stimulation of the median nerve there is a negative cortical discharge after 20 ms, followed by a positive discharge after about 25 ms. This cortical primary complex (the potential components are designated according to their polarity and the average latency in a normal collective as N20 and P25) is relatively stable against external influences, for example, the effects of drugs or narcotics. At the same time a spinal response can be obtained with electrodes over the spinous process of C7 or C2.

A three-peaked negative discharge is found here in normal volunteers, and the peaks N11, N13, and N14 correspond to the posterior root, a posterior horn generator, and a lemniscal brainstem generator. The latency difference between N13 and N20 is known as the central transmission time. It represents the conduction of the sensory impulse from the spinal cord to its arrival at the cortex (Fig. 5.45).

In unilateral lesions which also affect the sensory pathway there is a reduced amplitude of the cortical primary complex of the SEP with a normal spinal (C7) potential. With extensive lesions there is a decline in the cortical potential which is not necessarily preceded by a delay in the central transmission time (N13–N20). Brainstem and thalamic lesions lead to a prolongation of the brainstem transmission time; however, the cortical primary complex may also decay (Noel and Desmedt 1975; Fig. 5.46).

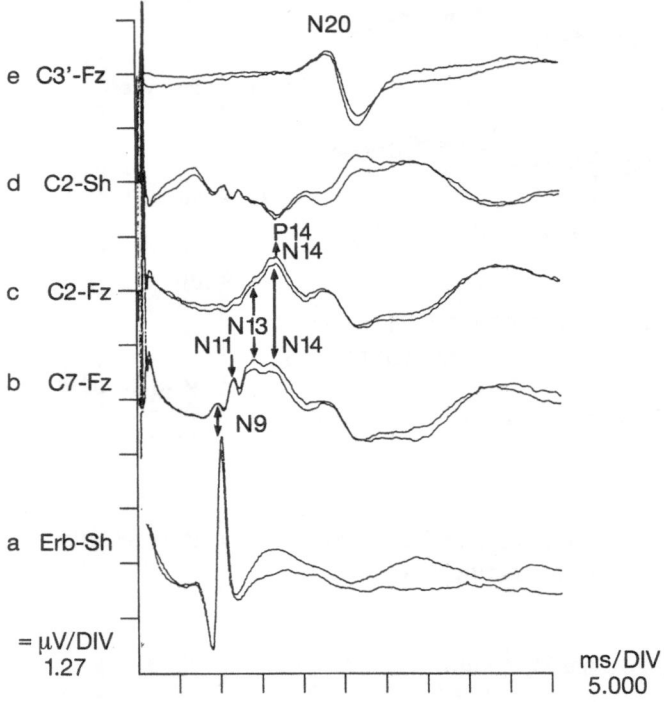

Fig. 5.45. a Erb potential, **b–d** spinal, **e** cortical

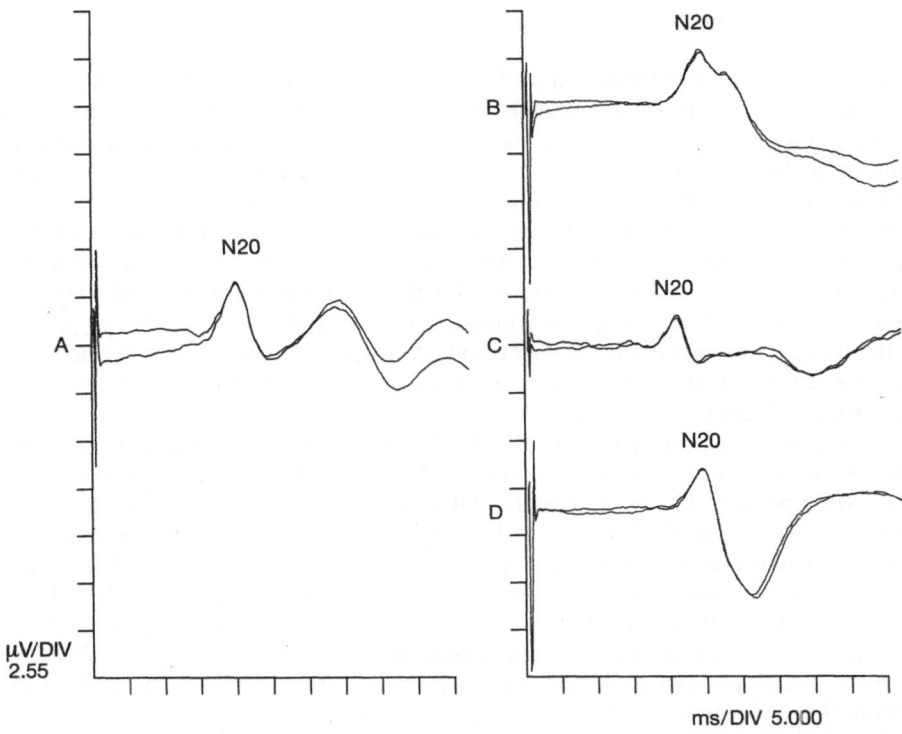

Fig. 5.46 A–D. Median SEPs (cortical) in ischemic infarcts. **A** Normal finding. **B–D** Pathologic findings

5.4.3 Topographic EEG Analysis ("Brain Mapping")

Advances in technical facilities, especially the rapid developments in computer technology, have made available for clinical application the topographic analysis of electrical cerebral activity, including EPs, which was previously the exclusive province of research programs. With the currently available equipment, for instance, zones of corresponding potential magnitudes (amplitude, frequency, polarity difference, etc.) can be analyzed like a map over time, in order to allocate the electrical cerebral activity in site and temporal course to its possible sources. While there are already numerous experimental and psychological studies describing the use of this technique, we still lack comprehensive concepts for clinical application, although initial results, mainly in the psychiatric field, are hopeful (John et al. 1988). In the field of cerebrovasular diseases there are interesting possibilities, for example, studies linking cerebral activity to metabolism (Nagata et al. 1986) which describe a linear correlation between rCBF and oxygen metabolism in PET and separate bands of the EEG spectrum (positive correlation with alpha activity, negative with delta activity). Again, various approaches to the use of this technique for monitoring during neuroradiologic and vascular surgical procedures have been realized without a definitive assessment of its value being possible so far.

5.4.4 Transcranial Magnetic Stimulation

Transcranial motor stimulation with an electromagnetic stimulator (Merton and Morton 1980), but lately increasingly often with a magnetic stimulator (Barker et al. 1985), makes it possible to obtain information about the function of central nervous motor pathways. The method is based on the stimulation of motor cortical areas through the intact skull. The reactions are recorded as in clinical electromyography by needle or surface electrodes from the limb muscles: latencies and potential amplitudes and form are assessed against normal values and in comparison of the two sides. Spinal stimulation, relatively simple with the electrical stimulator but somewhat more difficult with the magnetic stimulator (in which the nerve roots are probably stimulated), presents the possibility of calculating a central transmission time for the motor pathway if the synapse time for relay from the pyramidal tract to the motor neurone is deducted.

This method is currently in wide use, but it has not yet been possible to determine what additional definitive information can be obtained by this examination. Just as the SEPs provide no essential additional information when an unequivocal sensory disorder already exists clinically, so the simple demonstration of a motor disturbance by means of the motor potentials constitutes no genuine gain in information if there is obvious hemiparesis. However, one can think of certain fields in which additional information may be obtained in stroke patients by means of the motor potentials. This is the case with patients who, for neuropsychological reasons, cannot be subjected to an exact testing of power because they are aphasic-apraxic or show neglect, or their limited consciousness hinders precise testing of muscle function. There are probably also possibilities for obtaining information about prognosis of rehabilitation via the reappearance of initially decayed potentials and the type of changes in partially deranged motor potentials. However, all these assumptions still call for exact clinical assay and validation.

As transcranial magnetic stimulation constitutes no special stress, and the examination itself is not painful, a wide application of the method may be expected in future.

5.5 Cerebral Angiography

5.5.1 Indications for Angiography

Cerebral angiography is indicated only when – on the basis of the clinical examination and history, competently performed ultrasound studies, and a qualitatively adequate CT examination – it may be assumed that the result of the study will lead to therapeutic implications. These must also be applicable to the individual patient. This means, for instance, that in a patient with a high-grade symptomatic carotid stenosis for whom angiography is proposed, the operability for a planned carotid endarterectomy must also exist. The same applies to the introduction of anticoagulant or other pharmacologic regimes. Thus, if age, previous illness, risk factors, or operative risk in the individual case argue against the introduction of an otherwise appropriate treatment, angiography is to be avoided. In general, therapeutic implications arise only in patients exhibiting reversible symptoms or progressive symptoms. Sporadic

TIAs in the case of normal Doppler ultrasound are not an indication for immediate angiography; here the decision for angiography is made, if at all, only when the neurologic and medical (laboratory and cardiac) diagnosis has been concluded.

Table 5.8. Indications for angiography in cerebral ischemias

	Suspected diagnosis from clinical, CT, and Doppler ultrasound examination	*Possible therapeutic consequences*[a]
Carotid territory	High-grade hemodynamically active or embolizing carotid stenoses and occlusions	Operation (endarterectomy), possibly heparin, ASA
	Supraocclusional middle cerebral embolism	Thrombolysis, heparin
	Suspected pseudo-occlusion of internal carotid	Operation
	Progressive insult without extracranial carotid stenosis; suspected siphon or middle cerebral stenosis; embolism or occlusion	Heparin, coumarin (thrombolysis)
	Spontaneous or traumatic dissection of internal carotid	Heparin
	Suspected acute multiple emboli with good regression	Heparin, coumarin, antibiotics (valve replacement)
	Suspected Moya-Moya disease	?
	Suspected fibromuscular dysplasia	?
	Suspected angiitis	Cortisone, antibiotics, tuberculostatics, immunosuppression
	Differential diagnosis from sinus thrombosis, herpes simplex encephalitis	
Vertebrobasilar territory	Suspected basilar thrombosis/embolism or intracranial vertebral stenosis	Thrombolyis, heparin, coumarin
	Subclavian stenosis or occlusion	Operation, PTA
	Suspected bilateral high-grade stenosis or occlusion of vertebral origin	PTA, operation
	Monitoring of treatment	
	Diagnostic angiography without therapeutic implications to clarify spontaneous course and prognosis (?)	

[a] The lines of treatment listed constitute a subjective choice. In doubtful cases, and in view of the low complications rate of arterial DSA, the indications can be widened to embrace the diagnostic and prognostic aspects. However, consideration should always be given to the prospect of the therapeutic usefulness of the angiography findings. *PTA,* Percutaneous transluminal angioplasty.

Table 5.8 presents a subjective listing of the indications for angiography in reversible or progressive stroke with the possible therapeutic implications. It should be borne in mind that fibrinolytic treatment is still experimental (see p. 180), and that despite the negative results of the EC-IC bypass study there may still be indications for the bypass operation in quite a few cases. Many diseases that are not attributable to arterial ischemic lesions may initially manifest with the features of a progressive insult. In these cases, angiography may become necessary for purposes of differential diagnosis (sinus thrombosis, hemorrhagic encephalitis). In view of the relatively low complication rate of arterial digital subtraction angiography the indications for angiography can sometimes be extended, for example, to obtain information on the spontaneous course and prognosis of ischemic infarcts.

5.5.2 Technique of Angiography

Transfemoral angiography using selective catheterization makes it possible to demonstrate all the supra-aortic vessels selectively via one puncture site. In rare cases retrograde brachial angiography is performed. On the left side it provides a demonstration of the vertebrobasilar territory free from superimposition. Sometimes direct access via the axillary artery may be chosen to show the vertebral artery.

As well as depicting and documenting the origins of the great cervical vessels, the carotid bifurcation and the intracranial vessels are shown in special series. The anteroposterior view of the carotid bifurcation is improved by slight rotation of the head by 25°, which usually prevents superimposition of the bifurcation by external carotid branches. On films a simultaneous two-plane portrayal is preferred to reduce the amount of contrast. Angiography of the aortic arch is carried out to elucidate an arteritis involving the origins of the supra-aortic vessels or a dissection, but not with the aim of assessing the individual vessels supplying the brain. The amount of contrast used for this is greater than that required for sequential and selective depiction of the individual vessels. Digital subtraction angiography of the cerebral vessels should be performed only intra-arterially. Venous digital subtraction angiography with a large bolus of contrast is risky, and the resolution is inadequate.

The toxicity of the contrast medium has been reduced in recent years. Anaphylactic reactions are certainly unpredictable but can be controlled by the usual measures. Transient toxic complications, such as cortical blindness, are rarely seen with the new contrast media. Yet cerebral angiography, especially in patients with vascular diseases, is not a risk-free investigation. In transfemoral angiography, minor (mainly local) complications occur in about 1% of cases and more severe complications, including fatalities, in 0.5%. Therefore it is absolutely necessary to have precise indications and to explain the possible complications to high-risk patients with cerebrovascular disease.

The use of digital intra-arterial subtraction angiography calls for good cooperation by the patient (no respiratory excursion during the angiography series) or intubation anesthesia. This is essential for results of sufficient quality. If angiography has been decided on, the optimal quality of imaging must be aimed at; it is not reasonable to expose the patient even to the small risk of angiography without ensuring optimal technical performance of the examination.

Occasionally the conventional technique with serial film subtraction is thus still needed. A technically inadequate angiography provides no additional information and can even mislead the investigator. We request patients to fast prior to angiography. Any polycytemia is compensated by isovolemic hemodilution. The exact clotting state must be known. The catheter is perfused with heparinized Ringer's solution. Patients examined with a view to possible surgical procedures are prepared as for an operation.

5.5.3 Illustrative Angiographic Findings

Figure 5.47 shows a normal intracranial arterial phase of a common carotid representation in anteroposterior and lateral view, and Fig. 5.48 presents the later phases after injection into the right internal carotid. There is excellent filling of the arteries of the other hemisphere via the leptomeningeal collaterals.

Figure 5.49 illustrates a vertebrobasilar angiogram after injection into the left vertebral artery in hemiaxial and lateral views. Figure 5.50 shows a normal angiographic series of the carotid bifurcation. Figure 5.51 demonstrates three different degrees of stenosis of the internal carotid: an ulcerated stenosis of about 80%, a short subtotal stenosis of the internal carotid in the region of its origin, and a long filiform stenosis with less contrast of the distal carotid segment. Figure 5.52 presents a stenosis of the carotid siphon; such a stenosis is inaccessible to carotid surgery.

Pseudo-occlusion is the highest degree of internal carotid stenosis. In normal serial angiography only the proximal stump of the internal carotid is still visible, while in a prolonged series a very narrow collapsed internal carotid can be found using the subtraction technique. Pseudo-occlusion probably carries a high risk of embolism. Even when definitive carotid occlusion has occurred, a distal lumen can still be kept patent via an ascending pharyngeal anastomosis with the intrapetrosal portion of the internal carotid which produces a slow flow in the cerebral part of the internal carotid and may lead to ipsilateral embolism. If one suspects either pseudo-occlusion of the internal carotid or an acute obstruction with possible supraocclusional embolism (positive middle cerebral artery sign at CT), angiography should be performed not only on the affected internal carotid but also on the opposite side, in order to obtain information about collateralization via the anterior communicating artery (cross-filling).

In acute internal carotid occlusion, the depiction of contralateral flow can be used to demonstrate the upper border of the obstruction by retrograde filling from the carotid siphon. Most cases of embolic occlusion occur in branches of the middle cerebral artery; embolism of the anterior cerebral artery is uncommon. They are discovered when there is flow impairment in the middle cerebral artery. Embolic occlusions of the posterior cerebral artery as an expression of embolism of the posterior circulation are very often found at the division into the internal occipital and temporo-occipital arteries.

If there is suspicion of vasculitis, all the intracranial vascular territories must be investigated. The demonstration of multilocular lesions of the intracranial vessels with segmental narrowing, vascular interruptions, and stenoses is characteristic of arteritis. Vasculitic lesions are often found in the pars circularis of the posterior

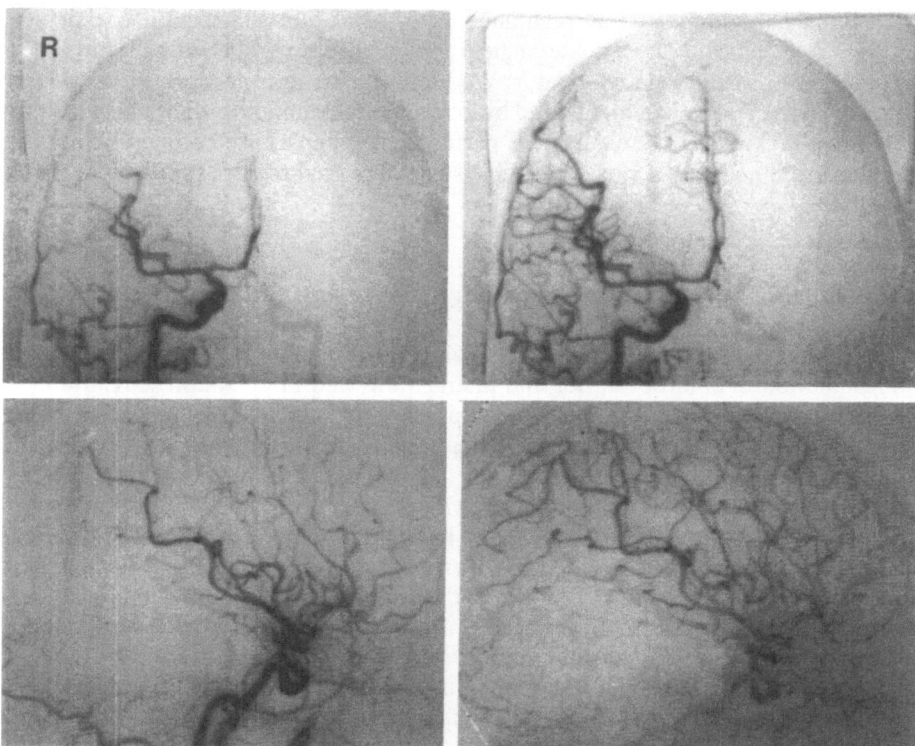

Fig. 5.47. Common carotid angiography showing the internal and external carotid branches, arterial phase, anteroposterior and lateral views. Normal angiogram in arterial digital subtraction angiography

cerebral artery. Carotid siphon stenoses, often bilateral, may also be the expression of vasculitis. A rare disease associated with intermittent ischemic symptoms is the Moya-Moya syndrome, which consists of multiple vascular lesions of the circle of Willis on uncertain etiology (Fig. 5.53).

In fibromuscular dysplasia spontaneous dissection occurs in a relatively large number of cases, and these act as causes of embolic insults. Fibromuscular dysplasia presents in the angiogram with a quite characteristic change in the vessel wall, marked by alternating dilated and constricted segments (the "pearl necklace") and aneurysm formation (Fig. 5.54). Strokes which occur in close temporal association with a head injury arouse suspicion of a traumatic carotid dissection (Fig. 5.55). In some cases, carotid dissection can also develop bilaterally. Proximal annular stenoses of the vertebral origin (Fig. 5.56) are rare sources of emboli. Arteriosclerotic lesions of the vertebral artery, on the other hand, do act as a source of cerebral emboli, which lead to a transient brainstem disturbance, sometimes also to an embolic basilar occlusion or to the uni- or bilateral posterior cerebral insults described above. Unilateral complete occlusion of the vertebral artery can be tolerated without clinical deficit, but if the obstruction is situated at the origin of the posterior inferior cerebellar artery, a

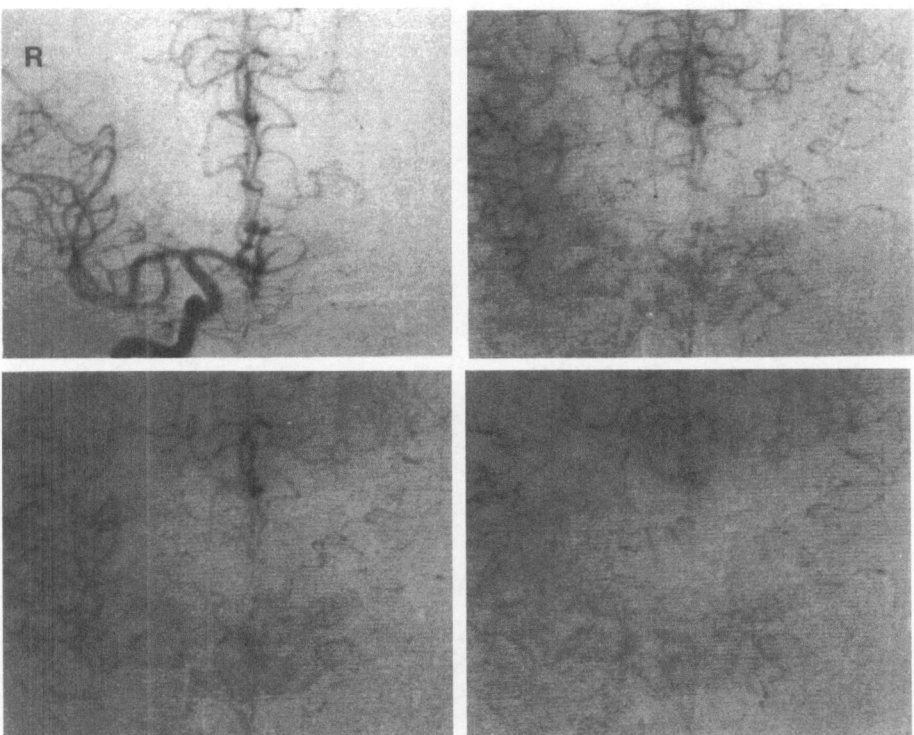

Fig. 5.48. Right internal carotid angiography with excellent collateral filling. Both anterior cerebral arteries are filled via the right internal carotid; in addition, the left middle cerebral territory is filled with only slight delay via leptomeningeal anastomoses

territorial infarct of this vessel results. Even bilateral vertebral occlusions can be tolerated if there is good collateralization via the carotid flow territory. However, there is in these patients a risk of basilar thrombosis, as shown in Fig. 5.57. The clinical features and classification of basilar occlusions are discussed in detail in Sect. 4.1.2.3. Figure 5.58 presents the angiographic findings in a subclavian steal syndrome (see p. 68). Two angiographic phases, one early and one late, are superimposed so that the vertebral artery (shown in white) corresponds to the retrograde perfused vertebral artery, via which the steal mechanism takes place.

5.5.4 Interventional Neuroradiology

5.5.4.1 Percutaneous Transluminal Angioplasty

To date there are only very few indications for percutaneous transluminal angioplasty (PTA) of vessels supplying the brain. The basic principle of PTA is that a stenosed vessel can be dilated by an intraluminal balloon. Reasonable indications include high-

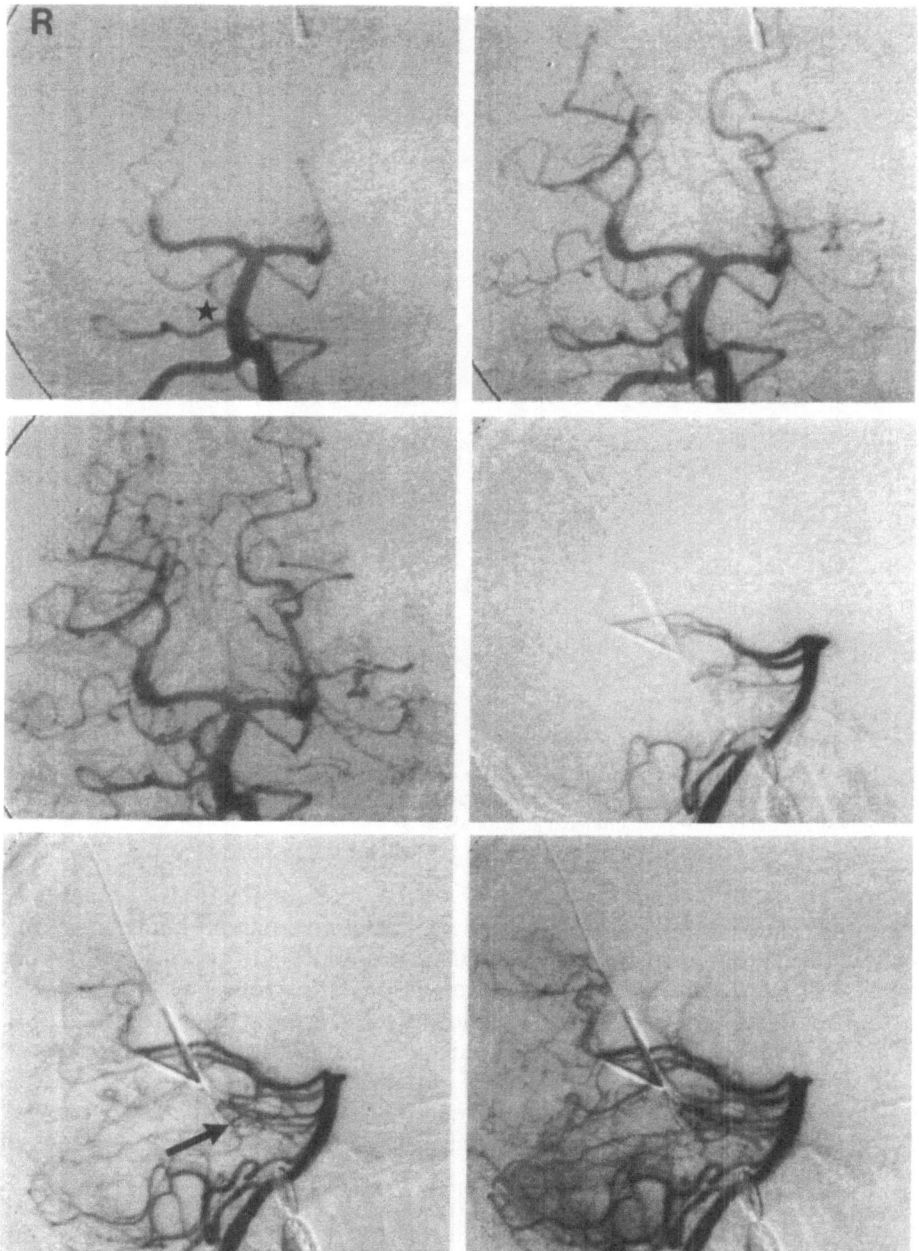

Fig. 5.49. Example of a vertebrobasilar angiogram, arterial phase, anteroposterior and lateral views. The stripe artifact which is not completely eliminated from the digital subtraction angiogram is due to the electrode and cable used for simultaneous neurophysiologic monitoring. The findings are those of a normal variant with a large-caliber AICA (*asterisk*) on the right but a typical course of the PICA on the left. Note the complete filling of both posterior cerebral arteries and the good portrayal of the long circumferential arteries (*arrow*)

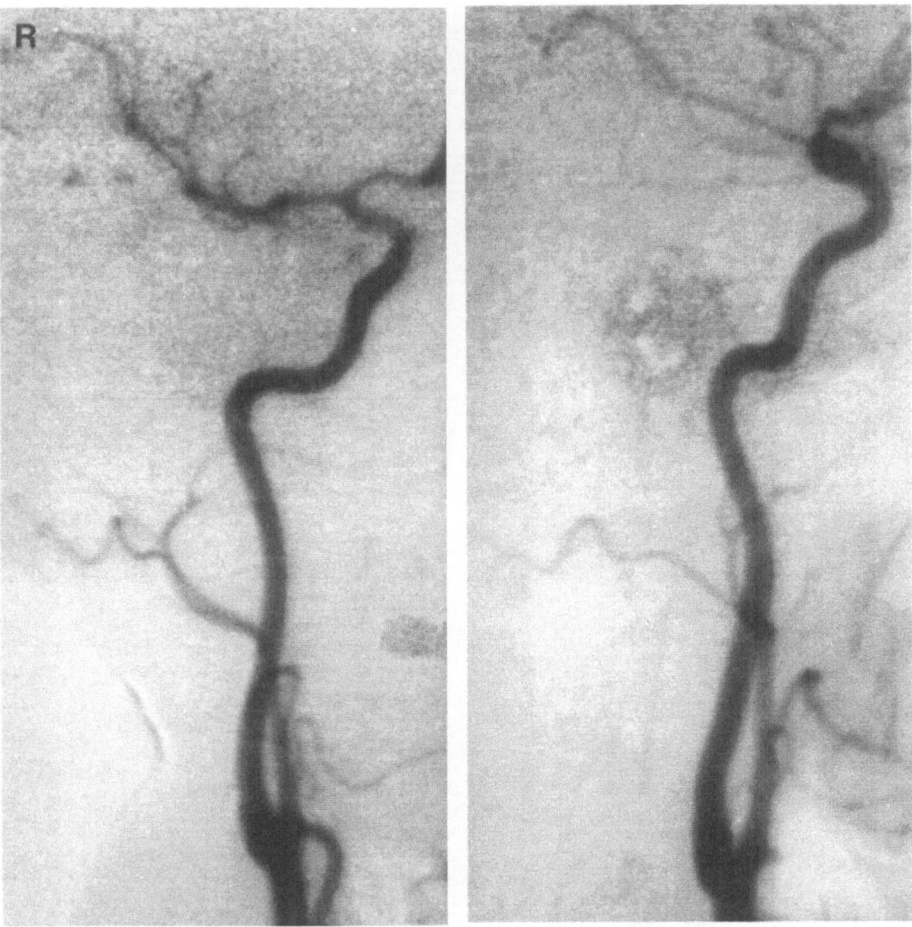

Fig. 5.50. Carotid bifurcation: normal findings with basal course of internal carotid artery

grade proximal vertebral artery stenosis at its origin with contralateral occlusion as well as a clinically manifest subclavian steal syndrome with proximal subclavian stenosis. Only in very few cases is PTA even considered for postoperative distal stricture after carotid endarterectomy. We consider dilation of an arteriosclerotic and possibly embolizing stenosis of the carotid contraindicated because of the major risk of embolism. Small series have been reported on PTA in the carotid (Theron et al. 1987) and the vertebrobasilar circulation (Higashida et al. 1987), the latter mostly in cases of delayed vasospasm following subarachnoid hemorrhage.

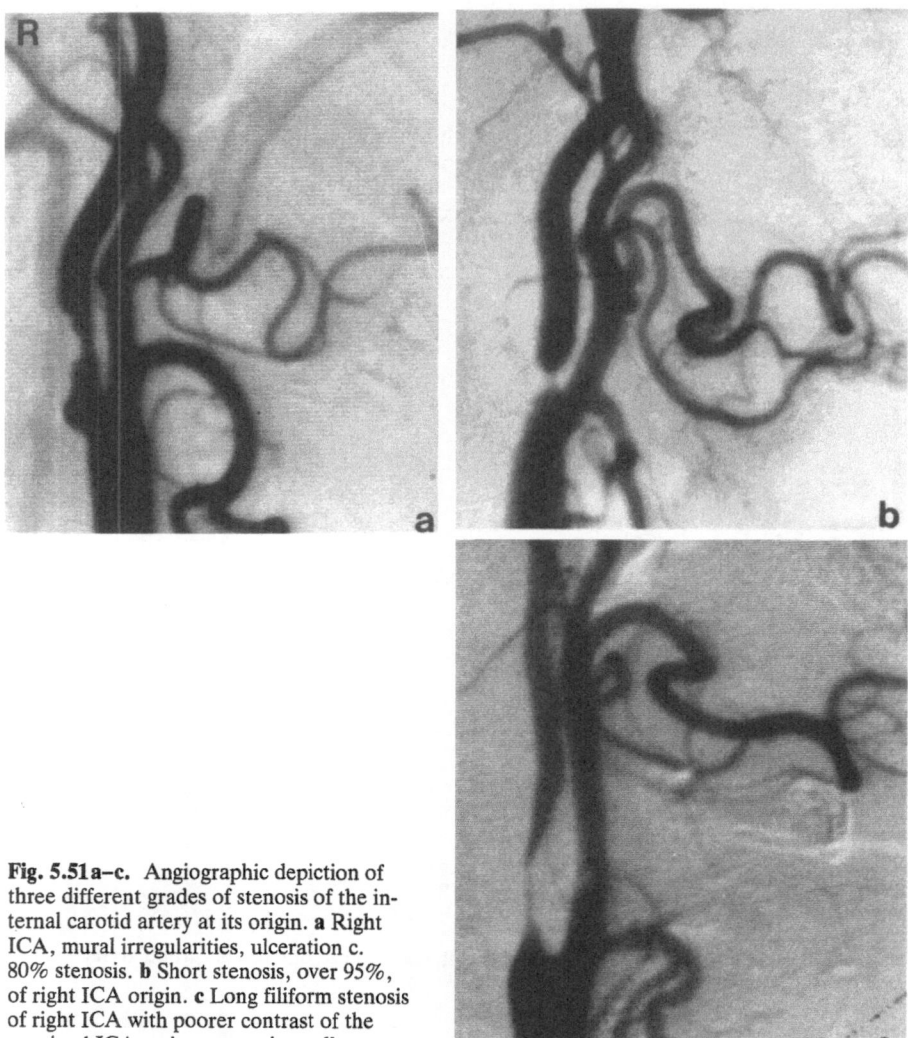

Fig. 5.51a–c. Angiographic depiction of three different grades of stenosis of the internal carotid artery at its origin. **a** Right ICA, mural irregularities, ulceration c. 80% stenosis. **b** Short stenosis, over 95%, of right ICA origin. **c** Long filiform stenosis of right ICA with poorer contrast of the proximal ICA and commencing collapse

5.5.4.2 Local Fibrinolytic Therapy

The possibility of local, intra-arterial administration of fibrinolytic agents in the acute obstruction of intracerebral vessels has been discussed and attempted since 1982 (Zeumer et al. 1982, 1985). The method has been successfully employed for vertebrobasilar occlusions (Hacke et al. 1988) and also in the anterior circulation. This method presupposes very early referral of the patient, a complete team available for neuroradiologic intervention, and possibly a neurologic intensive care unit. Results have been encouraging and have been confirmed at various centers with small

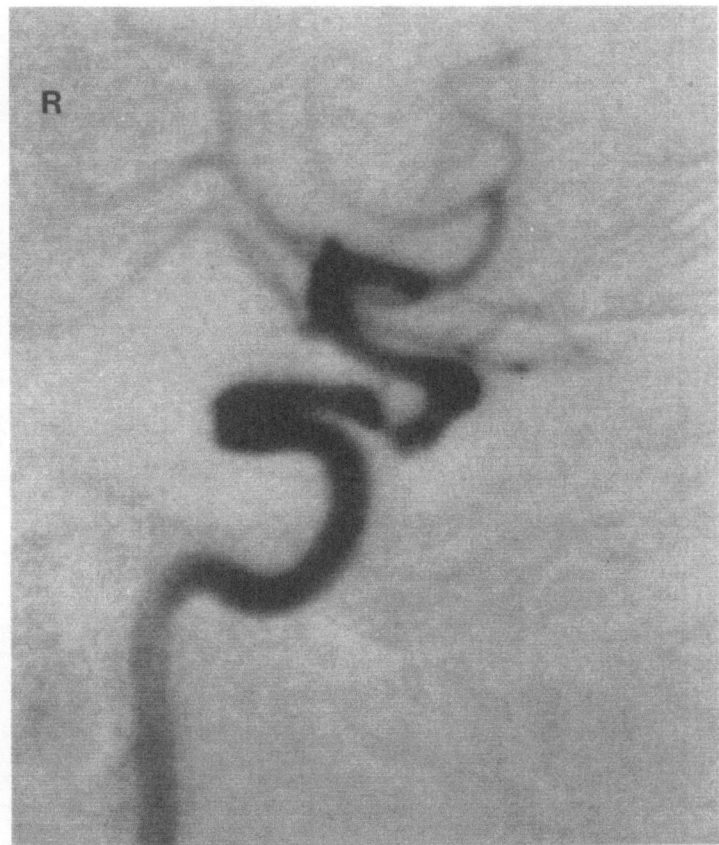

Fig. 5.52. Angiographic findings in carotid siphon stenosis in the intracranial segment (C2 segment)

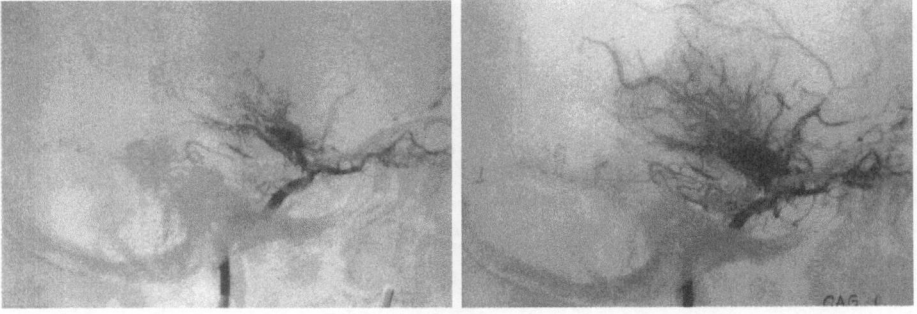

Fig. 5.53. Angiographic appearances in Moya-Moya syndrome with high-grade stenosis of the left ICA after origin of the ophthalmic artery and an extensive rete mirabile

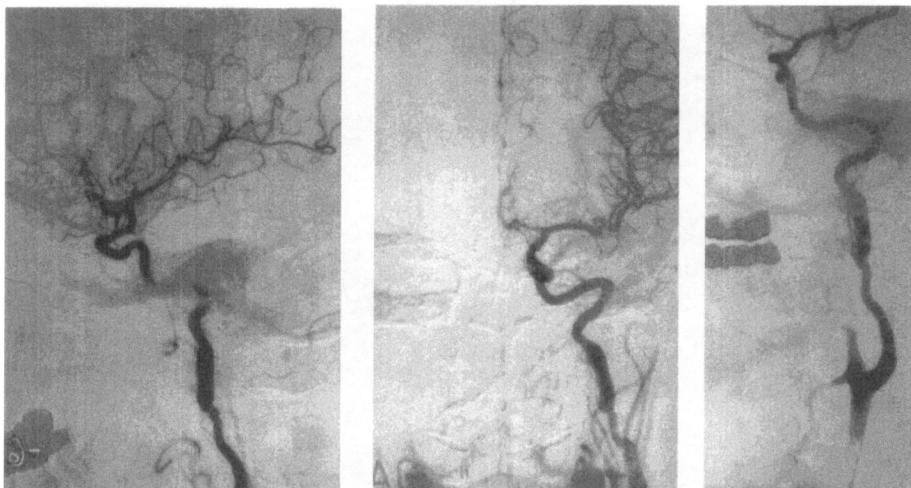

Fig. 5.54. Angiography of carotid aneurysm in fibromuscular dysplasia

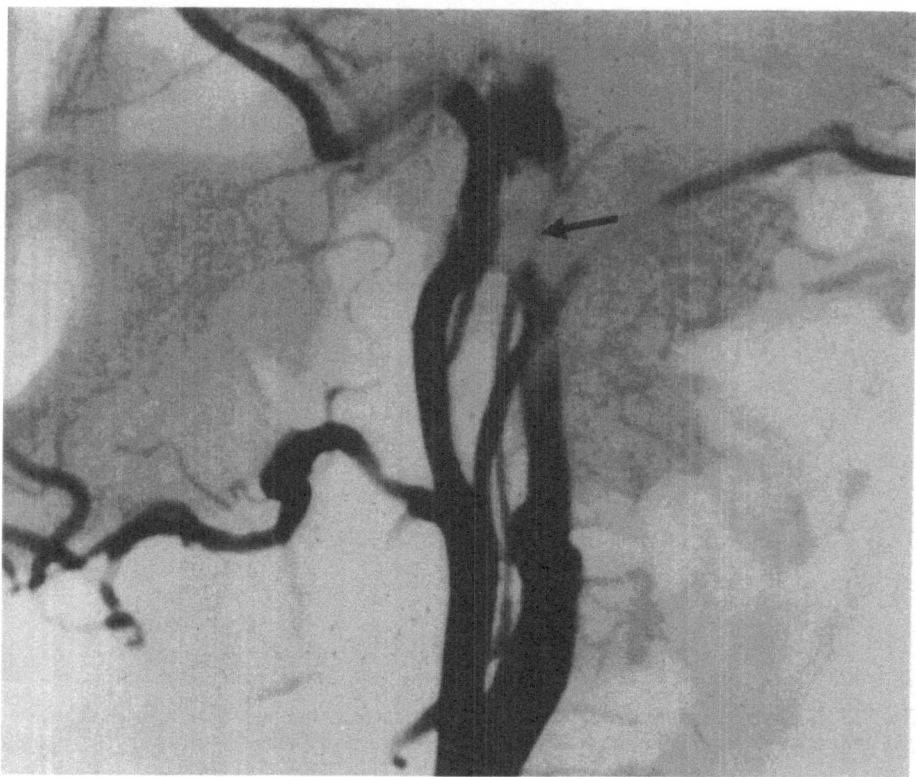

Fig. 5.55. Traumatic dissection of internal carotid at the skull base after cervical whiplash injury (*arrow*)

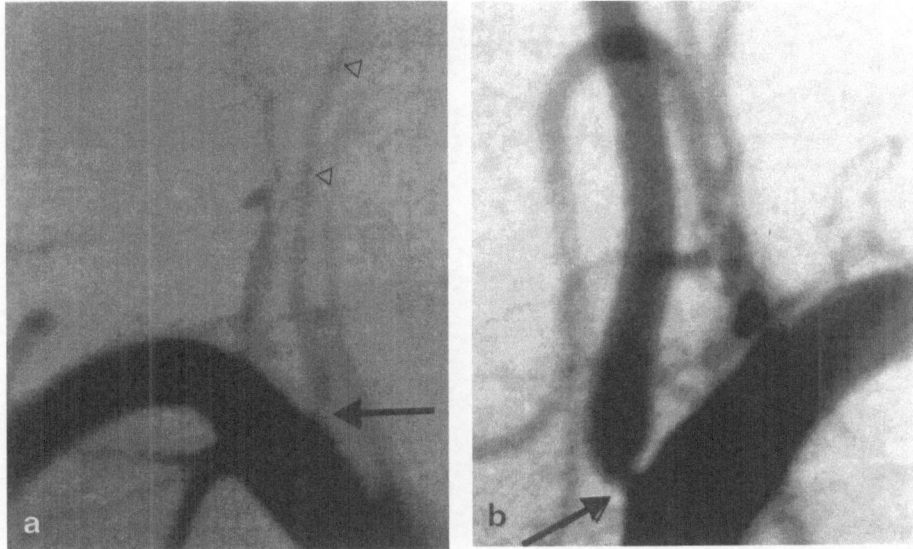

Fig. 5.56. a Subtotal vertebral origin stenosis, right (*arrow*) with very faint contrast in cervical portion of vertebral (*triangle*). **b** About 90% annular vertebral origin stenosis, left, with slight poststenotic dilatation

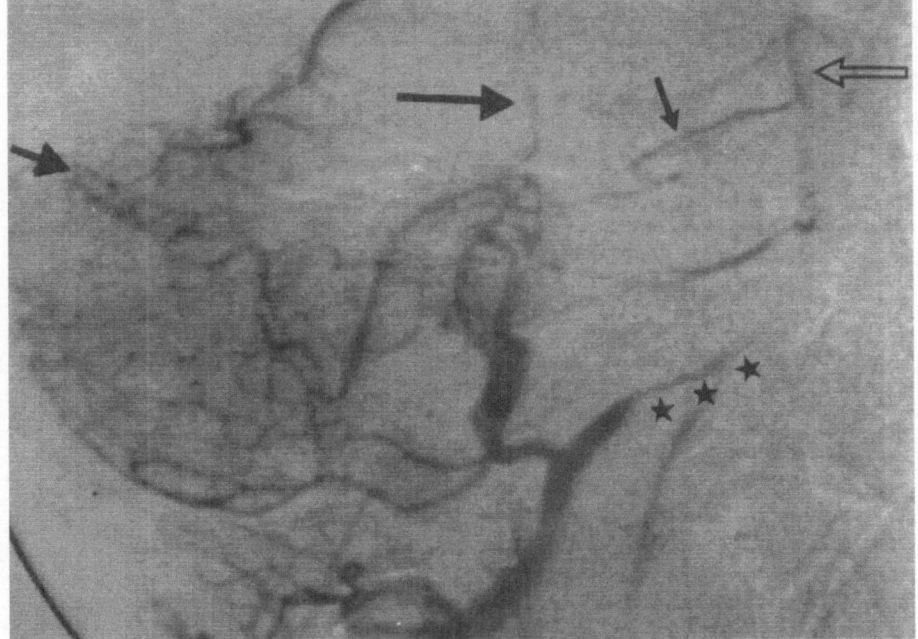

Fig. 5.57. Extensive arteriosclerotic stenosis of right vertebral artery before confluence at basilar artery (*stars*). An extensive leptomeningeal anastomotic plexus has been established with the SCA via the large-caliber PICA (*arrows*). The basilar artery is only slightly filled with contrast (*open arrow*)

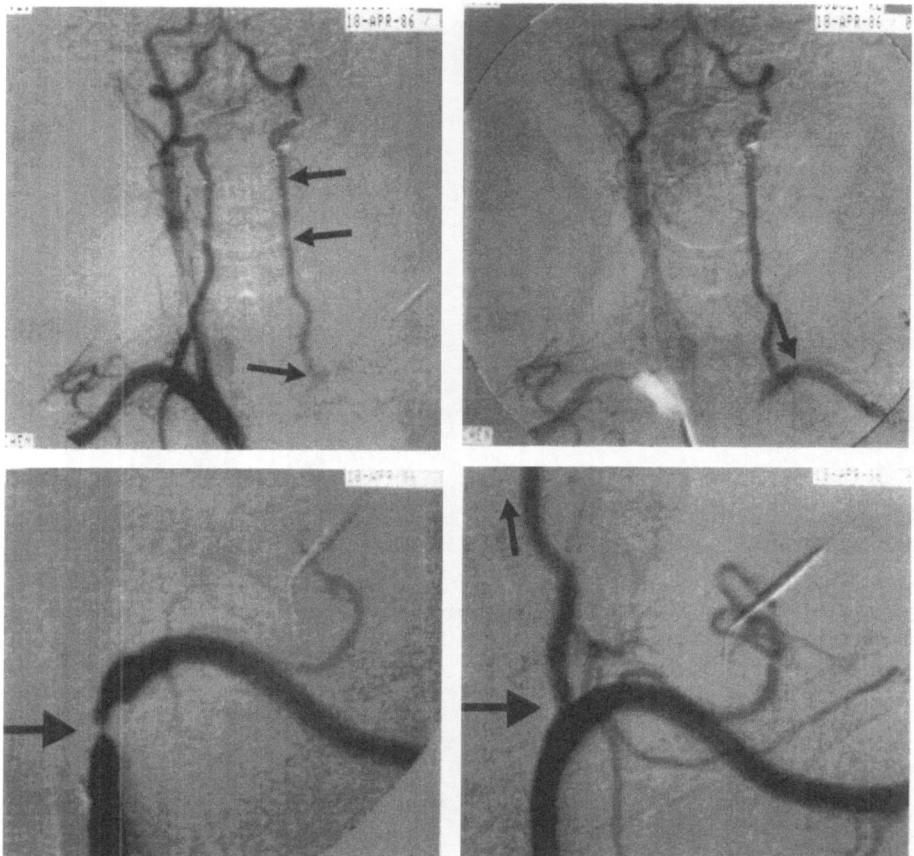

Fig. 5.58. Illustration of a subclavian steal syndrome with high-grade subclavian stenosis, left. In the *upper parts* of the figure the vertebrovertebral steal is well shown after injection of the right subclavian artery; the left subclavian artery is filled via the left, retrograde-filled vertebral artery (*small arrows*). Orthograde filling takes place after successful dilatation of the vertebral artery

numbers of patients. However, this therapeutic approach entails special requirements if it is to be used as a routine technique. Therefore it is not discussed in detail here, although the results are referred to in Sect. 6.2.3.2.

References

Aaslid R (1986) Transcranial Doppler sonography. Springer, Vienna New York
Aminoff MJ (1981) Electrodiagnosis in clinical neurology. Churchill Livingston, New York
Arbeille P, Lapierre F, Pourcelot L (1985) Evaluation des sténoses carotidiennes par les ultrasons. Encycl Méd Chir (Paris) Radiodiagnostic III, 32210, A09, 1
Awad I, Modic M, Little JR, Furlan AV, Weinstein M, et al. (1986) Parenchymal lesions in transient ischemic attacks: correlation of computed tomography and magnetic resonance imaging. Stroke 17:399

Barker AT, Jalinous R, Freeston IL (1985) Noninvasive magnetic stimulation of the human motor cortex. Lancet i:1106

Barnett HJM, Boughner DR, Taylor DW, Cooper PE, Kostuk WJ, Nichol PM (1980) Further evidence relating mitral-valve prolapse to cerebral ischemic event. N Engl J Med 302:139

Baron JC, Bousser MG, Rey A, Guillard A, Comar D, Castaigne P (1981) Reversal of focal "misery-perfusion syndrome" by extra-intracranial arterial bypass in hemodynamic cerebral ischemia. A case study with 15 O positron emission tomography. Stroke 12:454

Biller J, Adams HP, Johnson MR, Kerber RE, Toffol GJ (1986) Paradoxical cerebral embolism: eight cases. Neurology 36:1356

Blackwood W, Hallpike JF, Kocen RS, Mair WGP (1969) Atheromatous disease of the carotid arterial system and embolism from the heart in cerebral infarction: a morbid anatomical study. Brain 92:897

Bogousslavsky J, Regli F (1984) Cerebral infarction with transient signs (CITS): do TIAs correspond to small deep infarcts in internal carotid artery occlusion? Stroke 15:536

Bogousslavsky J, Fox AJ, Barnett HJM, Hachinski VC, Vinitski S, et al. (1986) Clinico-topographic correlation of small vertebro-basilar infarct using magnetic resonance imaging. Stroke 17:929

Bradley WG, Waluch V, Brant-Zawadzki M, Yadley RA, Wyoff RR (1984) Patchy, periventricular white matter lesions in the elderly: a common observation during NMR imaging. Noninvas Med Imaging 1:35

Brant-Zawadzki M, Norman D (1987) Magnetic resonance imaging of the central nervous system. Raven, New York

Brant-Zawadzki M, Solomon M, Newton TH, Weinstein P, Schmidley J, et al. (1985) Basic principles of magnetic resonance imaging in cerebral ischemia and initial clinical experience. Neuroradiology 27:517

Brant-Zawadzki M, Weinstein P, Bartkowski H, Moseley M (1987) MR imaging and spectroscopy in clinical and experimental cerebral ischemia: a review. AJR 148:579

Büdingen HJ, Reutern G-M, Freund H-J (1982) Doppler-Sonographie der extrakraniellen Hirnarterien. Thieme, Stuttgart

Cerebral Embolism Task Force (1986) Cardiogenic brain embolism. Arch Neurol 43:71

Cerebral Embolism Task Force (1989) Cardiogenic brain embolism. The scond report of the Cerebral Embolism Task Force. Arch Neurol 46:727

Chatrian GF, Shaw CW, Leffmann H (1964) The significance of periodic lateralized epileptiform discharges in EEG: an electro-encephalographic and pathological study. Electroencephalogr Clin Neurophysiol 17:177

Chiappa KH, Ropper AH (1982) Evoked potentials in clinical medicine. N Engl J Med 306:1140

Christian W (1982) Klinische Elektroencephalographie, 3rd edn. Thieme, Stuttgart

Daffertshofer M (1988) Grundlagen und Wertigkeit frequenzanalytischer Untersuchungen von Dopplersignalen der Arteria carotis interna. Dissertation, Düsseldorf

Desmedt JE (1980) Clinical uses of cerebral, brainstem and spinal somatosensory evoked potentials. Karger, Basel

Dougherty JH, Simmons JD, Parker J (1986) Subcortical ischemic disease: clinical spectrum and MRT correlation. Stroke 17:146

Eidelberg D, Johnson G, Barnes D, Tofts PS, Deply D, et al. (1988) ^{19}F NMR imaging of blood oxygenation in the brain. Magn Reson Med 6:344

Elster AD (1988) Cranial magnetic resonance imaging. Churchill Livingstone, New York

Ewing JR, Branch CA, Helpern JA, Smith MB, Butt SM, et al. (1989) Cerebral blood flow measured by NMR indicator dilution in cats. Stroke 20:259

Ferbert A, Buchner H, Brückmann H, Zeumer H, Hacke W (1988) Evoked potentials in basilar artery thrombosis. Electroencephalogr Clin Neurophysiol 69:136

Frackowiak RSJ (1985) Pathophysiology of human cerebral ischemia. Studies with position tomography and ^{15}oxygen. In: Sokoloff L (ed) Brain imaging and brain function. Raven, New York, p 139

Gelmers HJ Krämer G, Hacke W, Hennerici M (1989) Zerebrale Ischämien. Springer, Berlin Heidelberg New York Tokyo

Gibbs JM, Wise RJS, Leenders KL, Jones T (1984) Evaluation of cerebral perfusion reserve in patients with carotid artery occlusion. Lancet I:310

Hacke W (1986) Clinical relevance of multimodal assessment of brainstem functions in severe vascular brainstem lesions. In: Kunze K, Zangemeister WH, Arlt A (eds) Clinical problems of brainstem disorders. Thieme, Stuttgart, p 101

Hart RG, Tegeler CH (1986) Hemorrhagic infarction on CT in the absence of anticoagulant therapy. Stroke 17:558

Heiss W-D (1984) Methoden zur Untersuchung der zerebralen Hämodynamik. In: Paal G (ed) Therapie der Hirndurchblutungsstörungen. Edition Medizin, Weinheim, p 203

Heiss W-D (1989) Der ischämische Insult. Dtsch Ärztebl 86:30

Hennerici M, Neuerburg-Heusler D (1988) Gefäßdiagnostik mit Ultraschall. Thieme, Stuttgart

Hennerici M, Rautenburg W, Schwartz A (1987) Transcranial Doppler ultrasound for the assessment of intracranial arterial flow velocity, part 1: examination technique and normal values. Surg Neurol 27:439

Hennerici M, Herzog H, Rautenberg W, et al. (1988) Cerebral blood flow and metabolism in patients with asymptomatic carotid artery occlusion studied by positron-emission-tomography. J Neurol 235: S33

Higashida RT, Hieshime GB, Tsai FY, Halbach VV, Norman D, et al. (1987) Transluminal angioplasty of the vertebral and basilar artery. Am J Neuroradiol 8:745

Hinshaw DB, Thompson JR, Hasso AN, Casselmann ES (1980) Infarctions of the brainstem and cerebellum: a correlation of computed tomography and angiography. Radiology 137:105

Hornig CR, Dorndorf W, Agnoli AL (1986) Hemorrhagic cerebral infarction – a prospective study. Stroke 17:179

Huber P (1979) Zerebrale Angiographie für Klinik und Praxis, 3rd edn. Thieme, Stuttgart

John ER, Pritchard LS, Friedman J, Easton P (1988) Neurometrics: computer-assisted differential diagnosis of brain dysfunctions. Science 239:162

Karbowski K (1974) Das Elektroenzephalogramm im epileptischen Anfall. Huber, Bern

Katzmann R, Pappius HM (1973) Brain electrolytes and fluid metabolism. Williams and Wilkins, Baltimore

Kertesz A, Black SE, Nicholson L, Carr T (1987) The sensitivity and specificity of MRI in stroke. Neurology 37:1580

Kety SS, Schmidt CF (1948) The nitrous oxide method for the quantitative determination of cerebral blood flow in man: theory, procedure and normal values. J Clin Invest 27:476

Kopecky SL, Gersh BJ, McGoon MD, et al. (1987) The natural history of lone atrial fibrillation. N Engl J Med 317:669

Krayenbühl H, Yasargil G, Huber P (1979) Zerebrale Angiographie für Klinik und Praxis. Thieme, Stuttgart

Kretschmann HJ, Weinrich W (1986) Neuroanatomy and cranial computed tomography. Thieme, Stuttgart

Kuwert T, Hennerici M, Langen K-J, Herzog H, Rota E, Aulich A, Rautenberg W, Finenlager LE (1990) Compensatory mechanisms in patients with asymptomatic carotid artery occlusion. Neurol Res 12:89

Lechat P, Mas JL, Lascault G, et al. (1988) Prevalence of patent foramen ovale in patients with stroke. N Engl J Med 318:1148

Levine SR, Washington JM, Jefferson MF, Kieran SN, Moen M, et al. (1987) "Crack" cocaine-associated stroke. Neurology 37:1849

Lindegaard K-F, Bakke SJ, Aaslid R, Nornes H (1986) Doppler diagnosis of intracranial artery occlusive disorders. J Neurol Neurosurg Psychiatry 49:510

Lowitzsch K, Maurer K, Hopf HC (1983) Evozierte Potentiale in der klinischen Diagnostik. Thieme, Stuttgart

Macchi PJ, Grossmann JM, Gomon JM, Goldberg HI, Zimmermann RA, et al. (1988) High field MR imaging of cerebral venous thrombosis. J Comput Assist Tomogr 10:10

Mattle H, Grolimund P, Huber P, Sturzenegger M, Zurbrüggd HR (1988) Trancranial Doppler sonographic findings in middle cerebral artery disease. Arch Neurol 45:289

Merton PA, Morton HB (1980) Stimulation of the cerebral cortex in the intact human subjects. Nature 285:227

Mohr JP (1986) Stroke Data Banks. Stroke 17:171

Mull A, Aulich A, Hennerici I (1990) Transcranial Doppler ultrasonography vs. angiography for assessment of the vertebrobasilar circulation. J Clin Ultrasound 18:539

Nadjmi M, Piepgras V, Vogelsang H (1981) Kranielle Computertomographie. Thieme, Stuttgart

Nagata K, Tagawa K, Shishido F, Uemura K (1986) Topographic EEG correlates of cerebral blood flow and oxygen consumption in patients with neuropsychological disorders. In: Duffy FH (ed) Topographic mapping of brain electrical activity. Butterworths, Boston, p 357

Nakada T, Kwee IL, Card PJ, Matwiyoff NA, Griffey BV, et al. (1988) Fluorine-19 NMR imaging of glucose metabolism. Magn Reson Med 6:307

Noel P, Desmedt JE (1975) Somatosensory cerebral evoked potentials after vascular lesions of the brain-stem and diencephalon. Brain 98:113

Olszewski J (1982) Subcortical arteriosclerotic encephalopathy. Review of literature on the so-called Binswanger's disease and presentation of two cases. Wld Neurol 3:359

Padget DH (1944) The circle of Willis, its embryology and anatomy. Comestock, Ithaca

Poeck K (1985) Klinische Neuropsychologie. Thieme, Stuttgart

Powers WJ, Raichle ME (1985) Positron emission tomography and its application to the study of cerebrovascular disease in man. Stroke 16:361

Powers WJ, Press GA, Grubb RL, Gado M, Raichle ME (1987) The effect of hemodynamically significant carotid artery disease in the hemodynamic states of the cerebral circulation. Ann Intern Med 106:27

Ramadan NM, Deveshwar R, Levine SR (1989) Magnetic resonance and clinical cerebrovascular disease. An update. Stroke 20:1279–1283

Rautenberg W, Hennerici M (1988) Pulsed Doppler assessment of innominate artery obstructive diseases. Stroke 19:1514

Reneman RS, Merode T van, Hick P, Hoeks APG (1986) Cardiovascular application of multi-gate pulsed Doppler systems. Ultrasound Med Biol 12:357

Ross MA, Biller J, Adams HP jr, Dunn V (1986) Magnetic resonance imaging in Wallenberg's lateral medullary syndrome. Stroke 17:542

Rothrock JF, Lyden PD, Hesselink JR, Brown JJ, Healy ME (1987) Brain magnetic resonance imaging in the evaluation of lacunar stroke. Stroke 18:781

Salgado E, Weinstein M, Furlan AV, Modic MJ, Beck GJ, et al. (1986) Proton magnetic resonance imaging in ischemic cerebrovascular disease. Ann Neurol 20:502

Scharff RE, Hennerici M, Bluschke V, Lück J, Kladetzky RG (1982) Cerebral ischemia in young patients: is it associated with mitral valve prolapse and abnormal platelet activity in vivo? Stroke 13:454

Steinke W, Klötzsch C, Hennerici M (1990) Carotid artery disease assessed by colour Doppler flow imaging. AJNR 11:259

Stöhr M, Dichgans J, Diener HC, Buettner UW (1982) Evozierte Potentiale. Springer, Berlin Heidelberg New York

Theron J, Raymond J, Casasco A, Cortheoux F (1987) Percutaneous angioplasty of atherosclerotic and postsurgical stenosis of carotid arteries. AJNR 8:495

Tomsick TA, Brott TG, Olinger CP, Barsan W, Spilker J (1989) Hyperdense middle cerebral artery: incidence and quantitative significance. Neuroradiology 31:312

Waxman SG, Toole JF (1983) Temporal profile resembling TIA in the setting of cerebral infarction. Stroke 14:433

Whisnant JP (1982) Multiple particles injected may all go to the same cerebral artery branch. Stroke 13:720

Widder B (1985) Dopplersonographie der hirnversorgenden Arterien. Springer, Berlin Heidelberg New York

Wollschlaeger G, Wollschlaeger PB (1974) The circle of Willis. In: Newton TH, Potts D (eds) Radiology of the skull and brain: angiography II. Mosby, St Louis, p 1171

Zeumer H (1985) Survey of progress: vascular recanalizing techniques in interventional neuroradiology. J Neurol 231:287

Zeumer H, Ringelstein EB (1987) Computed tomography patterns of brain infarctions as a pathogenetic key. In: Poeck K, Ringelstein EB, Hacke W (eds) New trends in diagnosis and management of stroke. Springer, Berlin Heidelberg New York, p 75

Zeumer H, Hacke W, Ringelstein B (1983) Local intraarterial thrombolysis in vertebrobasilar thrombembolic diseases. Am J Neuroradiol 4:401

Zülch KJ (1985) The cerebral infarct. Pathology, pathogenesis, and computed tomography. Springer, Berlin Heidelberg New York

6 Treatment and Prophylaxis

6.1 General Treatment

6.1.1 Associated Systemic Diseases

Following a stroke, the patient's neurologic deficit may be most impressive, but his treatment and prognosis depend largely upon accompanying systemic disorders. Acute treatment, for instance, must take into consideration such things as cardiovascular disorders (myocardial infarction, valve defects, arrhythmias, hypertension), disorders of renal function, and diabetes mellitus. The early detection and treatment of such systemic problems can help to prevent complications that would be difficult to control later. Thus, in a patient with latent heart disease hypervolemic therapy with low molecular weight dextran may in fact elicit right heart failure and pulmonary edema instead of helping the patient.

6.1.2 Airways, Oxygenation, and Pulmonary Function

Ensuring good oxygenation of the blood and a normal, preferably rather low, p_aCO_2 to avoid a steal effect are the bases of any treatment for stroke. Although neither of these factors has an effect in the structurally damaged ischemic region, they are important for maintaining turnover in the marginal zone of the insult, the penumbra. In addition, a low p_aCO_2 leads to a fall in intracerebral pressure by reducing the intracerebral blood volume. Oxygenation of the blood is improved by administering $1–2 \, l \, O_2$/min via a nasal tube, a light sedative if there is marked hyperventilation, and bronchospasmolytics.

In examining the stroke patient, attention should be paid to pathologic respiratory patterns. In patients with impaired consciousness after brainstem infarcts, in basilar artery thrombosis, or in a large middle cerebral infarct there may be an early and urgent indication for intubation and mechanical ventilation. Intubation is best performed under brief anesthesia together with a muscle relaxant to avoid a reflexive rise in intracerebral pressure during the intubation. With troubles in swallowing and risk of aspiration a gastric tube should be passed early. In cases of severe infarct the use of a central venous catheter is recommended for exact adjustment with measurement of the central venous pressure. If ventilation becomes necessary, one should ensure that this is initially without positive end-expiratory pressure (PEEP) to minimize the venous backflow. Despite having good p_aCO_2 and 40% O_2 in the inspired air, many patients with recent strokes do not attain an adequate p_aCO_2, presumably because of shunting in the alveolar vessels. In these cases, adequate sedation with volume-controlled respiration, slight PEEP, and possibly prolongation of the inspiratory period are helpful; an increase in the O_2 concentration of inspired air, however, has only a short-term and dubious effect.

6.1.3 Heart

Acute cerebral ischemias may have effects on cardiac function which, together with the resulting ECG changes, cardiac arrhythmias, and sometimes even raised serum enzyme levels, suggest a previous myocardial infarction (Norris et al. 1979). Nevertheless, not all secondary cardiologic phenomena after cerebral ischemias should be regarded as being "centrally provoked." There is a high coincidence of myocardial infarction, sometimes not particularly impressive clinically, with cerebral ischemias. Digitalization is recommended only with obvious signs of heart failure. Normal rhythm should be restored by means of drugs or cardioversion; these considerations require consultation with a cardiologist. This is also the case in matters related to pacemaker care.

Prophylactic administration of antibiotics is not indicated. If embolizing inflammatory heart disease is suspected, broad antibiotic therapy immediately after taking a blood culture is necessary with penicillin (4×10^6 IU/day) plus a staphylococcal penicillin such as oxycillin (3×5 g) and an aminoglycoside, the dosage being adapted to renal function. Disseminated intravascular coagulation is treated by antithrombin III replacement, low-dose heparin (200 IU/h), and shock treatment.

6.1.4 Hypertension

While the conventional treatment of acute stroke used to call for reducing blood pressure, the problem of hypertension is currently tackled less aggressively. It is known that hypertension may be precipitated following an acute cerebral ischemia and can persist for several days (Wallace and Levy 1980). In the context of pathophysiologic considerations, it is evident that a high-normal blood pressure is desirable after an ischemia; obviously, however, substantially raised blood pressure values are to be avoided. Systolic values over 220 mmHg or diastolic values over 110 mmHg constitute an indication for early drug treatment, but even here the reduction in blood pressure should not be too drastic. The concept of high-normal blood pressure refers to systolic values not exceeding 160–170 mmHg and diastolic values 95 mmHg (Brott and Reed 1989).

The postischemic reflex hypertension usually subsides, and within a few days one sees a return to the initial level, which in most patients is one of mild hypertension.

For the reduction of a substantially raised pressure, nifedipine, given either orally or by infusion, is the drug of first choice. Antihypertensive agents of vasodilator and ganglion-blocking type are initially less appropriate.

Optimization of cardiac output with high-normal blood pressure and a normal heart rate is one of the essentials of stroke management. Central venous pressure should be maintained at around 8–10 cmH$_2$O, and its monitoring provides early warning of a volume deficiency (osmotherapy) or overhydration, either of which may have negative effects on cerebral perfusion.

Many patients with long-standing hypertension have rather normotensive values in the first days after stroke attack. However, the Bayliss effect (see p. 22), which maintains a relatively constant cerebral perfusion pressure despite variations in systemic blood pressure, often fails after infarction. Hence a positive effect from a slight rise in systemic blood pressure may be expected in these cases. Marked hypotension should lead to a search for a noncerebral cause, such as myocardial infarction, pulmonary embolism, internal hemorrhages, volume or protein deficiency, or sepsis.

6.1.5 Diabetes Mellitus

Many stroke patients are diabetics. Sometimes the diabetes is discovered only after an ischemic insult has developed. A preexisting diabetic metabolic status may deteriorate drastically during the acute phase of the disease, and temporary insulin treatment may then become necessary. Maintaining high glucose levels is not advantageous in acute strokes, for the problem is not one of reduced glucose supply to the brain cells but poor glucose utilization resulting from the lack of oxygen. The glucose level is related to the lactate acidosis and therefore contributes to the tissue damage (see p. 28; Pulsinelli et al. 1983). In some treatment centers it is still customary to give corticosteroids to all stroke patients. However, a positive effect of these drugs has never been demonstrated, even with space-occupying ischemic insults, and no effect can thus be expected even in cytotoxic edema. Furthermore, corticosteroids threaten aggravation of the diabetic metabolic status. The routine use of corticosteroids is therefore contraindicated.

6.1.6 Water and Electrolyte Balance

Aggressive dehydration as well as uncontrolled hypervolemia should be strictly avoided in stroke patients. In cases of intracerebral pressure the aim should be a slightly negative balance (about 200–300 ml negative balance daily). Electrolytes should be monitored at short intervals for replacement as required; if insulin is administered intravenously, consideration should be given to the increased potassium requirement. Determination of the osmolality in serum and urine helps to detect the development of diabetes insipidus, which may also be indicated by hyponatremia. Overhydration can increase the cerebral edema and lead to pulmonary edema and cardiac decompensation.

6.1.7 Other Measures

Epileptic Attacks and Hypoxic Myoclonias (Lance and Adams 1963):
The incidence of vascular epilepsies in the first 2 years is estimated at about 5%.
Partial (focal) or secondary generalized epileptic attacks may occur even in the acute
phase. Treatment is with clonazepam (2 mg i. v.) or diazepam (10–20 mg i. v.),
followed by rapid loading with phenytoin (e. g., a short infusion of 750 mg), there-
after 300–750 mg daily orally or by infusion. Myoclonias (see p. 73) can likewise be
treated in the acute phase with clonazepam via a perfusor (approximately 6–10 mg
daily), 5-hydroxytryptophane (100–300 mg), or trihexyphenidyl orally (2–10 mg
daily).

6.1.8 General Care

In the acute phase many patients are unable to swallow or can do so only with
difficulty. This can be ascertained early with a spoonful of water or an ice cube.
Control of bladder emptying may be lost, so that a catheter or a suprapubic tube must
be inserted; early bladder training can shorten the time these measures are needed. In
cases of constipation, laxatives should be given for a short period.
There is an increased risk of venous thrombosis and pulmonary embolism in severe
pareses. Treatment with low-dose heparin (5000 IU subcutaneously two or three
times daily) provides adequate prophylaxis (Gelmers 1980). A recent cerebral
infarction is not a contraindication.
The prognosis depends greatly on the early institution of intensive physiotherapy;
during the acute phase this should be carried out twice daily if possible and should
include respiratory exercises and exercises to prevent venous thrombosis and
contractures. Simple exercises of this kind can be instituted by the nursing staff in
intensive care units and in general wards. Frequent changes of position are needed in
any case to prevent decubital ulceration and to support ventilation.

6.2 Special Treatment in the Acute Phase

6.2.1 Preliminary Remarks on the Treatment of Ischemic Cerebral Infarcts

As yet, there are only two effective measures for the prevention of cerebral ischemias,
and treatment in the acute phase still lacks any medical or surgical modality that
clearly meets the standards of modern scientific investigation. The reason for this
alarming state lies largely in the numerous methodologic weaknesses of most
prophylactic and therapeutic studies.
The various pathogenetic factors that may be involved in the etiology of stroke could
not be studied as long as the methodologic requirements were lacking. The studies
were often conceived and carried out before the advent of CT; little attention has
likewise been paid to developments in ultrasound diagnosis and angiographic
technique. Also other questions, such as identification of the affected vascular
territory, have repeatedly led to problems: How can a prospectively planned study of

carotid endarterectomy yield meaningful results if patients with symptoms of the vertebrobasilar circulation are included? Might such an operation help patients with a systemic disease of the small vessels (lacunes) and the incidental finding of a low-grade carotid stenosis? What effect would hemodilution have in a patient whose infarcts are due to cardiac emboli? How useful are anticoagulants in patients whose problem is a hyalinosis of the small intracerebral vessels?

Future therapeutic studies will need to investigate different patient groups to assess accurately the effectiveness of various single and combined therapeutic measures. The treatment concept that results from these studies would be theoretically based upon etiopathogenetic considerations. While these still require testing for their practical importance, such considerations already suggest practicable approaches to a differential therapy of ischemic infarcts.

6.2.2 Drugs to Improve Perfusion of Ischemic Brain Tissue

The theoretical basis of this therapeutic approach is improvement of the cerebral microcirculation.

6.2.2.1 Measures to Improve the Rheologic Properties of the Blood

Blood viscosity is determined largely by the hematocrit value. In healthy volunteers the cerebral perfusion is reduced with an excessive hematocrit value and is increased by venesection. Patients with signs of neurologic deficit due to cerebral ischemia may have a high hematocrit value (often over 50%).

It has been shown that the size of the infarct on CT is correlated with the hematocrit value (Harrision et al. 1981). On the other hand, there is a risk that the reduction in oxygen-binding capacity of the blood may become critical if the hematocrit is too low. However, it has been shown that, even with a hematocrit level of 30%, optimal oxygen supply is still possible by means of primary increase in cardiac output and CBF, at least in young healthy persons. Older persons can also tolerate a hematocrit of around 40% by increasing cardiac output. The hematocrit value can be reduced by various methods, all of which are based on the principle of hemodilution (Gottstein and Held 1969).

Hemodilution

Hemodilution can be obtained in three different ways: isovolemic, hypovolemic, and hypervolemic dilution (Table 6.1).

In isovolemic hemodilution a given volume of blood (e.g., 500 ml) is replaced by an equal amount of fluid, whereas in hypovolemic dilution the blood volume is replaced only in part. The latter is advisable in patients with heart failure and hypertension. Hypervolemic hemodilution, involving an increase in volume, is the most aggressive form of the three and carries a risk of increased intracranial pressure; it therefore calls for intensive patient monitoring.

Table 6.1. Guide to hemodilution treatment in cerebral infarction (combinations are possible)

Type of treatment	Indication
Hypervolemic 1000 ml LMD or HES i. v. daily for 2–5 days	Hematocrit < 40%, no cardiac or renal failure
Hypervolemic with venesection 250–500 ml venesection daily for 2 days; plus 500 ml LMD or HES i. v. daily for 2–5 days	Hematocrit > 40%, no cardiac or renal failure
Isovolemic 250–500 ml venesection daily for 2 days; plus 250–500 ml LMD or HES i. v. in 2 h for 2 days	Hematocrit < 40%, 250 ml; hematocrit > 40%, 500 ml (in cardiac or renal failure)
Hypovolemic 250–500 ml venesection daily for 2 days, no replacement	Hematocrit < 40%, 250 ml; hematocrit > 40%, 500 ml

LMD, 10% low molecular weight dextran 40; HES, hydroxyethyl starch 6%.

In some European countries, solutions of low molecular weight dextran (dextran 40) or hydroxyethyl starch (HES 6%–10%) are still widely employed for replacement. The disadvantage of dextran is that some 0.5% of patients show hypersensitivity reactions of the anaphylactic type. These may be largely avoided by an initial hapten inhibition with 20 ml dextran-1 (Promiten); autologous plasma is a good alternative. The results of therapeutic studies conducted to date are controversial, but there appears to be a predominance of negative results (Table 6.2). A prospective randomized study intended to test the effectiveness of aggressive hypervolemic hemodilution with HES under intensive medical monitoring (Swan-Ganz catheter) had to be discontinued prematurely because of increased mortality in the treated group (Hemodilution in Stroke Study Group 1989). The results of this study gave rise

Table 6.2. Results of hemodilution treatment for cerebral infarction

Authors	Patients Ht/Co[a]	Commence-ment (h)	Period	Effect
Gilroy et al. (1969)	63/59	24–72	10 days	+
Spudis et al. (1973)	30/29	24	21 days	0
Kaste et al. (1976)[b]	30/20	24	21 days	0
Matthews et al. (1984)	52/48	?	6 months	0
Strand et al. (1984)	52/50	48	28 days	+
Scand. Coop. Study (1987)	183/190	48	3 months	0
Italian Coop. Study (1988)	633/634	12	6 months	0
HSSG (1989)[c]	45/43	24	3 months	0

[a] Ht, hemodilution treatment (dextran 40); Co, controls.
[b] Simultaneously treated with glucocorticosteroids.
[c] Treatment with pentastarch, a colloid solution of hydroxyethyl starch.

to much controversy. While the authors maintain that a subgroup of patients can be identified in whom hypervolemic hemodilution is helpful (Hemodilution in Stroke Study Group 1989), the results are seen by von Kummer et al. (1989) as confirming their view that no significant positive effect can be expected from hemodilution regardless of how this is performed. Recently, two further multicenter, randomized studies on isovolemic hemodilution have been reported (Scandinavian Stroke Study Group 1987; Italian Acute Stroke Study Group 1988) which also found no positive effects in the hemodilution groups. A subanalysis in the Scandinavian study showed, in fact, that patients with deep ischemic infarcts did rather worse on hemodilution.

The results of treatment studies conducted up to now have been controversial (Table 6.2). This method of treatment makes sense, if at all, only if begun very early. Nevertheless, hemodilution is still the standard treatment in many centers, particularly in Germany. A pathologically defensible indication exists in infarcts which are caused or enhanced by a raised hematocrit or raised blood viscosity.

It has been shown that erythrocyte deformability, which is determined largely by the blood viscosity, is influenced by various drugs such as pentoxyfylline, or piracetam; however, these in vitro effects do not seem to be accompanied by particularly impressive clinical improvement in the most recent studies in patients (Hsu et al. 1988).

6.2.2.2 Vasopressor Drugs

In normotensive patients, inducing hypertension has been considered as a method of improving cerebral perfusion pressure (Wise et al. 1972), although systematic clinical studies are not available. The advantages of any therapeutic effect must be weighed against the risks of hemorrhage or increased cerebral edema. This method may be employed under careful medical monitoring in individual cases that are characterized by hemodynamically induced ischemias, fluctuating symptoms, and low blood pressures. The particular drugs to be considered for such treatment are dopamine and dobutamine.

6.2.2.3 Vasodilators

Vasodilators were used widely until a few years ago, but investigations up to now have shown only very slight if any effect (Table 6.3). Because of this, and because of the risk of inducing a steal effect, the use of vasodilators must now be considered obsolete (Olesen and Paulson 1971).

6.2.2.4 Aminophylline

In view of the pathologic vascular reactions in the region of the penumbra, treatment with vasoconstrictor drugs may be preferable in order to obtain the opposite of a steal phenomenon, the counter-steal phenomenon. Although this is an experimentally measurable mechanism, it is not yet clear whether it has any clinical relevance.

Table 6.3. Effect of vasodilators on the cerebral perfusion. (From Cook and James 1981)

Drug	Effect	
	Parenteral	Oral
Papaverine	+	Weak +
Cyclandelate	+/−	Weak +
Hexobendine	+	0
Isoxsuprine	−	0
Ergoid mesylate	−/0	0
Betahistine	+	Weak +
Vincamine	+/0	0
Nicotinic acid	−/0	0
Cinarizine	0	0

+, increased cerebral blood flow; −, decreased; 0, no effect.

Aminophylline is a drug with vasoconstrictor effects on the cerebral vessels and has been used in a number of centers now for many years. However, no difference between aminophylline therapy and placebo could be demonstrated in a prospective double-blind study (Britton et al. 1980). It may be that a favorable effect on the penumbra could be obtained by the early initiation of this treatment, directly after the appearance of the ischemic syndrome. As with hemodilution, further studies are needed.

6.2.2.5 Prostacyclin

Prostaglandin metabolism was discussed above (Sect. 2.4.2) as an important factor in the development of ischemic cell damage. While the use of prostacyclin in myocardial infarction leads to a marked reduction in the size of the infarct (Ribeiro et al. 1981), no influence has been shown on infarct size or cerebral perfusion in cerebral infarction. Favorable results of prostacyclin infusions in open studies were not confirmed in a randomized double-blind study (Hsu et al. 1987; Table 6.4).

Table 6.4. Results of prostacyclin infusion in cerebral infarct

Authors	Patients	Commenced	Period	Effect
Gryglewski et al. (1983)	10	1–5 days	2 months	+
Miller et al. (1984)	7	24 h	1 month	(+)
Martin et al. (1985)	16/16	24 h	14 days	0
Hsu et al. (1987)	43/47	24 h	1 month	0

6.2.3 Drugs to Affect the Blood Clotting Mechanism

6.2.3.1 Anticoagulants

Warfarin (Coumadin) is a competitive inhibitor of vitamin K and blocks the formation of the vitamin K-dependent factors in the extrinsic coagulation pathway (II, VII, IX, X) as well as proteins C and S. Coumarin treatment is monitored by the prothrombin time (Quick's test).

Heparins comprise a group of mucopolysaccharides whose anticoagulant effect is exerted after binding to antithrombin III via inactivation of factors VIIIa, IXa, Xa, and XIa as well as thrombin and plasmin. Antithrombin III is activated in the presence of thrombin. It has been debated whether particular groups of heparins with uniform molecular weights (low molecular weight heparins) may have stronger antithrombotic properties.

The results of early clinical studies of anticoagulation after cerebral infarction were generally not accepted because of methodologic limitations and the fear of hemorrhagic complications. However, the clinical importance of complications was probably overestimated in the past. In contrast to experimental conditions, there is only a slight risk of deterioration even in secondary hemorrhages. About 20% of ischemias develop secondary hemorrhages without coagulation; these follow a clinically silent course but are visible on CT. As seen in Table 6.5, the risk of cerebral hemorrhage during anticoagulant treatment is 4%–18% annually; 2%–9% of these complications have a fatal outcome. The most important additional risk factor is hypertension. The rationale for anticoagulation therapy with heparin has recently been the subject of controversy. On the one hand, Phillips (1989) and Scheinberg (1989) reject the indication for heparinization in any type of ischemic infarct because of the possible risk and the absence of controlled studies; on the other, Miller and Hart (1988) consider acute anticoagulation, in the absence of any proven therapy, to be a reasonable and necessary treatment in a range of specific situations. Phillips (1989) and Scheinberg (1989) point to the risks of hemorrhage and heparin-induced thrombopenia and to the slight but confirmed platelet-activating effects of heparin. The argument that heparin acts only as an anticoagulatory and not as a fibrinolytic enzyme (and that the reduction in stroke size after cerebral embolism is therefore

Table 6.5. Anticoagulation in acute cerebral ischemia

Authors	Patients AC Co	Period (months)	Strokes AC Co	Percentage of deaths AC Co	Hemorrhage AC Co
Marshall and Shaw (1960)	26 25	1.5–6	23 20	12 8	12 4
Baker (1961)	56 62	9–13	10 9	10 3	18 5
Baker et al. (1962)	72 60	10–16	42 27	8 8	10 7
Hill et al. (1962)	66 65	28–31	33 29	8 1	11 0
Howell et al. (1964)	103 92	34–42	1 22	1 7	8 2
Enger and Boyesen (1965)	51 49	23–39	8 16	2 6	6 0

AC, anticoagulants; Co, controls.

relatively minor) can be countered by the evidence of reduction of renewed embolus formation. Moreover, there is no general agreement as to the time at which full heparinization should be instituted, nor whether this should be influenced by the observed size of the infarct. Larger infarcts undoubtedly carry a greater risk of (spontaneous) systemic bleeding (Okada et al. 1989). Heparin does not add to this risk and is thought to have a negative influence on the extent of the hemorrhage. It is usually recommended to begin anticoagulation therapy only several days after the larger infarction, if a repeat CT scan shows no hemorrhagic transformation (Cerebral Embolism Task Force 1989). Initiating ths therapy, however, means that there is no longer any possibility of preventing additional thrombus growth at the site of embolism.

We regard the following indications for early anticoagulation therapy:

1. Slowly progressive arterial thrombosis with the picture of a progressive insult (Table 6.6).
2. Cardiac cerebral emboli. Earlier retrospective studies showed a relatively high incidence of recurrent embolism, but this was not confirmed in prospective series; thus, no therapeutic effect was shown unequivocally in these studies (Tables 6.7, 6.8). Patients with atrial fibrillation and previous stroke are reportedly at high risk of recurrent stroke, and long-term anticoagulant prophylaxis is generally recommended. The risk of stroke in younger patients (under 50–60 years) with atrial fibrillation but without overt cardiovascular or cerebrovascular disease barely exceeds that in the general population (Kopecky et al. 1987). In view of the presumed time of anticoagulation and the annual increase in warfarin-associated complications, the use of long-term anticoagulation cannot be justified. Even long-term therapy with platelet-aggregation inhibitors in patients with rheumatic atrial fibrillation is still under evaluation. A recent trial (Petersen et al. 1989) failed to clarify the question due to a number of methodologic limitations.
3. High-grade intracranial stenoses, especially in the vertebrobasilar system and the proximal middle cerebral artery.
4. Carotid and vertebral dissection.
5. High-grade carotid stenoses with varying symptoms.
6. Proven heparin-sensitive coagulapathies, such as protein C deficiency.

Table 6.6. Anticoagulants in progressive infarction ("stroke in evolution")

Authors	Patients AC Co	Period (months)	Percentage of Further progression AC Co	Deaths AC Co
Carter et al. (1961)	38 38	6	32 50	7 17
Fisher (1961)	51 49	7	14 40	8 14
Baker et al. (1962)	61 67	12–15	23 46	8 15
Millikan (1965)	181 60	12	20 52	7 40

AC, anticoagulants; Co, controls.

Table 6.7. Early recurrence of cardiogenic embolism without anticoagulants

Authors	Patients	Period (days)	Embolism (%)
Retrospective			
Szekely (1964)	46	28	4
Furlan et al. (1982)	30	7	17
Koller (1982)	38	7	8
Bass (1983)	30	30	10
Sage and Uitert (1983)	59	14	2
Prospective			
Calandre et al. (1983)	15	7	0
CESG (1983)[a]	21	14	9
Lodder and van der Lugt (1983)	18	14	0
Santamaria et al. (1983)	109	7	4

[a] CESG, Cerebral Embolism Study Group.

Table 6.8. Recurrent embolism and hemorrhage after early anticoagulation (cardiogenic cerebral emboli)

Authors	Patients		Recurrences		Hemorrhages[a]	
	AC	Co	AC	Co	AC	Co
Calandre et al. (1983)	25	17	0	1	(3)	(2)
CESG (1983)[b]	24	21	0	2	0 (0)	2 (0)
Lodder and van der Lugt (1983)	21	18	2	0	2 (0)	0 (0)
Lodder et al. (1988)	70	50	14	9	3	0
Petersen et al. (1989)	335	336/336[c]	5	20/21	23	8/6

[a] In parentheses, those with clinical deterioration.
[b] CESG, Cerebral Embolism Study Group.
[c] 672 patients served as controls; 336 were treated with aspirin (75 mg/day) and 336 received placebo.
AC, anticoagulants; Co, controls.

Anticoagulation can be achieved most rapidly by the intravenous infusion of heparin, usually after giving an initial bolus of 3000–5000 IU. Regulation is obtained by means of the partial thromboplastin time, which is maintained at 2–2.5 times the normal value; this is done preferably by long-term infusion using a pump with 10000–15000 IU over 12 h until adequate inhibition of coagulation is obtained. The daily dosage required for this is 20000–40000 IU. If the decision is made for long-term anticoagulation, this is achieved with anticoagulants of the warfarin type in the usual way. Evidence that low-dose anticoagulation may be effective in embolizing cardiac diseases does not eliminate the need to monitor for minor side effects and complications.

Contraindications to the use of anticoagulants include hypertension, hemorrhagic tendency, peptic ulcers, severe diabetic retinopathy, old age (over about 70 years), inadequate patient compliance (as in alcoholism or dementia), or inadequate facilities for supervision. Views concerning the appropriate duration of this treatment vary, but it is usually limited to 6–12 months and is then replaced by platelet-aggregation inhibitors.

6.2.3.2 Thrombolytics

Among drugs acting by thrombolysis a distinction can be made between intrinsic and extrinsic enzymes. Streptokinase is an example of an extrinsic substance, while intrinsic thrombolytic enzymes include urokinase, tPA, and scuPA. The latter two exert their effect predominantly at the thrombus.

Early studies on the systemic use of thrombolytics indicated a high risk of developing secondary hemorrhages (reviewed by del Zoppo et al. 1986; Sloan 1987). By analogy with the local infusion of thrombolytic agents in myocardial infarction, local thrombolysis has been employed since the early 1980s first for basilar thromboses and later also in the middle cerebral territory (Zeumer et al. 1982; Nenci et al. 1983; Zeumer 1985; Brückmann et al. 1987; del Zoppo et al. 1988; Hacke et al. 1988; Mori et al. 1988; Zeumer et al. 1989). Studies of the two largest groups reported to date found evidence of a positive clinical course toward recanalization (del Zoppo et al. 1988; Hacke et al. 1988). This, together with the fact that developments in gene technology have made thrombus-specific thrombolytics such as r-tPA available in adequate quantity, has led to tests of the early systemic use of such enzymes for basilar occlusions and in angiographically confirmed vascular occlusions in the carotid – middle cerebral region. What, if any, value is to be attached to this treatment is not currently known.

In any case, the overall efficacy of thrombolytic therapy in stroke patients remains to be established. In addition, there are many questions about the choice of agent and route of administration (intravenous tPA versus intra-arterial urokinase), the need for associated antiplatelet or anticoagulant therapy to prevent reocclusion, and the interval after stroke during which this therapy can be safely and effectively administered. While present practice limits thrombolytic therapy to the small subpopulation of stroke patients in whom arterial occlusion can be documented within the first few hours, the promise of effective treatment may encourage clinicians to early referral and evaluation of stroke patients and thus increase the number of candidates for thrombolysis. There is some evidence of an additive effect in thrombolytic treatment combined with drugs thought to be protective at the cellular level (De Ley et al. 1989). Thrombolytics are contraindicated if there is an increased risk of hemorrhage (anticoagulant treatment, menorrhagia, hemorrhagic colitis, or peptic ulcer). Severe hypertension (diastolic pressure above 100 mmHg) also constitutes a contraindication. The complications include hemorrhages, of which intracerebral bleeding is the most feared. Fresh-frozen or fresh plasma must be available for the control of systemic hemorrhagic complications. The treatment can be carried out only under conditions of intensive medical care and should be limited to cases of severe ischemia.

6.2.4 Drugs to Protect Ischemic Brain Tissue

Drugs used to influence the catabolic processes after an ischemic event constitute a very heterogeneous group and show a varied pharmacologic profile.

6.2.4.1 Barbiturates

Under experimental conditions barbiturates can reduce the infarct size by reducing the oxygen requirement if they are administered before or within 30 min of an induced ischemia. In healthy tissue they lead to vasoconstriction (counter-steal phenomenon, see p. 27). Barbiturates reduce the rate at which free fatty acids are liberated and neutralize free radicals. They further reduce the intracellular potassium concentration. Translation of this model into clinical practice is difficult, and reports of results are correspondingly meager. This treatment is frequently quite impracticable in patients with acute cerebral ischemia because of time restrictions. In one pilot study, patients with acute ischemia were given 1 g thiopentone every 8 h up to a total dose of 10 g. While this led to a decline in mortality, there was uncertainty about the neurologic state of the patients treated (Agnoli et al. 1979). In another study phenobarbitone was given in doses of 200–300 mg daily for 2 days without any effect (Yatsu and Coull, unpublished communication). The treatment of cerebral ischemia after cardiac arrest with thiopentone had no influence on mortality or on the severity of the neurologic deficit (Brain Resuscitation Clinical Trial Study Group 1986).

At present, barbiturate protection of patients with acute cerebral ischemia does not seem to be an advisable form of treatment, despite its interesting pharmacologic basis.

6.2.4.2 Calcium Antagonists

The concept that infarct size depends, among other things, upon a whole chain of processes precipitated by the influx of calcium ions into the cell may have important therapeutic implications now with the availability of drugs having calcium-antagonist action. Through the prophylactic or therapeutic use of such drugs, the development of an infarct may be prevented, delayed, or limited.

Calcium antagonists constitute a new class of drugs with special electrophysiologic properties. Some calcium antagonists, such as nimodipine, have a special affinity for the cerebral vessels. Like the barbiturates, a positive effect of this substance has been

Table 6.9. Calcium antagonists in ischemic stroke

Author	Patients T/C	21-day or 28-day death rate T (%)	C (%)	$p <$	Neurological outcome All	Major	Minor deficit
Gelmers (1984)	30/30	7	17	0.01	$p = 0.0001$ —		—
Gelmers et al. (1988)	93/93	9	20	0.05	$p = 0.01$	$p < 0.005$	$p = 0.653$
Martinez-Vila (1990)	82/82	15	17	n.s.	$p = 0.04$	$p < 0.05$	$p = 0.52$
Krämer et al. (1991)	239/243	6	9	n.s.	$p = 0.36$	$p < 0.03$	$p = 0.26$

In the first 3 studies start of treatment was within 24 h, the last study within 48 h.
T, treatment (nimodipine); C, controls; n.s., not significant.

demonstrated experimentally if employed within 60 min after the onset of the ischemia (Steen et al. 1985). Cerebral blood flow measurements show that nimodipine can improve tissue perfusion without evoking a steal effect (Gelmers 1982).

PET studies showed improved perfusion and metabolism of the ischemic brain area after nimodipine infusion (Hakim et al. 1989). Treatment with calcium antagonists that penetrate the brain but have only limited cardiovascular effects has been undertaken in a series of clinical trials. European investigators reported that the diphenylpiperazine derivative flunarizine may be useful from an experimental point of view, but there is little information about its role in acute brain infarction. Nimodipine, a potent dihydropyridine-type calcium antagonist has been used in most clinical trials (Gelmers 1984; Gelmers et al. 1988; Martinez-Vila 1989; Krämer et al. 1991). The results of the initial clinical studies with calcium antagonists during acute cerebral ischemia affords a glimmer of hope that these drugs will be clinically useful (Table 6.9). Among those who respond better to calcium antagonist therapy are stroke patients with major to severe neurologic deficits. The internal between stroke onset and treatment should be kept to under 24 h, probably to under 12 h.

6.2.4.3 Other Therapeutic Approaches

Free radicals play an important part in the genesis of ischemic cell damage (see Sect. 2.4.2). Substances that neutralize free radicals (so-called antioxidants or free radical scavengers) might therefore be employed as protective agents. Besides the barbiturates discussed above, vitamins C and E may have a protective effect, although clinical studies have not yet yielded any concrete results.

Naloxone is an endorphin antagonist. It influences calcium influx into the cell (see Sect. 6.2.4.2) and may also have antioxidant as well as lipid peroxidant effects. Single observations in patients after subarachnoid hemorrhage have shown that acute neurologic deficits disappear briefly after administration of naloxone. As the dose required for cerebral ischemias is five to ten times higher than that needed to antagonize the action of morphine, the possibility of severe complications (acute cardiac arrest) must be considered. A review of various experimental and uncontrolled clinical studies of naloxone in the treatment of acute infarct has been presented by Martinez-Arizala et al. (1989). A first study, in which a bolus injection of between 2.5 and 200 mg/m^2 body surface (average 160 mg) was given intravenously, followed by a 24-h infusion with half the bolus dose per hour, showed a favorable effect (Jabaily and Davis 1984) and justifies the conducting of a systematic study.

Antagonists to the N-methyl-D-aspartate (NMDA) group of glutamate receptors may offer a new perspective in the treatment of ischemic cerebral infarcts. A range of in vivo and in vitro experiments confirm the potential efficacy of this approach; these are reviewed by Albers et al. (1989). The theoretical basis of this treatment is the massive accumulation of extracellular glutamate in ischemia, which acts on the different neurones as an excitatory transmitter. This also leads to unphysiologic and energy-consuming activity of the endangered neurones, which accelerates their cellular destruction. NMDA receptor antagonists should prevent this neurotoxicity by blocking the cell receptors for glutamate. Clinical studies have not yet been published.

6.2.5 Drug Treatment of Ischemic Cerebral Edema

6.2.5.1 Corticoids

Raised intracranial pressure and massive displacement leading to transtentorial herniation constitute important causes of early mortality after cerebral infarction (e.g., "malignant" middle cerebral infarction). It is possible that corticoids could influence vasogenic cerebral edema (sealing of the "tight junctions" of the blood-brain barrier). However, cerebral edema in the early phase after stroke is predominantly cytotoxic edema and is not significantly influenced by corticoids. Nevertheless, a nonspecific pressure reduction can be obtained, especially with high doses, by means of the less marked dehydrating effect exerted on the healthy brain tissue. The disadvantage of high doses of corticoids is the effect on glucose metabolism. Both experimental and clinical studies have yielded controversial results (Table 6.10). The routine use of corticoids in patients with acute cerebral ischemia is not indicated, but in desperate cases in patients with territorial infarcts and large mass displacements treatment with dexamethasone in high doses may sometimes be used. The dosage in there cases is comparable to that for vasogenic edema in the vicinity of cerebral tumors or metastases (e. g., 80–120 mg dexamethasone i.v., followed by 16 mg 4–6 times daily in gradually decreasing dosage).

Table 6.10. Glucocorticosteroids in cerebral infarction

Authors	Patients	Commence-ment (h)[a]	Treatment Improved	Dead	Controls Improved	Dead
Dyken and White (1956)	36	24		76%		53%
Rubinstein (1965)	19	24		31%		66%
Patten et al. (1972)	31	24	67%	0%	41%	0%
Candelise and Spinnler (1972)	49	24		54%		40%
Bauer and Tellez (1973)	54	48	48%	19%	16%	34%
Candelise et al. (1975)	152	24	62%	38%	66%	34%
Norris (1976)	53	24	17%	27%	36%	19%
Santanbrogio et al. (1978)	66	24	44%	56%	44%	56%
Norris and Hachinski (1986)	113	24		28%		28%

[a] Commencement of treatment in hours after onset of ischemia.

6.2.5.2 Hyperosmolar Substances

On theoretical grounds, an effect on cytotoxic cerebral edema is to be expected from hyperosmolar agents such as hypertonic glucose, mannitol, sorbitol, urea, and glycerol solutions. This effect is based on the development of an osmotic gradient between the blood stream and brain and the extra- and intracellular space, with the blood-brain barrier functioning as a semipermeable membrane. However, after only a few hours an equilibrium exists on either side of the membrane, and the osmotic effect is lost. Shortly afterwards a rebound effect develops, leading to water uptake in the damaged parts of the brain with subsequent swelling. Moreover, the repeated

Table 6.11. Osmotherapy in cerebral infarction

Authors	Patients Tr/Co	Hours	Period	Effect
Glycerol				
Mathew et al. (1972)	29/25	72	14 days	+
Gelmers (1975)	50/50	12	28 days	0
Fritz and Werner (1975)	50/56	24	14 months	0
Gilzanz et al. (1975)	30/31	36	14 days	+
Larsson et al. (1976)	12/15	6	3 months	0
Frei et al. (1987)	41/20	24–32	6 months	0
Bayer et al. (1987)	85/88	48	12 months	0
Mannitol				
Candelise et al. (1975)	75/64	24	10 days	0
Santanbrogio et al. (1978)	28/32	24	10 days	0

Tr, treatment with glyceral or mannitol; Co, controls.

administration of the agent can lead to severe electrolyte disturbances, and the resulting hypervolemia can cause decompensation phenomena. The rebound effect and electrolyte disturbances are not of great importance in the continuous administration of glycerol.

As with the use of dexamethasone, osmotherapy should be limited to severe cases with mass displacements since clinical studies have not demonstrated any convincing effect (Table 6.11). The agents used include mannitol (25%, 200 ml) and glycerol (orally 1.5 g/kg body weight every 24 h and i.v. 1.2 g/kg body weight every 24 h). Nevertheless, like hemodilution, this is employed as standard treatment in some centers.

6.2.6 Treatment of Inflammatory Cerebral Vascular Processes

The treatment of inflammatory cerebral vascular diseases is directed at the underlying disorders, of which the involvement of the cerebral vessels is usually only a part.

6.2.6.1 Treatment of Immunovasculitis

According to current concepts, the various forms of immunovasculitis are based on relatively similar immunopathogenetic processes; immunosuppression is presently the treatment of choice. As soon as the diagnosis is confirmed (see Sect. 4.2.4), high-dose corticoid treatment (80–100 mg methylprednisone or comparable corticoids in equivalent dose) should be given. Progressive reduction in dose based on the clinical course and the ESR should only be made after several weeks. However, a maintenance dosage of 6–8 mg daily is often necessary even after normalization of the laboratory parameters. In most cases, this is associated with immunosuppression with azathioprine (approximately 2–2.5 mg/kg body weight each day), less often with the cytostatic cyclophosphamide. Interactions with allopurinol must be watched for, and if these occur, the dose of azathioprine must be reduced to one-fourth.

6.2.6.2 Treatment of Specific Infective Vasculitis

The treatment of specific infective forms of vasculitis depends on the organisms. They include the (rare) vasculitic form of cerebrospinal syphilis, the forms of tuberculous and bacterial meningitis, and those associated with opportunistic infections such as parasitoses (toxoplasmosis) and fungal infections. Direct vascular involvement is also possible in AIDS.

6.3 Prophylaxis of Cerebral Ischemia

6.3.1 Drug Prophylaxis

The drug prophylaxis of cerebral infarction after a TIA is based on two principles: platelet-aggregation inhibition and anticoagulation.

6.3.1.1 Platelet-Aggregation Inhibitors

Platelet-aggregation inhibitors influence the platelet-endothelium reaction. Numerous studies with acetylsalicylic acid (ASA), dipyridamole, and sulfinpyrazone have shown repeatedly that the occurrence of new TIAs and of cerebral and retinal (as also myocardial) infarcts is reduced. In most of the prospective randomized studies 1000–1300 mg ASA was given; gastrointestinal bleeding often occurred with this dose, however, the favorable therapeutic effect can be preserved while the incidence of side effects are reduced with a lower dose. A British study has confirmed this for a dose of 300 mg ASA daily, and theoretically this could be replaced by a further dose reduction to below 100 mg daily (UK TIA Study Group 1988); however, a Danish study in 1988 was unable to distinguish it from placebo in doses below 100 mg (Boysen et al. 1988). Dipyridamole (25 mg) plus ASA (330 mg) has been demonstrated to have a prophylactic effect similar to that of 1000 mg ASA. The efficacy of dipyridamole alone not yet been demonstrated; thus its usefulness as a substitute for ASA in patients with ASA intolerance remains unknown. Unfortunately, the administration of dipyridamole in addition to ASA has been of no definite value in trials of stroke prophylaxis. A meta-analysis of seven controlled trials comparing ASA and/or sulfinpyrazone or dipyridamole with placebo found the ASA combination therapy to have a significant benefit on stroke (Sze et al. 1988).

Ticlopidine is a new antiplatelet drug, the mechanism of which is not clear but may involve interference with fibrinogen binding to platelets. The prophylactic Ticlopidine Aspirin Stroke Study (Hass et al. 1989) entered over 3000 patients with TIA or minor stroke. Patients were given 1300 mg ASA or 500 mg ticlopidine and followed up for as long as almost 6 years. There was a 21% reduction in fatal or nonfatal strokes in the patients treated with ticlopidine compared with those treated with ASA. Interestingly, this protective effect appeared to be even greater in women than in men. In a therapeutic study, the Canadian-American Ticlopidine Study group (Gent et al. 1989) randomized over 1000 patients with recent cerebral infarction to receive either ticlopidine or placebo. Among the patients treated with ticlopidine there was a 30% reduction in stroke, myocardial infarction, and vascular death. These promising

Table 6.12. Platelet-aggregation inhibitors after TIA or infarct

Authors	Inclusion[a]	Dose (g)	Patients Tr	Co	Endpoint[b]	Result
Acetylsalicylic acid						
Fields et al. (1978)	TIA	1.3	88	90	TIA	+
					CS, D	0
Reuther and Dorndorf (1978)	TIA/RIND	1.5	29	29	TIA, CS	0
Fields et al. (1978)	TIA/CE	1.3	65	65	TIA, CS, D	0
Can. Coop. Study (1978)	TIA/RIND	1.3	144+[c]	156+[c]	TIA	+
			146	139	CS, T	+
Guiraud-Chaumeil et al. (1982)	TIA/RIND	1	147	155[d]	CS, D	0
Candelise (1982)	TIA	1	63	61[e]	TIA, CS, D	n.d.[f]
Bousser et al. (1983)	TIA (16%) & CS (84%)	1	198	204	CS	+
Sorensen et al. (1983)	TIA/RIND	1	101	102	CS, D	0
Swed. Coop. Study (1987)	CS	1.5	253	252	TIA, CS, D	0
UK TIA Study (1988)	TIA/RIND	0.3 or 1.2	606/815	814	CS, D	+[g]
Acetylsalicylic acid and dipyridamole						
American-Canadian Coop. Study (1985)	TIA	A + D/A[h]	448	442	CS, D	n.d.
ESPS (1987)	TIA/RIND/ CS	A + D[i]	1250	1250	CS, D	+[j]
Ticlopidine						
CATS (Gent et al. 1989)	CS	T[k]	525	528	CS, MI, D	+
TASS (Hass et al. 1989)	TIA/RIND	T/A[l]	1529	1540	CS, D	+

[a] Inclusion criteria: CS, completed stroke; CE, carotid endartesectomy.
[b] Endpoint: D, death; MI, myocardial infarction.
[c] Some patients treated with sulfinpyrazone.
[d] Control group treated with Hydergine (dihydroergotoxinmesilate).
[e] Control group treated with sulfinpyrazone.
[f] n. d., no difference.
[g] Treatment better than placebo; no information about dosage.
[h] Treatment: 1.3 g acetylsalicylic acid and 0.3 g dipyridamole vs 1.3 g acetylsalicylic acid.
[i] Treatment: 0.975 g acetylsalicylic acid and 0.225 g dipyridamole vs placebo.
[j] Combination of (i) better than placebo.
[k] Treatment with 250 mg ticlopidine twice daily, therapeutic study.
[l] Treatment with 250 mg ticlopidine twice daily versus 1.3 g aspirin, prophylactic study.

preliminary results are somewhat tempered by side effects, including dermatitis, diarrhea, and occasionally neutropenia. The exact role played by ticlopidine in the prevention of stroke must yet be determined, but it seems that ticlopidine can be used as a substitute for ASA in patients who do not tolerate the side effects of ASA. Dipyridamole and sulfinpyrazone, which can also be argued on theoretic grounds as having a favorable influence on platelet-aggregation inhibition, have shown no significant reduction of cerebral infarcts in clinical studies (Table 6.12).

6.3.1.2 Anticoagulants

The use of anticoagulants for the prevention of cerebral infarction has been suggested for a period of 2–3 months after the first TIA. In several hospitals treatment is planned to begin with anticoagulant therapy if the first attack did not occur over 2 months previously, subsequently changing over to a platelet-aggregation inhibitor. The difficulty in interpreting earlier studies (Table 6.13) was the impossibility at that time to select patients according to the etiopathogenesis and type of cerebral ischemia. The incidence of the most important side effect, secondary hemorrhage, has probably been overestimated. It was not possible to distinguish between the clinically unimportant hemorrhagic transformation of infarct tissue and the connected, possibly space-occupying, gross parenchymatous hemorrhage.

Table 6.13. Anticoagulants after TIA

Authors	Patients		Period	Percentage of cerebral infarcts	
	AC	Co	(months)	AC	Co
Fisher (1958)	29	23	30	3	34
Siekert et al. (1963)	175	160	60	4	32
Baker (1962)	24	20	20	4	25
Pearce et al. (1965)	17	20	12	5	10
Baker et al. (1966)	30	30	40	7	23
Friedman et al. (1969)	21	23	27	0	35
Toole et al. (1975)	21	56	46–56	29	13
Ollson et al. (1976)	163	124	21–25	0	15
Gallhofer et al. (1979)	42	40	20	8	21
Terent and Anderson (1980)	25	16	48	8	31

AC, anticoagulants; Co, controls.

6.3.2 Prophylactic Surgical Therapy

Vascular surgical procedures in cerebrovascular diseases are of a primarily preventive nature. They are intended to improve the hemodynamics in vascular occlusions or stenoses and to eliminate a source of cerebral emboli. Carotid thrombendarterectomy is performed to eliminate a stenosis in the neck, and EC-IC bypass is intended to create a collateral circulation for the vascular system distal to the site of flow obstruction.

6.3.2.1 Carotid Endarterectomy

Carotid endarterectomy (EA) can be carriet out under general or local anesthesia. Intraoperative monitoring of the anesthetized patient is possible by means of EEG, evoked potentials, transcranial Doppler sonography, and regional cerebral blood flow, and serves essentially as an indication for an intraluminal shunt. Of course, its use has been the subject of controversy, as has been the use of monitoring in general, for all these measures relate only to the hemodynamic aspect of operative complications. The operation itself usually takes the form of an open "shelling out" plastic procedure, in which early or delayed cerebral emboli are the most common of severe complications. Occasionally, the vagus and hypoglossal nerves are (usually reversibly) damaged by pressure lesions. The indication for a one-stage bilateral surgical procedure is nowadays largely ignored.

No reliable indication for carotid EA exists as yet (Krämer et al. 1986), which is remarkable in view of the great number of operations performed annually. This is due to the fact that up to now there have only been two, small prospective randomized studies comparing the benefits and the risks of this procedure, both with negative results. The currently most common indication is in patients after TIA when an ipsilateral carotid stenosis is demonstrable; this is based mainly on retrospective and nonrandomized series. Nonstenosing plaque formation is only rarely a valid indication for surgery. The indications are also very variable in the presence of existing arteriosclerotic vascular lesions in other parts of the body, especially before major vascular surgery on the heart and large arteries of the body. Here, too, no proven clinical data exist to provide rational indications for prophylactic carotid EA.

Improved diagnosis by means of better angiographic technique and contrast media have led in recent years to a markedly reduced incidence of surgical complications and a reduction in complications in certain centers. Nevertheless, findings regarding the spontaneous course of asymptomatic carotid stenoses (Hennerici et al. 1982; Roederer et al. 1984) have contributed to a drastic limitation of indications, at least in neurologically asymptomatic extracranial vascular lesions. Several prospective randomized studies have therefore been initiated to compare the usefulness of prophylactic carotid EA with drug therapy using platelet-aggregation inhibitors. Until the results of these studies are known, the risks and advantages of both forms of treatment must be weighed against the spontaneous course in the light of individual points of view and local conditions.

At present, it appears defensible to suggest surgery in patients when there is no marked restriction of life expectancy due to some other disease, and when the complication rate for permanent neurologic deficit with a surgical procedure is demonstrably less than 3%. Such conditions include the following:

1. In high-grade internal carotid stenoses after repeated transient disturbances of neurologic function, where a causal connection is seen after exclusion of other pathogenic mechanisms
2. In fluctuating neurologic symptoms without persistent deficit, when there is subtotal internal carotid stenosis
3. When, during the monitoring of a progressive, high-grade carotid stenosis with transient functional disorders or functionally unimportant persistent neurologic

deficit, the imaging techniques demonstrate a cerebral infarct (territorial or border zone)

4. In a similar situation as in (3) occasionally even in asymptomatic patients

6.3.2.2 EC-IC Bypass Operation

EC-IC bypass surgery was intended as a method for the prophylaxis of hemodynamically induced ischemias with intracranial vascular lesions. It involved making a connection between a branch of the superficial temporal artery and a pial branch of the middle cerebral artery. A range of bypass operations was also developed in the vertebrobasilar system. Special effectiveness was ascribed to procedures for carotid siphon stenoses, Moya-Moya syndrome, or proximal middle cerebral stenoses. Also patients who had previous TIAs or infarcts with only minor neurologic deficit and with extracranial internal carotid occlusion were considered as candidates.

The effectiveness of this operation was tested in an international, prospective randomized study (EC/IC Bypass Study Group 1985). No prophylactic effect of this treatment was demonstrated, either overall or in any specific subgroups. In fact, certain patient groups in whom, on the basis of pathophysiologic considerations, a prophylactic effect seemed promising even fared significantly worse than comparable groups treated with drugs alone. This study has attracted a number of criticisms; for example, CT findings and thus certain etiopathogenetic aspects were not considered since the investigation began in 1977. Further objections were directed against the large number of patients selected by the centers and allocated primarily to surgical treatment, thus perhaps introducing a selection bias. Until further study resolves these questions, there is no reliable indication for EC-IC bypass operations in the prophylaxis of cerebral ischemia.

6.3.2.3 Surgical Treatment of Space-Occupying Cerebellar Infarcts

Extensive, secondarily space-occupying, territorial infarcts of the cerebellum, usually infarcts in the PICA or SCA territories, may give rise to an obstructive hydrocephalus by secondary displacement of the foramina of Luschka and Magendie or pressure on the aqueduct brought about by secondary edema. An added risk is that of subtentorial or tonsillar herniation. Clinically, these developments are manifested by increasing disturbance of consciousness some 2–4 days after the onset of the initially benign symptoms; one also notes secondary brainstem signs and increasing respiratory failure. Monitoring evoked potentials aids in localizing the lesion. Therapeutically, osmotherapy combined with controlled artificial respiration and hyperventilation is often unsuccessful in influencing the life-threatening state. Combined osteoplastic decompression operation of the posterior cranial fossa, with enlargement of the foramen magnum plus external ventricular drainage of CSF, may be life saving and result in an excellent prognosis of the cerebellar infarct (Keidel 1984; Heros 1982; Auer et al. 1986).

6.3.2.4 Other Surgical Procedures

Aortic Arch Surgery (Ostial Stenoses)

The aortic arch syndrome refers to extensive arteriosclerotic lesions of the ostia of the vessels arising from the aortic arch. This involves various bypass operations as well as indirect endarterectomy. Endarterectomy of the brachiocephalic trunk is difficult and tedious and is fraught with numerous complications. Reocclusions appear to be less common than in procedures on the internal carotid.

Subclavian Steal Syndrome

The clinical and pathophysiologic features of the subclavian steal syndrome are described on p. 68. The demonstration of a manifest subclavian steal syndrome using Doppler sonography or radiology, with subclavian stenosis or occlusion, is not in itself an adequate indication for the operation (Hennerici et al. 1988). The syndrome of intermittent ischemia of the arm or the extremely rare vertebrobasilar neurologic features due to the steal meachnism may favor surgery. Here, both percutaneous angioplasty (Brückmann et al. 1986) and subclavian-carotid transposition (Edward and Mulherin 1984) have been suggested.

Kinking and Coiling

The genesis and significance of elongation, kinking, and coiling of the internal carotid artery are obscure. Apart from arteriosclerotic dilation and fibromuscular dysplasia, the demonstration of coiling in childhood leads one to think also of a congenital origin.
These findings are generally regarded as harmless and no longer call for surgery. It has been suggested that kinking without stenosis may be associated with increased thrombogenicity so that treatment with platelet-aggregation inhibitors is conceivable.

Transluminal Angioplasty

Transluminal angioplasty, which is comparable in technique and equipment to angioplasty of the coronary arteries, should be considered only for the arteries supplying the brain in stenoses of high-grade bilateral vertebral origin or contralateral vertebral occlusion, as well as in manifest subclavian steal syndromes (Brückmann et al. 1986). After the first positive results with transfemoral catheter-laser thrombendarterectomy in the heart, the technique has now also been performed in sporadic cases on the carotids. Since the maximum size of the particles developed by the laser-induced tissue evaporation is only 7 µm, there should be virtually no risk of cerebral embolism (Lammer et al. 1986). Whether this technique can replace even part of the surgical carotid endarterectomy must remain an open question, especially since the indications for carotid operation are themselves controversial.
The use of these techniques in the carotid arteries offers the attractive possibility of reducing the lesion in the same sitting as performing an angiogram, without the risks of general anesthesia and with the prospect of early hospital discharge for the patient.

The possibility of downstream embolization of dislodged fragments, observed in 5% of peripheral angioplasties, however, is the major cause of concern. This concern may be exaggerated if the experience of Theron et al. (1987) is representative. These authors reported all procedures in six patients with atherosclerotic lesions and five patients with recurrent stenosis after endarterectomy. Heparin was administered and temporary balloon occlusion performed in the internal carotid distal to the site of angioplasty. After the procedure, the carotid was thoroughly aspirated, then flushed. No obvious macroscopic material was found in the aspirated blood, nor was any material found on microscopic examination. Dilation was performed successfully in six patients, and no complications occurred. On the other hand, this procedure seems to be applicable only to hemodynamically irrelevant, well-collateralized lesions as it requires ballon occlusion for several minutes, a procedure which is not tolerable in patients with hemodynamic risk. First case reports have been published about revascularizing, transarterial measures for high-grade, intracranial stenoses and spasms in vertebrobasilar regions (Higashida et al. 1987).

6.4 Rehabilitation in Cerebrovascular Diseases[1]

Rehabilitation measures such as physiotherapy and speech training are necessary even during the acute phase. The curative treatment and specific rehabilitation measures to be carried out in connection with inpatient stay are discussed below. As with drug treatment, here too there are no confirmed, unequivocal empirical findings on the value of particular techniques (e.g., physiotherapy, visual field training). An improvement in aphasia from specific speech therapy compared with the spontaneous outcome has recently been reported (Poeck et al. 1988).

The aim of neurologic rehabilitation is to achieve the greatest possible extent of physical and psychological independence of the patient after a lesion of the central or peripheral nervous system. This calls for a scrupulous rehabilitation program, which in turn requires as detailed a picture as possible of the patient's pattern of derangement. In acute neurology the clinical and instrumental diagnosis is aimed at the nosologic localization of a clinical picture and determining its causes; however, in rehabilitation neurology the diagnostic survey must provide a complete picture of both the lost and the residual capacities of the patient, and in terms of performance relevant to everyday life.

In addition to aspects of disturbed motor performance (paresis) or planning (apraxias) and possible motor-plus features (spasticity, rigor, involuntary movements), such a survey includes an exact account of the perception performance of memory, ability to concentrate, conceptual thought, and especially the ability to communicate (speech disturbance, aphasia). Assessment of the mental state is also important. Again, depressive moods and disordered motivation are very common in cerebrovascular diseases, and disorders of attention and the ability to concentrate are virtually always present. The social setting of the patient must always be included in the planning of rehabilitation measures. The full extent of independence which the patient might

1 This section was written by Dr. Volker Hömberg, Director, Neurologic Treatment Center, Düsseldorf University, Hohensandweg 37, 4000 Düsseldorf 13, FRG.

attain in light of the pattern of impairment is often not achieved due to lack of attentiveness by his relatives. Analysis of the patient's home conditions is essential in providing aids relevant to daily life and avoiding aids which the patient cannot use. To assess the degree of independence during neurologic rehabilitation, some have used so-called independence scores, for example, the Barthel index (Barthel and Mahoney 1965). In addition, we have developed our own scores for assessing motor functions which facilitate transfer of the neurologic findings into an everyday context (Table 6.15).

Developing a disturbance profile is indispensable to the planning of further treatment and includes a complete neuropsychologic, speech disorder, and psychiatric diagnosis. This takes about 1 week.

6.4.1 Planning of Neurologic Rehabilitation

The various strategies for restoring function after irreversible damage to the central nervous system are listed in order of decreasing preference in Table 6.14. Restitution of the damaged tissue is impossible. The first approaches by transplantation of autologous monaminergic tissue into the brain for the restitution of function of widely projected transmitter systems (e. g., in Parkinson's or Alzheimer's disease) are still in the domain of experimental medicine and must be critically evaluated before possible therapeutic application (Joynt and Gash 1987).

It is more realistic to attempt functional improvement by "awakening" alternative structures in the vicinity of the damaged brain tissue. This rationale is also adopted in the controversial area of visual field training (Zihl and von Cramon 1985); through systematically eliciting saccadic eye movements within the scotoma the extent of the outer limits of the visual field can often be enlarged, and a marked improvement in visual orientational behavior in the disturbed visual field can almost always achieved. The suggested mechanism of this therapeutic approach is that, after damage to visual projection areas, connected visual association areas can contribute to the restoration of perception performance. Another example of the vicarious intercession of undisturbed cerebral areas is the so-called melodic intonation therapy (Sparks et al. 1974) used in aphasia therapy. In global aphasias an amazing facilitation of speech performance can often also be obtained if the patient attempts to sing instead of speak. This facilitation is probably achieved by activation of undamaged areas of the subdominant hemisphere.

The most common strategy in neurologic rehabilitation consists of working out with the patients ways in which to compensate for the loss of a function. In the simplest case this may be a walking aid, but in complex cases it may be necessary to use very

Table 6.14. Rehabilitation strategies for the restoration of function, in order of decreasing preference

1. Restitution of damaged tissue
2. "Awakening" of alternative structures
3. Learning of "rerouting" strategies
4. Managing using technical aids
5. Replacement using technical aids

Table 6.15. Score for assessment of motor functions

Hand motor score	Points	Arm motor score	Points
1. Fist closure		*1. Positioning of hand*	
Impossible	0	– Paralyzed arm + unstable shoulder	0
Power < 10% of other side	1	– Stabilization of shoulder and mass	
Power < 50% of other side	2	movements possible (e.g., hemispastic elbow	
Power normal	3	flexion)	1
		– Planned placing of forearm from shoulder	
2. Fist opening		and elbow on horizontal surface in one of 4	
Impossible	0	quadrants of a sheet of paper	2
Visible extension	1	– Free placement of forearm in space	3
Complete (paretic) extension	2	– Free placement of forearm and free choice of	
Normal	3	wrist position	4
			max = 4
3. Pinch (dice grasp)			
Impossible	0	*2. Load carrying*	
Dice with 5 cm edge	1	– Impossible	0
Dice with 1 cm edge	2	– Passive load carrying only	1
Dice with 0.5 cm edge	3	– Active load carrying without use of hand	2
		– Active load carrying using hand without	
4. Independent finger movement (finger-thumb		active letting go	3
opposition)		– Normal	4
Impossible	0		
One finger with associated movement	1	**Lower limb motor scope**	
One finger without associated movement	2		
Normal (at least 3 fingers without associated		*1. Standing leg function*	
movement)	3	– Absent	0
		– No weight shift possible	1
5. Undoing a nut from a screw (reciprocal		– Healthy leg can be lifted but step cannot be	
synergy)		taken	2
Impossible	0	– Step possible on level surface	3
Possible	1	– Weight shift on stair climbing without follow-	
		up step	4
6. Syringe pressing (simple synergy)			max. = 4
Impossible	0	*2. Leg-swing function*	
Possible	1	– Absent	1
		– Advance possible only with ground contact	1
7. Writing with pencil (state thickness)		– Advance possible on flat surface without	
Holding pencil impossible	0	ground contact	2
Line or scribble possible	1	– Advance possible by over a foot-length on	
Scribbled writing	2	level surface without ground contact	3
Normal writing	3	– Advance on stairs possible	4
			max. = 4
8. Writing speed			
Slower than usual	0	*3. Foot raising*	
Normal	1	– Impossible	0
		– Minimally possible while lying down	1
		– Incomplete foot raising in walking	2
		– Complete foot raising but incomplete foot	
		rolling	3
		– Normal foot raising	4
			max. = 4

complex technologic aids, such as computer-based communication aids or environmentally controlled aids in tetraparetic patients. These also include the use of functional electric stimulation, a pattern-repeated muscle stimulation in patients with upper motor neurone lesions for the restoration of standing, walking, or grasping functions. Here, muscle groups are stimulated in a planned sequence via surface electrodes or electrodes implanted in the muscle or nerve trunk to replace the absent supranuclear regulation (Mauritz 1986). These techniques also remain largely in the experimental stage. Their use requires very precise indications and very careful choice of patients. An important problem is that practically all these systems still work in an unregulated "open loop" mode and can only very inadequately imitate natural motor behavior with sensory feedback. Moreover, the use of these techniques is often problematic for the patients as a great deal of time is required for maintenance of the trained state of the stimulated muscles. One must always consider to what extent the use of such a technique makes economic sense for the individual patient.

6.4.2 Choice and Planning of Treatment

The use of neurologic rehabilitation measures always presupposes the collaboration of a team of therapists that includes physiotherapists, ergotherapists, speech therapists, neuropsychologists, and often also engineers. It is important for the outcome of the rehabilitation measures in a patient that the treatment program be worked out by the team together, that the treatment objectives in separate fields be clearly harmonized, and that the program be monitored and modified after an interval of several weeks. The therapeutic techniques most used in neurologic rehabilitation are the so-called exercise techniques whose rationale consists either of reestablishing a lost function or developing and practicing systematic "rerouting" strategies with the patient. Here, a pragmatic approach based on the actual lesional state of the patient makes more sense than pursuing ideologically based concepts or programs of physiotherapy. This is especially the case since – despite a supposed orientation to neurophysiologic findings – these often involve merely spinal reflex mechanisms and ignore newer concepts of the regulation of motor control. Comparative studies of physiotherapeutic methods have usually shown no significant difference in efficacy (e.g., Logigian 1985; Palmer et al. 1986).

6.4.3 Efficiency Monitoring and Predictive Factors for Results of Treatment

The basic prerequisite for critical monitoring of the efficiency of neurologic rehabilitation measures is the employment of quantitative methods for assessing movement, including the functional scores described above. When such methods are employed in prospective studies, such as in the course of stroke rehabilitation, a marked increase in independence and individual motor functions can be demonstrated (e. g., Heller et al. 1987; Heinemann et al. 1987). The rate of improvement varies greatly with the severity of the disturbance, and it is extremely difficult to define favorable or unfavorable predictive factors. In a recently published multivariate analysis of improvement characteristics in stroke rehabilitation (Heinemann et al. 1987), the authors found no significant relationship to the age of the patient, site of the hemispheric lesion, or degree of handicap at the beginning of treatment. Neuroradiologic findings also do not usually provide any significant predictive factors. We have recently begun to examine the predictive value for the ultimate rehabilitation results in hemiparetic patients which is offered by quantitatively measuring the integrity of corticospinal efferents using magnetic stimulation of the motor cortex. There is a significant correlation between the final functional state of patients as measured by the Barthel index and the deficits, divided into three grades of severity, as measured by cortical stimulation at the initiation of treatment.

6.4.4 New Techniques in Neurologic Rehabilitation

Reference should be made to two techniques in the treatment of motor disorders which are not yet widespread but may be very helpful in the facilitation of voluntary movement. The first is the above-mentioned functional electric stimulation. This sometimes leads to a marked reduction in spasticity and is particularly helpful in reducing tonus in the early phase so as to reinstate voluntary movements (Hömberg 1988). This stimulation can be supplemented by the use of EMF biofeedback techniques which allow patients, especially with marked afferent disturbances, to reinstate voluntary motor functions by hearing or seeing the EMG signals. Obviously, a prerequisite for this is the preservation of residual motor power in the limb. The effectiveness in stroke patients of this operant conditioning by the biofeedback approach has been repeatedly documented (e.g., Brudny et al. 1974, 1976; Basmajian 1979). A comparison of the use of this technique with conventional physiotherapy showed that a combination of the two methods gives the best results (Inglis et al. 1984). It is also possible to combine the EMG biofeedback technique directly with electrostimulation, so that increasing supportive electrical stimulation is applied with a greater magnitude of the EMG signal feedback (Fields 1987).

Another interesting new approach to neurologic rehabilitation is the use of microcomputer programs in neuropsychological treatment. The use of computers has the advantage over classical retraining programs in rehabilitative neuropsychology that the severity of the exercise demands is continuously adjusted to the patient's current performance; thus an optimal level of motivation is always maintained, and both frustrating excessive demands and tedious inadequate demands are avoided. Moreover, the use of this technique allows continuous recording of exercise progress and the formulation of a very versatile training program (Hömberg and Halsband 1988). We have recently developed a technique that allows the incorporation of video information about the life situation into a microprocessor-regulated program via an appropriate interface. This permits the production of a better program and one more suited to the current disability of the patient. Moreover, it has now become possible, through the introduction of so-called expert systems, to rapidly develop and modify specific program modules adapted to the individual patient, available even to therapists unpracticed in computer program language (Rass et al. 1988). As attitude measurements made by us have shown (Steinhoff and Hömberg 1988), use of the computer has been very well received by patients. However, a prerequisite is consistently supportive care by psychologically trained personnel during the computer training. The use of this technique permits an intensivization of training but does not achieve any economy in personnel.

Finally, some examples of interesting techniques should be mentioned that combine exercises with drug treatment. As has been shown in animal experiments, the administration of amphetamines after a lesion of the motor cortex has a definitely accelerating effect on recovery of motor function (Feeney et al. 1982). The effectiveness of amphetamines in combination with physiotherapy has also been demonstrated recently in a small sample of stroke patients (Crisostomo et al. 1988).

Another interesting use of drugs in combination with exercise techniques is the administration of cholinergics, especially the oral administration of physostigmine in combination with systematic memory training (McLean et al. 1987). While studies on the influence of cholinergics on memory functions without accompanying systematic training showed inconsistent findings and no significant evidence of clinical improvement, this study showed definite effects for the first time. We have observed the effectiveness of such an approach in some patients with global amnesia treated by physostigmine and memory training in combination. Perceptual or motor neglect, i. e., disregard of one or other part of the body or part of the perceptual space, is often a very disturbing feature in patients with cerebrovascular lesions of both the right and left hemispheres. Alleviation of this neglect by means of exercise techniques is often only transitory.

Data from animal experiments showing involvement of the ascending dopaminergic systems in the frontal and limbic cortex have recently been followed by evidence in man that perceptual spatial neglect can be positively influenced by the administration of dopamine agonists (bromocriptine). This certainly constitutes an interesting pharmacologic approach, but one that needs further testing of its efficacy.

Finally, it must also be pointed out that many patients with cerebrovascular insults show marked depressive symptoms; these should be treated with oral antidepressants after appropriate psychodiagnostic confirmation. It has been shown in a prospective study (Reding et al. 1986) that the employment of antidepressants in depressive stroke patients leads to a definite improvement in rehabilitation results.

References

Agnoli A, Palene N, Ruggieri S, Leonardis G, Benzi G (1979) Barbiturate treatment of acute stroke. Adv Neurol 25:269

Albers GW, Goldberg MP, Choi DW (1989) N-Methyl-D-aspartate antagonists: ready for clinical trial in brain ischemia? Ann Neurol 25:398–403

American Canadian Co-operative Study Group (1985) Persantin-aspirin trial in cerebral ischaemia. Stroke 16:406

Asplund K, Eriksson S, Hägg E (1986) Multicenter trial of hemodilution in acute ischemic stroke. Acta Neurol Scand 73:530

Auer LM, Auer T, Sayamal (1986) Indications for surgical treatment of cerebellar hemorrhage, and infarction. Acta Neurochir (Wien) 79:74

Baker RN (1961) An evaluation of anticoagulant therapy in the treatment of cerebrovascular disease. Report of the Veterans Administration Cooperative Study of Atherosclerosis. Neurology 11:132

Baker RN, Broward JA, Fang HC (1962) Anticoagulant therapy in cerebral infarction. Neurology 12:823

Barthel D, Mahoney F (1965) Functional evaluation. The Barthel index. State Med J 2:61

Basmajian JV (1979) Bio-feedback: principles and practice for clinicians. Williams and Wilkins, Baltimore

Bass E (1983) Anticoagulation in cerebral embolism. Can J Neurol Sci 10:32

Bauer RB, Tellez H (1973) Dexamethasone as treatment in cerebral vascular disease. II. A controlled study in acute cerebral infarction. Stroke 4:547

Bayer AJ, Pathy MSJ, Newcombe R (1987) Double-blind randomized trial of intravenous glycerol in acute stroke. Lancet I:405

Bousser MG, Eschwege E, Haguenau M (1983) "AICLA" controlled randomized trial of aspirin and dipyridamole in the secondary prevention of athero-thrombotic cerebral ischemia. Stroke 14:5

Boysen G, Soelberg Sørensen P, Jutzler M, Andersen AR, Boas J, Olsen JS, Joensen P (1988) Danish very-low-dose aspirin after carotid endarterectomy trial. Stroke 19:1211

Brain Resuscitation Clinical Trial Study Group (1986) Randomized clinical study of thiopental loading in comatose survivors of cardiac arrest. N Engl J Med 314:397

Britton M, DeFaire U, Helmers C, Miah K (1980) Lack of effect of theophylline on the outcome of acute cerebral infarction. Acta Neurol Scand 62:116

Brott T, Reed RL (1989) Intensive care for acute stroke in the community hospital setting. The first 24 hours. Stroke 20:694–697

Brückmann H, Ringelstein EB, Buchner H, Zeumer H (1986) Percutaneous transluminal angioplasty of the vertebral artery: a therapeutic alternative to operative reconstruction of proximal vertebral artery stenosis. J Neurol 233:336

Brückmann H, Ferbert A, Del Zoppo GJ, Hacke W, Zeumer H (1987) Acute vertebral basilar thrombosis: angiologic-clinical comparision and therapeutic implications. Acta Radiol 369:38

Brudny J, Korein J, Levidow L, Grynbaum BB, Lieberman A, Friedmann LW (1974) Sensory feedback therapy as a modality of treatment in central nervous system disorders of voluntary movement. Neurology 24:925

Brudny J, Korein J, Grynbaum BB, Friedmann LW, Weinstein S, Sachs-Frankel G, Belandres PV (1976) EMG feedback therapy: review of treatment of 114 patients. Arch Phys Med Rehabil 57:55

Calandre L, Ortega JF, Berbejo F, Portera A (1983) Cerebral embolism and anticoagulation. Neurology 33:1103

Canadian Cooperative Study (1978) A randomized trial of aspirin and sulfinpyranzone in threatened stroke. N Engl J Med 299:53

Candelise L (1982) A randomized trial of aspirin and sulfinpyrazone in patients with TIA. Stroke 13:175

Candelise L, Spinnler H (1972) Dexamethasone and stroke. Med J Aust 2:335

Candelise L, Colombo A, Spinnler H (1975) Therapy against brain swelling in stroke patients, a retrospective clinical study on 227 patients. Stroke 6:353

Carter AP (1961) Anticoagulant treatment in progressive stroke. Br Med J II:70

Cerebral Embolism Study Group (1983) Immediate anticoagulation of embolic stroke: a randomized trial. Stroke 14:668

Cerebral Embolism Task Force (1989) Cardiogenic brain embolism. The second report of the Cerebral Embolism Task Force. Arch Neurol 46:727–743

Cook P, James I (1981) Cerebral vasodilators. N Engl J Med 305:1560

Crisostomo EA, Duncan PW, Propst M, Dawson D, Davis JN (1988) Evidence that amphetamine with physical therapy promotes recovery of motor function in stroke patients. Ann Neurol 23:94

De Ley G, Weyne J, Demeester G, Stryckmans K, Goethals P, et al. (1989) Streptokinase treatment versus calcium overload blockade in experimental thrombembolic stroke. Stroke 20:357–361

Del Zoppo GJ, Zeumer H, Harker LA (1986) Thrombolytic therapy in acute stroke: possibilities and hazards. Stroke 17:595

Del Zoppo GJ, Ferbert A, Otis S, Brückmann H, Hacke W, Zyroff A, Arke LA, Zeumer H (1988) Local intra-arterial fibrinolytic therapy in acute carotid territory stroke. A pilot study. Stroke 19:307

Duke RJ, Bloch RF, Turpie AG, et al. (1986) Intravenous heparin for the prevention of stroke progression in acute partial stable stroke: a randomized controlled trial. Ann Intern Med 105:825–828

Dyken M, White PT (1956) Evaluation of cortisone in the treatment of cerebral infarction. JAMA 162:1531

EC/IC Bypass Study Group (1985) Failure of extracranial-intracranial arterial bypass to reduce the risk of ischemic stroke. N Engl J Med 313:1191

Edward WH, Mulherin JL (1985) The surgical reconstruction of the proximal subclavian and vertebral artery. J Vasc Surg 2:634

Enger E, Boyesen S (1965) Long-term anticoagulant therapy in patients with cerebral infarction. Acta Med Scand 178 [Suppl 438]:1

ESPS Group (1987) The European stroke prevention study. Lancet II:1351

Feeney DM, Gonzales A, Law WA (1982) Amphetamine, haloperidol, and experience interact to affect rate of recovery after motor cortex injury. Science 217:855

Fields RW (1987) Electromyographically triggered electric muscle stimulation for chronic hemiplegia. Arch Phys Med Rehabil 68:407

Fields WS, Lemak NA, Frankoski RF, Hardy RJ (1978) Controlled trial of aspirin in cerebral ischemia. II. Surgical group. Stroke 9:309

Fisher CM (1961) Anticoagulant therapy in cerebral thrombosis and cerebral embolism. A national cooperative study. Neurology 11:119

Fleet WS, Valenstein E, Watson RT, Heilman KM (1987) Dopamine agonist therapy for neglect in humans. Neurology 37:1765

Frei A, Cottier C, Wunderlich P, Ludin E (1987) Glycerol and dextran combined in therapy of acute stroke. Stroke 18:373

Friedman GD, Wilson S, Mosier JM (1969) Transient ischemic attacks in a community. JAMA 210:1428

Fritz G, Werner I (1975) The effect of glycerol infusion in acute cerebral infarction. Acta Med Scand 198:287

Furlan AS, Cavalier SJ, Hobbs RE (1982) Hemorrhage and anticoagulation after non-septic embolic brain infarction. Neurology 32:280

Gallhofer G, Ladurner G, Lechner H (1979) Prognosis of prophylactic anticoagulant treatment in ischemic stroke. Eur Neurol 18:145

Gelmers HJ (1975) Effect of glycerol treatment on the natural history of acute cerebral infarction. Clin Neurol Neurosurg 78:277

Gelmers HJ (1980) Effects of low-dose subcutaneous heparin on the occurrence of deep vein thrombosis in patients with ischemic stroke. Acta Neurol Scand 61:313

Gelmers HJ (1982) Effect of nimodipine on postischemic cerebrovascular activity, as revealed by measuring regional cerebral blood flow. Acta Neurochir (Wien) 63:283

Gelmers HJ (1984) The effects of nimodipine on the clinical course of patients with acute ischemic stroke. Acta Neurol Scand 69:232

Gelmers HJ, Gorter K, de Weerdt CJ, Wiezer JHA (1988) A controlled trial of nimodipine in acute ischemic stroke. N Engl J Med 318:203

Gent M, Blakely JA, Easton D, Ellis DJ (1989) The Canadian-American ticlopidine study (CATS) in thromboembolic stroke. Lancet I:1260

Gilroy J, Barnhardt MI, Meyer JS (1969) Treatment of stroke with dextran 40. JAMA 210:293

Gilzanz V, Rebollar JL, Buencuerpo J, Chantres MT (1975) Controlled trial of glycerol versus dexamethasone in the treatment of cerebral oedema in acute cerebral infarction. Lancet I:1049

Gottstein U, Held K (1969) Effekt der Hämodilution nach intravenöser Infusion von niedermolekularen Dextranen auf die Hirnzirkulation des Menschen. Dtsch Med Wochenschr 94:522–526

Gryglewski RJ, Nowak S, Kosta-Trabka E, Kusmiderski J, Dembinska-Kiec A, Bieron K, Basita M, Blasczyk B (1983) Treatment of ischemic stroke with prostacyclin. Stroke 14:197

Guiraud-Chaumeil B, Rascol A, David J, Boneu B, Clanet M, Bierme R (1982) Prévention des récidives des accidents vasculaires cérébraux ischémiques par les anti-agrégants plaquettaires. Resultats d'un essai thérapeutique controlé de 3 ans. Rev Neurol (Paris) 138:367

Hacke W, Zeumer H, Ferbert A, Brückmann H, del Zoppo GJ (1988) Intra-arterial thrombolytic therapy improves outcome in patients with acute vertebobasilar occlusive disease. Stroke 19:1216

Hakim AM, Pokrupa RP, Wolfe LS (1984) Preliminary report on the effectiveness of prostacyclin in stroke. Can J Neurol Sci 11:409

Hakim AM, Evans AC, Berger L, Kuwabara H, et al. (1989) The effect of nimodipine on the evolution of human cerebral infarction studied by PET. J Cereb Blood Flow Metab 9:523

Harrison MJG, Pollock S, Kendell BE, Marshall J (1981) Effect of haematocrit on carotid stenosis and cerebral infarction. Lancet II:114

Hass WK, Easton DJ, Adams HP, Pryse-Phillips W (1989) A randomized trial comparing ticlopidine hydrochloride with aspirin for the prevention of stroke in high-risk patients. N Engl J Med 321:501

Heinemann AW, Roth EJ, Cichowski K, Betts HB (1987) Multivariate analysis of improvement and outcome following stroke rehabilitation. Arch Neurol 44:1167

Heller A, Wade DT, Wood VA (1987) Arm function after stroke: measurement and recovery over the first three months. J Neurol Neurosurg Psychiatry 50:714

Hemodilution in Stroke Study Group (1989) Hypervolemic hemodilution treatment of acute stroke. Results of a randomized multicenter trial using pentastarch. Stroke 20:317–323

Hennerici M, Rautenberg W, Mohr S (1982) Stroke risk from symptomless extracranial arterial disease. Lancet II:1180

Hennerici M, Hülsbömer HB, Hefter H, Lammerts D, Rautenberg W (1987) Natural history of asymptomatic extracranial artery disease. Brain 101:777

Hennerici M, Klemm C, Rautenberg W (1988) The subclavian steal phenomenon: a common vascular disorder with rare neurologic deficits. Neurology 38:669

Heros RC (1982) Cerebellar hemorrhage and infarction. Stroke 13:106–109

Hill AB, Marshall J, Shaw DA (1962) Cerebrovascular disease: trial of long-term anticoagulant therapy. Br Med J II:1003

Hömberg V (1989) Rehabilitation in spastic syndromes – nonpharmacological ways of treatment. In: Emre M, Benecke R (eds) Spasticity. Parthenon, Cornforth, p 97

Hömberg V, Halsband U (1988) Die Problematik der Interpretation von Trainingsverläufen bei computergestützter kognitiver Rehabilitation. In: Computer helfen heilen (in press)

Howell DA, Talow SFT, Feldman S (1964) Observations on anticoagulant therapy in thrombo-embolic disease of the brain. Can Med Assoc J 90:611

Hsu CY, Faught RE, Furlan AJ, et al. (1987) Intravenous prostacyclin in acute nonhemorrhagic stroke: a placebo-controlled double-blind trial. Stroke 18:352

Hsu CY, Norris JW, Hogan EL, et al. (1988) Pentoxifylline in acute nonhemorrhagic stroke. A randomized placebo-controlled double-blind trial. Stroke 19:716

Inglis J, Donald MW, Monga TN, Sproule M, Young MJ (1984) Electromyographic biofeedback and physical therapy of the hemiplegic upper limb. Arch Phys Med Rehabil 65:755

Italian Acute Stroke Study Group (1988) Haemodilution in acute stroke: results of the Italian haemodilution trial. Lancet I:318

Jabaily J, Davis JN (1984) Naloxone administration to patients with acute stroke. Stroke 15:36

Joynt RJ, Gash DM (1987) Neural transplants: are we ready? Ann Neurol 22:455

Kaste M, Fogelolm R, Waltimo R (1976) Combined dexamethasone and low-molecular-weight dextran in acute brain infarction: Double blind-study. Br Med J II:1409

Keidel M, Galle G, Wiedmayer J, Taghavy A (1984) Der maligne Kleinhirninfarkt. Fortschr Neurol Psychiatr 52:277–283

Keltern JG (1986) Heparin induces thrombocytopenia. Hemostaseolagy 16:173–186

Koller RL (1982) Recurrent embolic cerebral infarction and anticoagulation. Neurology 32:283

Kopecky SL, Gersh BJ, McGoon MD (1987) The natural history of lone atrial fibrillation. N Engl J Med 317:669

Krämer G, Busse O, Warlow C, Hopf HC (1986) Aktueller Stand gefäßchirurgischer Eingriffe bei zerebrovaskulären Erkrankungen. 2. Karotis-Thrombendarterektomie. Aktuel Neurol 13:188

Krämer G, Tettenborn B, Aichner F, Schmutzhard E, Schwantz A, Busse O, Hornig C, Ladurner G (1991) Nimodipine in acute ischemic stroke. Results of the Nimodipine German Austrian stroke trial (to be published)

Lammer J, Asher PW, Choy DSJ (1986) Transfemorale Katheter-Laser-Thrombendarterektomie (TEA) der Arteria carotis. Dtsch Med Wochenschr 111:607

Larsson O, Marinovich N, Barber K (1976) Double-blind trial of glycerol therapy in early stroke. Lancet I:832

Lodder J, Lugt PJM van der (1983) Evaluation of the risk of immediate anticoagulant treatment in patients with embolic stroke of cardiac origin. Stroke 14:42

Lodder J, Dennis MS, Raak van L, Jones LN, Warlow CP (1988) Cooperative study on the value of long term anticoagulation in patients with stroke and non-rheumatic atrial fibrillation. Br Med J I:1435

Logigian MK, Samuels MA, Falconer J (1983) Clinical exercise trial for stroke patients. Arch Phys Med Rehabil 64:364

Marshall J, Shaw DA (1960) Anticoagulant therapy in acute cerebrovascular accident. A controlled trial. Lancet I:995

Martin JF, Handy N, Nicholl J (1985) Double-blind controlled trial of prostacyclin in cerebral infarction. Stroke 16:386

Martinez-Arizala A, Holaday JW, Reed W (1989) Is there a role for naloxone in the treatment of stroke? Crit Care Med 17:839–840

Martinez-Vila E, Matias Guiu J, Guillen F, Bigorra J, Martinez-Lage JM (1989) A placebo controlled trial of nimodipine in the treatment of acute ischemic cerebral infarction. In: Hartmann A, Kuschinsky W (eds) Cerebral ischemia and calcium. Springer, Berlin Heidelberg New York, pp 358–366

Martinez-Vila E, Guillèn F, Villanueva JA, Matias Guiu J, Bigorra J, Gil P, Carbonell A, Martinez-Lage JM (1990) A placebo controlled trial of Nimodipine in the treatment of acute ischemic cerebral infarction. Stroke 21:1023

Mathew NT, Rivera VM, Meyer JS, Charney JZ, Hartmann A (1972) Double-blind evaluation of glycerol therapy in acute cerebral infarction. Lancet II:1327

Matthews WB, Oxbury JM, Grainger KM, Grenhall RC (1976) A blind controlled trial of dextran-40 in the treatment of ischemic stroke. Brain 99:193

Mauritz KH (1986) Restoration of posture and gait by functional neuromuscular stimulation (FNS). In: Bles W, Brandt T (eds) Disorders of posture and gait. Elsevier, Amsterdam, p 367

McDowell F, McDevitt E (1965) Treatment of the completed stroke with long-term anticoagulant: six and one-half years experience. In: Millikan CH, Siekert RG, Whisnant JP (eds) Cerebral vascular diseases. Fourth Princeton Conference. Grune and Stratton, New York, p 185

McLean A, Stanton KM, Cardenas DD, Bergerud DB (1987) Memory training combined with the use of oral physostigmine. Brain Injury 1:145

Miller VT, Hart RG (1988) Heparin anticoagulation in acute brain ischemia. Stroke 19:403

Miller VT, Coull BM, Yatsu FM, Shah AB, Beamer NB (1984) Prostacyclin infusion in acute cerebral infarction. Neurology 34:1431

Millikan CH (1965) Anticoagulant therapy in cerebrovascular disease. In: Millikan CH, Siekert RG, Whisnant JP (eds) Cerebral vascular diseases. Fourth Princeton Conference. Grune and Stratton, New York, p 183

Nenci GG, Gresele P, Taramelli M, Agnelli G, Signorini E (1983) Thrombolytic therapy for thromboembolism of vertebrobasilar artery. Angiology 34:561

Norris JW (1976) Steroid therapy in acute cerebral infarction. Arch Neurol 33:69

Norris JW, Hachinski VC (1986) High dose steroid treatment in cerebral infarction. Br Med J 292:21

Norris JW, Hachinski VC, Meyers MG, Callow J, Wong T, Moore RW (1979) Serum cardiac enzymes in stroke. Stroke 10:548

Okada Y, Yamaguchi T, Minematsu K, Miyashita T, Sawada T (1989) Hemorrhagic transformation in cerebral embolism. Stroke 20:598

Oleson J, Paulson OB (1971) The effect of intra-arterial papaverine on regional cerebral blood flow in patients with stroke or intracranial tumor. Stroke 2:148

Olson JE, Müller R, Berneli S (1976) Long-term anticoagulant therapy for TIAs and minor strokes with minimum residuum. Stroke 7:444

Palmer FB, Shapiro BK, Wachtel RC, et al. (1986) The effects of physical therapy on cerebral palsy. N Engl J Med 318:803

Patten BM, Mendell J, Bruun B, Curtin W, Carter S (1972) Double-blind study of the effects of dexamethasone on acute stroke. Neurology 22:377

Pearce JM, Gubbay SS, Walton JN (1965) Long-term anticoagulant therapy in transient cerebral ischaemic attacks. Lancet I:6

Petersen P, Boysen G, Godtfredsen J, Andersen ED, Andersen B (1989) Placebo-controlled, randomised trial of warfarin and aspirin for prevention of thromboembolic complications in chronic atrial fibrillation. Lancet I:175

Phillips JS (1989) An alternative view of heparin anticoagulation in acute focal brain ischemia. Stroke 20:295

Poeck K, Huber W, Willmes K (1988) Outcome of intensive language therapy in aphasia. Brain

Pulsinelli WA, Levi DE, Sgisibee B, Scherer P, Plum F (1983) Increased damaged after ischemic stroke in patients with hyperglycemia with or without established diabetes mellitus. Am J Med 74:540–544

Rass D, Behrends U, Hömberg V (1988) Autorensystem mit Video-Interface: Erstellung kognitiven Trainingsmaterials. In: Computer helfen heilen (in press)

Reding MJ, Ortho LA, Winter SW, Fortuna IM, Di Ponte P, McDowell FH (1986) Antidepressant therapy after stroke. A double blind trial. Arch Neurol 43:763

Reuther R, Dorndorf W (1978) Aspirin in patients with cerebral ischemia and normal angiograms or non-surgical lesions. Results of a double blind trial. In: Breddin K, Dorndorf W, Loew D, Marx R (eds) Acetylsalicylic acid in cerebral ischemia and coronary heart disease. Schattauer. Stuttgart, p 97

Ribeiro LGT, Brandon TA, Hopkins DG, Reduto LA, Taylor AA, Miller RR (1981) Prostacyclin in experimental myocardial ischemia: effects on hemodynamics, regional myocardial blood flow, infarct size and mortality. Am J Cardiol 47:835

Roederer GO, Langlois YE, Jager KA, et al. (1984) The natural history of carotid arterial disease in asymptomatic patients with cerebral bruits. Stroke 15:605

Rubinstein MK (1965) The influence of adrenocortical steroids on severe cerebrovascular accidents. J Nerv Ment Dis 141:291

Sage JL, Uitert RL van (1983) Risk of recurrent stroke in patients with atrial fibrillation and non-valvular heart disease. Stroke 14:537

Santamaria J, Graus F, Peres J (1983) Cerebral embolism and anticoagulation. Neurology 33:1104

Santanbrogio S, Martinotti R, Sardella F, Porro F, Randazzo A (1978) Is there a real treatment of stroke? Clinical and statistical comparison of different treatments in 300 patients. Stroke 9:130

Scandinavian Stroke Study Group (1987) Multicenter trial of hemodilution in acute ischemic stroke. I. Results in the total patient population. Stroke 18:691

Scheinberg P (1989) Heparin anticoagulation. Stroke 20:173

Siekert RG, Whisnant JP, Millikan CH (1963) Surgical and anticoagulant therapy of occlusive cerebrovascular disease. Ann Intern Med 58:637

Sloan MA (1987) Thrombolysis and stroke: past and future. Arch Neurol 44:748

Sorensen PS, Pedersen H, Marquardsen J (1983) Acetylsalicylic acid in the prevention of stroke in patients with reversible cerebral ischemia. Stroke 14:5

Sparks R, Helm N, Albert M (1974) Aphasia rehabilitation resulting from melodic intonation therapy. Cortex 10:303

Spudis EV, de La Torre E, Pikula L (1973) Management of completed strokes with dextran-40. A community hospital failure. Stroke 4:895

Steen PA, Gisvold SE, Milde JH, Newberg L, Scheithauer BW, Lanier WL, Michenfelder J (1985) Nimodipine improves outcome when given after complete cerebral ischemia in primates. Anesthesiology 62:406

Steinhoff C, Hömberg V (1988) Interaktion Patient Computer: Versuch einer Einstellungsmessung. In: Computer helfen heilen (in press)

Strand T, Asplund K, Eriksson S, Hagg E, Lithner F, Wester PO (1984) A randomized controlled trial of hemodilution therapy in acute cerebral stroke. Stroke 15:980

Swedish Cooperative Study (1987) High dose acetylsalicyl acid after cerebral infarction. Stroke 18:325

Sze PC, Reitman D, Pincus M, Sachs HS, Chalmers T (1988) Antiplatelet agents in secondary prevention of stroke. Stroke 19:436

Szekely P (1964) Systemic embolism and anticoagulant prophylaxis in rheumatic heart disease. Br Med J I:1209

Terent A, Anderson B (1980) The outcome of patients with transient ischemic attacks and stroke treated with anticoagulants. Acta Med Scand 208:359

Theron J, Raymond J, Casasco A, Courtheoux F (1987) Percutaneous angioplasty of atherosclerotic and postsurgical stenosis of carotid arteries. AJNR 8:495

Toole JF, Janeway R, Choi K (1975) Transient ischemic attacks due to atherosclerosis. A prospective study in 160 patients. Arch Neurol 32:5

UK TIA Study Group (1988) United Kingdom transient ischaemic attack (UK-TIA) aspirin trial. Br Med J 296:316

von Kummer R, Back T, Scharf J, Hacke W (1989) Stroke, hemodilution, and mortality. Stroke 20:1286

Wallace JD, Levy LL (1980) Blood pressure after stroke. JAMA 246:2177

WHO Task Force on Stroke and Other Cerebrovascular Disorders (1989) Recommendations on stroke prevention, diagnosis and therapy. Stroke 20:1407

Wilson BA (1987) Rehabilitation of memory. Guilford, New York

Wise G, Sutter R, Burkholder J (1972) The treatment of brain ischemia with vasopressor drugs. Stroke 3:135

Zeumer H (1985) Survey of progress: vascular recanalizing techniques in interventional neuroradiology. J Neurol 231:287

Zeumer H, Hacke W, Kolmann HL, Poeck K (1982) Lokale Fibrinolysetherapie bei Basilaris-Thrombose. Dtsch Med Wochenschr 107:728

Zeumer H, Freitag HJ, Grzyska U, Neunzig HP (1989) Local intraarterial fibrinolysis in acute vertebrobasilar occlusion. Technical developments and recent results. Neuroradiology 31:336

Zihl J, Cramon D von (1985) Visual field recovery from scotoma in patients with postgeniculate damage. Brain 108:335

Subject Index